Health and Development

Health and Development

The Millennium Perspectives

Edited by

K. Gangadharan

RAWAT PUBLICATIONS

Jaipur • New Delhi • Bangalore • Hyderabad • Guwahati

ISBN 978-81-316-0405-2

Published by
Prem Rawat for **Rawat Publications**
Satyam Apts, Sector 3, Jawahar Nagar, Jaipur 302 004 (India)
Phone: 0141 265 1748 / 7006 Fax: 0141 265 1748
E-mail: info@rawatbooks.com
Website: www.rawatbooks.com

New Delhi Office
4858/24, Ansari Road, Daryaganj, New Delhi 110 002
Phone: 011 2326 3290

Also at *Bangalore, Hyderabad* and *Guwahati*

Typeset by Rawat Computers, Jaipur
Printed at Chaman Enterprises, New Delhi

Contents

Section II
Health and Development: Issues and Strategies

Section III
Equity and Health

Preface

Health an
socio-econ
improveme
socio-econ
improved
awarene
services
improvem
acceptan
product o
one of th
status d
diseases, m
major chan
malaria
the epide
lemp

Rom
consequ
physical ina
are also
be over

Preface

Health and development is highly relevant in the present global socio-economic environment. In the development approach, improvement in health status is viewed primarily as a product of socio-economic development. By definition, development implies improved nutrition, hygienic living and working conditions, greater awareness of health problems and wider accessibility to health care services, which have a favourable affect on health status of the people. Improvements in health status as well as health care are treated as integrated components of the development process. Since health is a product of multivariate production process, in which medical care is just one of the many inputs, the impact of the state intervention on health status depends on its overall socio-economic policies. Infectious diseases, maternal and perinatal conditions continue to contribute to a major chunk of morbidity at the global level. In addition to tuberculosis, malaria and HIV/AIDS, the developing countries have been witnessing the epidemics of re-emerging infectious diseases like dengue, leptospirosis and chicungunia.

Rapid urbanization, industrialization, changes in lifestyle and consequent hike in risk factors such as tobacco use, unhealthy diet and physical inactivity caused a rise in global burden of chronic illness. There are also overriding environmental and mental health issues that cannot be overlooked. The double burden of communicable and non-communicable diseases thus present a formidable challenge on the already resource-limited health systems of different countries. The policy reform measures introduced at the global level also resulted in the steady erosion of funds set apart by the government for preventive and curative care packages. These multifaceted problems calls for a development approach on basic health care.

Health has a predominant role in improving GDP per capita and poor health reduces GDP per capita by reducing labour productivity and relative size of the labour force. The core objective bringing out this volume on 'Health and Development' is to discuss the lessons of health care development, examine the emerging issues and analyse the current strategies followed to tackle the basic issues in the health care sector. The internationally agreed Millennium Development Goals have pointed out specific targets for health. Investment in health care will lead to relieving people from poverty, sickness and distress. In the changed environment as part of reforms, it requires to be revived whether the share of the public subsidies in the health sector is progressive or not. The attainment of United Nations Millennium Development Goals relatively the health within the time frame will require heavy investment in health, especially in public, primary health care. The hike in morbidity load in developing countries recently is mainly due to the depletion of environmental quality and rise in urbanization. So, the health hazards in the urban areas as part of urbanization and environmental threats needs special attention. Infection, diseases, maternal and perinatal conditions continue to contribute a major chunk of morbidity and mortality at the global level. We are also undergoing rapid epidemiological and demographic transition and this is reflected in the rising burden of chronic new communicable diseases.

The present volume is the outcome of the two days International Conference on 'Health and Development: Issues, Strategies and Options' organized by the Department of Applied Economics, Kannur University during 22nd and 23rd October 2008. The conference succeeded in bringing together scholars, teachers, health economists, public health persons, social scientists and NGO experts in the areas of social health to discuss the health and development issues, share experiences and deliberate on strategies to build capacity to identify and respond to the health needs of the people and also suggest suitable policy lines for the health planners, policy maker and administrators. The Indian Council of Medical Research, New Delhi, and the University Grants Commission, New Delhi sponsored the conference. We finally received twenty revised papers after the conference. I hope that this volume will prove to be an enriching and authentic work for the students of health economics and will be a useful reading text for the research scholars, teachers, public health personnel, administrators, policy makers and planners in the health care sector.

First of all, I would like to express my thanks to all the contributors of the papers and delegates of the conference for their valuable contributions. All my colleagues in the department extended their help, cooperation and support in the completion of the exercise. I would like to particularly convey my thanks to K.P. Vipin Chandran who worked very hard during the course of the conference and also took charge of all typing and record keeping assistance both during the course of the conference and at the preparation of the manuscript. My thanks are also due to Rawat Publications, Jaipur for efficiently bearing the responsibility for the publication of the book.

K. Gangadharan

Contributors

Ankush Agrawal, Research Scholar, Indira Gandhi Institute of Development Research (IGIDR), Mumbai.

K. Anbu, Lecturer, Department of Social Work, Pondicherry University, Puducherry.

V. Anitha, Lecturer, P.G. and Research Department of Economics, S.N. College, Sivagiri, Varkala, Kerala.

R. Annapoorani, Professor of Economics, Avinashilingam University for Women, Coimbatore, Tamil Nadu.

Saumya Chand, Research Scholar, Department of Economics, Faculty of Social Sciences, Banaras Hindu University, Varanasi.

Malathy Duraisamy, Professor, Indian Institute for Technology, Chennai.

P. Duraisamy, Professor, Department of Econometrics Madras University, Chennai.

K. Gangadharan, Reader and Head, Department of Applied Economics, Kannur University, Kannur, Kerala.

B.N. Ghosh, Professor of Economics, Department of Economics, Eastern Mediterranean University, North Cyprus and Director (Hon.), Centre for the Study of Human Development, Leeds (UK).

K. Govindarajalu, Professor of Economics, Bharathiar University, Coimbatore.

Anns Issac, Research Scholar, Centre of Social Medicine and Community Health, Jawaharlal Nehru University, New Delhi.

B.S. Mishra, Manager-Health, Bharat Integrated Social Welfare Agency (BISWA), Sambalpur, Orissa.

Manju S. Nair, Lecturer, Department of Economics, University of Kerala, Thiruvananthapuram.

Anand Parihar, Senior Research Officer, Global Adult Tobacco Survey-India, International Institute for Population Sciences, Mumbai.

Usha Ram, Associate Professor, Department of Public Health and Mortality Studies, International Institute for Population Sciences, Mumbai.

S. Ramaswamy, Professor and Head, Gandhigram Rural University, Gandhigram, Tamil Nadu.

J. Sacratees, Lecturer, Manonmaniam Sundaranar University, Tirunelveli, Tamil Nadu.

G. Sathis Kumar, Research Scholar, Gandhigram Rural University, Gandhigram, Tamil Nadu.

M.H. Suryanarayana, Professor, Indira Gandhi Institute of Development Research (IGIDR), Mumbai.

Sabu Thomas, Lecturer in Politics, Government College, Madappally, Vadakara, Kerala.

K.E. Vaidyanathan, President, Indian Association of Social Sciences and Health (IASSH), Chennai.

V. Vijayalakshmi, Research Scholar, Department of Sociology, Pondicherry University, Puducherry.

K.V. Vinesh Kumar, Project Fellow, UGC MRP, Department of Applied Economics, Kannur University, Kerala.

K.P. Vipin Chandran, Research Scholar, Department of Applied Economics, Kannur University, Kannur, Kerala.

Introduction

K. GANGADHARAN

There is complex interrelationship between health and development; it is certainly not a one-way relationship, and there are surely reciprocal and synergistic elements to it. It has long been acknowledged that the health status of the population in any particular place or country influences development. It can be a limiting factor, as generally poor individual health can lower work capacity and productivity; this can severely restrict the growth of economies. On the other hand, economic development can make it possible to finance good environmental health, sanitation and public health campaign, education and immunization, screening and health promotion and to provide broader-based social care for needy groups.

Both the concepts, health and development, are in any case difficult to define and almost impossible to quantify in way quite acceptable to all. But we are all aware that health status is changing with development and it is not invariably changing for the better. Life expectancy has increased the world over but the quality of life is under severe threat and there are large numbers of people in many countries for whom development has not led to health improvements. For example, many people, especially among the poor and particularly in the so-called Third World, are experiencing twin threats from infectious and chronic diseases. These problems are not confined solely to poor countries and retrenchment in public sector and overdomination of private sector and private health care. Expenditure is a common phenomenon which makes the public health care system a scarecrow.

Economic growth and development affect the health of the people by increasing their level of income and hence in the consumption, increasing goods and services. It means, there is a positive relationship between health and stages of economic growth and development but it is not always true. In this connection it is useful to note two important consequences of the improvement of health: demographic transition and epidemiological transition. As population become healthier, they also live long which is known as demographic transition. It occurs due to two reasons. First, when the health status of the individual improves, they live longer. Assuming given birth rate, the net addition to the population each year increases, increasing the share of older people in the total population. Second, the fertility rate may tend to decline due to better health and greater economic security. Of course, this has more indirect effect on the change in health status; as development proceeds, the pattern of diseases change which is known epidemiological transition. This has also two effects. First, when some diseases and good health are controlled or eliminated, the relative importance of other diseases increases as a matter of arithmetic. Second, as individuals live longer, diseases that only affect older individuals increase in absolute terms. Similarly, reduction in maternal mortality leads to a larger number of older women and to a greater prevalence of post-menopausal health problems.

Determinants of Health

The fact that the health status of a person is largely determined by chance, that health is perishable and lacks tradeability, does not rule out considering health being result of a production process. Health of an individual is complicated and multidimensional; and influenced by plethora of factors such as income of the person; pattern of educational attainment; population growth; density of population and age structure; abundance of natural resources; personal and government savings; physical capital stock; the geography, for example, the location and climate of a country; food; housing and sanitation; social practices; measures to control environmental hazards; and communicable diseases positively or negatively. Per capita income is highly correlated with indicators such as life expectancy and infant mortality, not only in between but also within countries, which is known as income-health linkage. This is because of two reasons. First, as income increases, it has become easier or cheaper to attain and maintain given level of health over time. Second, individual preferences have been changed over time and that for a given level of income, individuals have become more concerned about health. The close linkage between the two (income and health outcome) have not been fully appreciated.

Good health is not only an outcome of increasing income but is also a determinant of the other. Apart from governing the core of human well-being, health itself promotes development via increase in productivity and hence income, which is known as health income linkages. The improvement in health status of people is essential to sustain economic and social development. It is not difficult to imagine that healthier people tend to be more fit, strong, and energetic than unhealthy individuals and they add more value within the same time. The issue of health is of great importance both from the point of view of the individuals and the nation as well. The health status of a population is a reflection of the socio-economic development of the country and is shaped by a variety of factors – the level of income and standard of living, housing, sanitation, water supply, education, employment, health consciousness, personal hygiene and by the coverage, availability, accessibility and affordability of health care delivery services. It is widely accepted that the poor health status of low-income countries is the product of inadequate nutrition, lack of protected water supply and over crowded and unsanitary working conditions. Health is an important problem both in advanced and developing countries.

It was against this background to study the spatial, social and economic aspects of health and development, the Department of Applied Economics, Kannur University organized an international conference on 'Health and Development: Issues, Strategies and Options' on 22nd and 23rd October 2008. It was sponsored and funded by Indian Council of Medical Research and University Grants Commission, New Delhi. The conference was devoted to acquire a broad understanding of the linkage between health and development and succeeded in eliciting the basic issues and constraints connected with health and development and suggested policy measures for reducing the volume and intensity of these issues. Experts from multiple disciplines participated in the conference and presented their papers with subsequent in-depth discussions on each aspect of the subject. In all, twenty papers finally revised after the conference has been received from the experts belonging to multidisciplinary boundaries for publication. These papers are accordingly categorized into four sections and presented subsequently in the book. The major sub-themes are: (1) Health Care System and Policy; (2) Health and Development: Issues and Strategies; (3) Equity and Health; and (4) Health Status and Health Security.

I

Health Care System and Policy

B.N. Ghosh in his paper 'Rich Doctors and Poor Patients: Market Failure and Health Care Systems in Developing Countries' argues that, in developing countries, health care systems (HCS) have been facing the problem of market failure, implying that the fair rules of market principles do not apply and patients often become losers. Explaining the theoretical issues involved, the paper examines various causes of market failures in health care systems including: rent-seeking activities by doctors, asymmetric information between doctors and patients, between patients and insurance companies, and the oligopolistic behaviour of health care practitioners. The policy implications of the study suggest that in many cases, government intervention is essential to eliminate market failures in the health care systems in developing countries.

M.H. Suryanarayana in his paper 'Eleventh Five-Year Plan on Food Security: Estimates and Interpretations' examines the issue of food security in the wake of food inflation and its adverse implications for morbidity and health status. The Eleventh Five-Year Plan of the government of India too recognizes the need to ensure food security to provide a sustained solution to morbidity. However, there is much scope for reconsidering its assessment of the situation on food security in India. According to him one issue, which has not received due academic attention, is the inconsistency in methods used for comparative analysis of issues pertaining to food security and health status. While issues pertaining to food security are examined with reference to objective measures like average food grain consumption, calorie intake and calorie norms, those pertaining to morbidity are analysed on the basis of subjective perceptions and hence, estimates of morbidity. The calorie norms used for food security verification were developed in the 1950s/1960s and could be outdated and irrelevant with improvements in education, awareness, modes of production, hygiene and sanitation and standard of living. Hence, it would not make any sense to verify questions on food security with reference to outdated exogenous norms, presupposing that the expert knows the needs of the people better than the people themselves. Therefore, to ensure consistency in methods, Suryanarayana in his paper examined issues pertaining to food security with reference to people's own perception of having consumed adequate food. He provides profiles of food security based on objective measures as well as household perception on adequacy of food and raises certain issues pertaining to policy and research.

K. Gangadharan in his paper 'Policy Reforms and Health Care System in Kerala: Constraints and Optims' examined the crisis that occurred in the health care segment of Kerala especially with the era of liberalization and economic reforms. The enormous growth of private sector hospitals and clinics and neglect of public health centres, as scare-crows is an indication that the state sector is lagging far behind in the field of social reproduction. The paper provides solid database for the declining role of public sector and the dominating share of private sector in the health care scenario of Kerala. The study suggested some basic and fundamental policy measures for revamping public health care system like targeted information education and communication campaign for urban slums and rural poor on family planning and Reproductive and Child Health (RCH) services, environmental and health awareness programme with NGO participation, better nutrition, environmental and preventive health care programmes, taxation of private health care for funding public preventive health care services, and greater public investment in health sector.

II
Health and Development: Issues and Strategies

Malathy Duraisamy and **P. Duraisamy** in their paper 'Investing in Health: A Review of Measurement, Theory and Indian Evidence' provides an overview of health indicators, examine trends in some of the health indicators in India, present an economic theory which provides a framework for analysing household's demand for health and present empirical evidence based on household demand framework for India. According to them health is an important form of investment in human capital. Health is unobservable and several indicators are used to measure the health status of the population. Each measure has its usefulness and limitations. A careful examination of the measurement and issues related to the indicators is essential to appreciate the multidimensionality of health. A more important concern is to see what determines the health status of a population. Social scientists have contributed to this endeavour. Notable contributions have been made by economists in the analysis of various issues relating to health and health care. In this paper the production and demand for health within a household context has been examined using the household demand model.

K. Govindarajalu in his paper 'Government Expenditure on Health Care Provision in India' analyses the government health expenditure in India between 1995 and 2007. He has analysed the government expenditure on health care provisions and funding under National Rural Health Mission (NRHM). The overall picture of government spending on health reveals that the trend in the expenditure has been increasing in nominal terms but slow in real and per capita terms. However, the combined expenditure of both centre and state has shown the declining trend over the period. At the same time there has been an increasing trend in government health expenditure as per cent of GDP and also in the share of government health expenditure in total government expenditure during 2005 and 2007. It has been observed that this increasing trend is due to the introduction of NRHM launched in 2005. NRHM provides for a significant share in total state allocation. During 2006–07 there has been 20.58 per cent of NRHM allocation in the total state's allocation. The paper provides an in depth analysis of the trends in public expenditure on health especially with the post-and pre-NRHM periods.

'Emerging Health Scenario in India: Present Challenges and Future Strategies' by **R. Annapoorani** provides that the deplorable conditions of basic infrastructural facilities on the one side and lack of committed health personnel and health infrastructure on the other are the basic problems for the burgeoning health problems of the country. Health is an important aspect of human resource development and good health is considered as an integral element of development. With increased urbanization and changing environment, the changing nature of health problems has become a great concern for the world today. Therefore, out of ten millennium development goals, three goals emphasize on health. They are to reduce child mortality, improve maternal health and combat HIV/AIDS/malaria and other diseases. India is in the second stage of health transition characterized by high morbidity, though crude death rate decreased from 12.5 to 8.7 between 1981 and 2001. A comparative picture of India with other countries of the world indicates that India lags behind other developed countries in health indicators. Further, there is disparity in health indicators among the states and this is the cause for serious concern.

V. Anitha in her study on 'Cost of Treatment: A Study Based on Medical Pluralism' examines the cost of treatment under different systems of medicine like allopathy, ayurveda, homoeopathy, siddha, unani, naturopathy and yoga in the typical context of Kerala, a state identified for better health care development. The study found that there exists large disparity in the cost of treatment in different systems of medicine. The cost of allopathy is the highest in both rural and urban areas followed by that of ayurveda and homoeopathy. The average direct cost of treatment regarding acute illness as well as chronic illness under all the systems of medicine in urban areas is greater than that in rural areas. The average indirect cost of treatment under allopathy and ayurveda for chronic illness in urban areas is greater than that in rural areas while in the case of homoeopathy, the average indirect cost of acute illness as well as chronic illness in rural areas is greater than that in urban areas. The paper concludes by disclosing the fact that increasing burden of chronic and degenerative diseases in Kerala demands systematic expansion of medical pluralism, which has the potential to provide cost-effectiveness, accessibility, availability and equity in the field of health care.

K.P. Vipin Chandran in his paper 'Health-Related Millennium Development Goals in India: Realities and Challenges' focuses on the specific issues related to the health-related millennium development goals MDGs in India. The paper sets out three objectives and examines the progress regarding health-related MDGs and lastly suggests the policy initiatives and strategic approaches for achieving health-related millennium development goals in India. The paper provides that targets set in the National Health Policy, National Population Policy and the Eleventh Five-Year Plan are in tune with those under the MDGs. The NRHM is expected to provide the much-needed stimulus and strengthen the capacity of the health infrastructure towards attaining the MDGs by 2015. According to him the targeted programmes for vulnerable and marginalized groups are essential with increased public investment, especially in the education and health sectors.

J. Sacratees in his paper 'Economic Valuation of Impact of Air Pollution in Manali Industrial Area of Chennai, Tamil Nadu' estimates the welfare loss due to hazardous air quality of Manali Industrial Area of Chennai city, which is one of the fast developing metropolitan cities of South India. This area is surrounded with high industrial corridors and operating with heavy vehicles. The primary causes of air pollution are use of heavy vehicles and enormous chemical, thermal and petrochemical industrial operations. In fact, the Manali area is highly vulnerable area as far as air pollution is concerned. The study estimated the loss of welfare use of econometric methods like Logit and Tobit models in order to introduce willingness to pay to improve the quality of urban air pollution. The paper analysed how reducing air pollution could increase the monetary value of health benefits. Above all the economic costs associated with these health risks are also evaluated using available economic information. It enabled for the measure of calculation of cost of illness and man-days loss, wage loss, cost of medicine and cost of hospitalization due to air pollution etc. This paper addressed the current status and consequences of air quality, which causes concern in the developing countries.

'Availability of ICDS Facilities and Its Association with Child Nutrition in Rural India' by **Anand Parihar** and **Usha Ram** examined that nutrition is an important determinant of health. The first six years of life are the most crucial period of the life and have a great and lasting influence on the quality of life of a human being. This chapter is concerned with the basic rights of children under the age of six years, especially their right to nutrition, health and education. It focuses on the Integrated Child Development Services (ICDS) as a crucial means of protecting these rights. There are a number of factors, which affect child nutrition, either directly or indirectly. The study reveals that in rural India, about 26 per cent children are severely stunted whereas seven per cent children are severely wasted and eighteen per cent children are severely underweight. About forty-nine, seventy-nine and 54 per cent children are average among stunted, wasted and underweight. About thirty-two per cent of children living in rural India are severely stunted belonging to age group 25–36. Severe wasting is observed among children under 12 months of age whereas severe underweight children range between 13 and 48 months of age. Children belonging to scheduled caste, scheduled tribe or other backwards classes have relatively high levels of malnutrition according to all three measures. Children from scheduled tribes have the poorest nutrition status on almost every measure.

III
Equity and Health

Manju S. Nair in her paper 'Rich-Poor Divide in Health Status in India' examined on how the India's poorest people are faring, demonstrating the persistence and pervasiveness of inequalities in health using NFHS–III data. With the available data the author has revealed that the poorest people fare worse than the richest on a range of health outcomes including infant and childhood mortality and nutritional status and fertility indices. Widespread discrepancy exists in the use of health services like vaccination coverage, health care visits, maternity related services etc. In general, the poor in India are disadvantaged in all aspects of health. At the household level the poor are more vulnerable to disease because of a lack of financial resources, limited knowledge of and education on health matters, limited use of health services and inadequate nutrition. The paper categorically states that the poor are more likely to find that the health services are unavailable, inaccessible, too expensive or of relatively low quality. Governmental spending also may not benefit the poor because many governments allocate the highest proportion of their health budgets to urban hospitals, leaving rural residents without adequate health facilities. The study suggested that in the long term a comprehensive pro-poor approach will influence the multiple social and economic determinants of health disparities, improving access to vital services, opportunities and reducing discrimination and isolation.

Ankush Agrawal in the study 'Infant Mortality in India: Dimensions of Development' examines the distribution of infant mortality rates (IMR) in its spatial and temporal dimensions in India. Given the focus on the Millennium Development Goals (MDGs), it examines whether past trend behaviour would lend any support to the belief that its MDG target for child mortality is realizable. The study examined, inter alia, the pace of reduction and, convergence in IMR across states by sector. The study finds evidence for absolute convergence across the Indian states as well as convergence conditional on state per capita income.

'Gender Discrimination in Health Care' by **Saumya Chand** has provided a three dimensional analysis connected with the concept of gender and health care. First, to discuss the concept of gender preference and discrimination in nutrition and health care in Indian society and status of women's health in India. This part also, emphasizes on various socio-economic factors responsible for gender discrimination and impact of gender discrimination in health care facilities, especially on female mortality and sex ratio. The second part of the paper she emphasizes on the regional variations in the female mortality and sex ratio and provides a comparative picture on all-India bases. At the end of the paper she suggests some measures for improvization of better health facilities for women in India.

'Health of the Workers in Plantation Economy: A Study of Cardamom Plantations in Kerala' by **Anns Issac** examines the various dimensions of health of workers in cardamom plantations in Idukki district of Kerala. Plantation sector has significant role in Kerala in terms of both the number of people dependent on it for livelihood and in terms of its contribution to GDP. The study has been undertaken with an objective to understand the workers well-being in relation to changes in cardamom industry and to understand as to how workers negotiate their basic rights to health by looking into their material conditions. It also focuses on the dynamics of representation of plantation workers issues by various stakeholders.

'Poverty and Human Development in India: An Inter-State Analysis' by **K.V. Vinesh Kumar** provides various dimensions of poverty among the states in India with implications on human development. The utilization of health services is nearly twice in the southern states as compared to the northern states where mortality rate is higher. Improvement in health in India contributes in more poverty reduction and serves as an element of a pro-poor strategy. National governments too are rethinking about their health and development strategies to suit the poverty-health milieu. Dealing with poverty is not a new situation to India and her 60 years of health policy experience has had several strategies to deal with poverty-health nexus. The study proved that in those states where human development is high, the proportion of people below poverty line is very low and he advocates that better human development is the panacea for the removal of poverty.

G. Sathis Kumar and **S. Ramaswamy** in their paper 'Refugee Health Care: Policy Options and Strategic Directions' mainly addresses to the emerging issues in refugee health care and an attempt has been made to identify the policy options which necessitates the need of the health strategy for the refugee; and also examined the existing strategic and policy directions in refugee health care. The study is highly significant in the current global context as the world's refugee burden falls increasingly on developing countries. Current refugee phenomenon is characterized by large influxes from one developing country into another. Every year, millions of people around the world flee their homes, and become the victims of violence, and other circumstances including an environmental component – from rising sea level, to drought, to encroaching deserts. The study suggests for refugee communities to make strategic choices conducive to their health and better access for refugees to a range of health services to enhance the health services directed to the refugee's health, in partnership with community-based organizations, and governmental agencies.

IV
Health Status and Health Security

'Ageing of Population in India: Emerging Health Issues' by **K.E. Vaidyanathan** provides the various health consequences of ageing process and its implications for policy. He defined ageing of population as the process by which the proportion of elderly persons in the population increases as a result of continuous decline in fertility and mortality over the years. In 1990, the proportion of population over 60 years of age has been only 6.8 per cent, but this is likely to increase to 20.1 per cent by 2050. Moreover, the oldest old (80 years and over) is also expected to increase to 3.1 per cent in 2050 from about 0.4 per cent in 1990. In absolute terms the elderly population in India (60+) will increase from 76.7 million in 2000 to 302.5 million in 2050, which is a fourfold increase. The population of very old (80+) will increase from 6.1 million in 2000 to 47 million in 2050, almost an eightfold increase. The method adopted in the paper is to compare the situation in India with the situation in China and other countries with more advanced ageing. At the same time an attempt has been made to look at the situation in states like Kerala and Tamil Nadu, which are ahead of the rest of the states in the ageing process. The paper also provides that the ageing of population is taking place alongside the epidemiological transition in the country as reflected in the changing pattern of causes of death. There will be a decline in the share of communicable diseases as we move from the nascent stage of ageing to an advanced stage of ageing. The relative share of infectious and parasitic diseases will decline and the relative share of non-communicable diseases will increase. Non-communicable diseases like malignant neoplasm, diabetes mellitus, cardiovascular diseases and nutritional and endocrinal disorders will increase with the ageing of population. As a result of the shift towards chronic and degenerative diseases, there is a greater risk of disabilities among the elderly. The extended longevity of the elderly will comprise of years with chronic illnesses, the most common ailments being cardiovascular diseases, hypertension, diabetes, visual and hearing impairment, mental illnesses etc. Since women tend to live longer than men, the number of women will surpass the number of men among the elderly, and many of them will be widows who will depend upon their sons or daughters or public support systems for support. They are also likely to be more vulnerable to illnesses during old age. The paper provides proper recommendations for promoting the WHO framework of 'active ageing', where active ageing is defined as the process of optimizing opportunities for health, participation and security in order to enhance quality of life as people become aged.

B.S. Mishra in his paper 'Ensuring Health Services for the Poor through Sustainable Micro-Insurance: Experience of BISWA in Sambalpur, Orissa' reveals how an NGO acts as a safety net for health problems of the rural people through a micro insurance scheme. Health insurance is needed by both the people living below poverty line and those above it. The paper provides the in-depth analysis of how Bharat Integrated Social Welfare Agency (BISWA's) innovative approach of micro insurance+services benefited the rural people and how it could be gradually extended to a wider population of Sambalpur district of Orissa. In the paper he also suggests pluralistic and innovative model to reach out to members of SHGs, federations (clusters of SHGs), beggars and people with disability and opt for a sustainable development approach for pro-poor development in achieving MDG by 2015.

The paper 'Health Status of Elderly in Old-Age Homes' by **V. Vijayalakshmi** and **K. Anbu** aims to find the health status of elderly in an old-age home naming 'Volantariat' in Puducherry. It concentrates on the health care facilities provided by the old-age home. The paper reveals that India, like many traditional societies, today faces a unique situation in providing care for its elderly as the existing old-age support structures in the form of family, kith and kin, are fast eroding and the elderly are ill-equipped to cope alone with their lives in the face of infirmity and disability. The onus of caring for the elderly is therefore now much more on the state than the family and has necessitated the creation of adequate institutional support. Old-age homes are a necessity in the present day scenario as such it examines the working of one such old-age home at Puducherry.

Sabu Thomas in his paper 'The Politics of Health Security: Challenges of Neo-Liberal State: An Indian Perspective' reveals that the emergence of globalization undermined the very notion of a welfare state and replaced it with a soft state. This new state is characterized with liberalization, privatization and public private participation. It is conditioned by the themes of international funding agencies. According to him major challenge of globalization is the balancing between state as corporation and state as a guardian. The soft state is a service provider; a business concern – levying the services whenever and wherever possible.

In the Indian context this new paradigm shift shattered the edifice of our health policy. He also states that the inevitable pay-use policy, when implemented to health sector may result in many far reaching consequences, In the absence of a strong social security system the marginalized may become a prey to the health corporations. Even though the support of international agencies resulted in enhanced infrastructure, in the long run they cannot be maintained if they are not rewarding. He categorically identifies three major challenges in this context. They are health care input management crisis, infrastructure, professionals and policy process management crisis-employee management, beneficiary management and system maintenance, output crisis, social cost and political cost. This crisis forms the base of any future political discourse on health system in neo-liberal state. The main three remedial approaches suggested by him are protective guardian community approach – It postulates the community as the guardian of individual concerns, health security can be achieved by the decentralized activities of these communities. Alternative choice approach – New alternative choice should replace the traditional dependence system. The disease burden can be subjected and fought with alternative choices and finally the public-private partnership approach.

Conclusion

The population of the world has witnessed an unprecedented growth mainly over past five decades. The world population, which was 2.5 billion in 1950, has gone up to about 6.5 billion today and is expected to cross 8 billion mark by 2025. This hike in population has aroused much interest in the health and health status of the people around the globe. Every nation in the world is now faced with acute crisis in the health care sector and the usual depiction of crisis in public health is in terms of cost of care, quality of care, higher cost and lesser care, questions of affordability, rapidly rising prices and growing dissatisfaction about the availability of services. According to Henry Sigerist "Health is one of the goods of life to which man has a right; wherever this concept prevails the logical sequence is to make all measures for the protection and restoration of health accessible to all, free of charge; medicine like education is then no longer a trade, it becomes a public function of the State", Even the developed nations like America and Canada are faced with acute health care crisis and it is reflected in the form of lack of universal coverage and insurance, deteriorating quality and high cost of care, poor management, increasing expenditure for geriatric care etc.

In India, we have certain worrying features in our system. We account for 21 per cent of the global burden of disease and 25 per cent of maternal deaths take place in this country and the same may be true of neonatal mortality rate. Similarly, the share of total expenditure on public health system in India stands at a dismally low figure of 0.9 per cent of GDP. The people of the country are not protected against the high cost of health care and they are in the octopus hold of private health care providers. In this juncture any health system should see to it that the financial protection is extended against the catastrophic illnesses and the poor people who are really worst affected with high cost, are not constrained to seek care. So development agenda must be planned in such a way that the fruits of development must be able to percolate to the downtrodden, marginalized and vulnerable sections of the society without adversely affecting the health care accessibility, equity, quality along with a living environment promoting health.

Section I

Health Care System and Policy

1

Rich Doctors and Poor Patients

Market Failure and Health Care Systems in Developing Countries

B.N. GHOSH

As affirmed by the World Health Organization (WHO), health can be conceptualized as a state of complete physical, mental and social well-being. Thus, the concept of health includes the physiological as well as psychological dimensions of human life. Public health is a type of public good, or more precisely merit good, which is very critical for general social welfare. Body capital (the physical human body) is part and parcel of the human capital that determines the rate of growth of labour productivity and economic progress of a country. These days, in many developing countries, health planning, therefore, is made an integral part of general economic planning. Public health services are the services that are rendered by government institutions for the prevention and cure of diseases and also for the maintenance of the good health of the nation. Public health services are concerned mainly with dissatisfaction, discomfort, disease, disability and death (Sifford, 1977; Cullis and West, 1979: 12–13). Conventional wisdom, however, does not make any valid distinction between the health care systems and health care services in making theoretical and empirical analyses, although the two do not mean the same thing. Health care services are more concerned with all types of services that are needed for good health and the drug sector is generally excluded. The health care system is the totality of the health care protocol that includes all types of institutions, inputs and outputs that the system is dealing with. The present paper takes into consideration the broader view of health care by encompassing patients, doctors, insurance agents, drug manufacturers, drug policy, health institutions and health policy formulations by governments. Obviously, this includes more than just health care services.

It is believed that the market system brings about efficiency and equity and that it can automatically remove all types of distortions, inadequacies and problems (Ghosh, 2001). However, if one examines the state of the health care system (HCS) in developing countries, one does not fail to observe that it is neither efficient nor equitable. These HCSs have not been able to increase the supply of health care goods to meet demand; they have not been able to provide markets for many types of health care goods and services; they have not been able to reduce price differences of these products within and across countries, and they have not been able to reduce inequalities in the distribution of health care goods and services. What has gone wrong in the working of the HCS in many developing countries? Why cannot they function properly? Why and how have they failed? What is the alternative to market failure in the HCSs? All these questions are very relevant in public HCSs in developing countries. An attempt has been made in this paper to answer these questions in a straightforward manner as far as possible.

The present paper is related to a well-known debate that became prominent from the mid-1980s between the neo-liberal writers of the tradition of Chicago-Virginia Schools on the one hand and the more social democratic views of Rawls, Stiglitz and Sen, on the other, about the relative hazards of 'market failures' and 'government failures'. The social democratic tradition has castigated the unbridled role of the market and goes against the Chicago-Virginia School approach. This paper picks up the thread of this debate and supports the social democratic viewpoint.[1]

The paper is organized in the following way. The first section is an analysis of the syndrome of market failure. This will include a theoretical discussion on market failure, followed by an analysis of market failure in the HCS in developing countries. The next section delineates the major consequences of market failure in the HCS. The policy implications of the study focus on the importance of government intervention in the event of market failure in the HCS. These are elaborated in subsequent sections. The final section offers some conclusions.

The Syndrome of Market Failure

In understanding market failure, it is essential to start off the discussion with the concept of market. A market is an interactive socio-economic institution for facilitating the exchange of goods and services between prospective buyers and sellers. Markets provide an allocative mechanism whereby price signals indicate opportunities and directions for exchange. A market is a very critical, impersonal and neutral institution that makes possible exchanges of goods and services at prices set by it through the process of interactions of demand and supply. In a market, the price mechanism is used as an important signal for the demand and supply such that when the price is high, it is profitable to supply more, and at the same time, the consumers get a signal to decrease the demand, other things remaining the same. Given the supply and demand in the market in the short period, a particular price level becomes an equilibrium price at which both demand and supply would be equal and the market would be cleared. The market is cleared automatically by the forces of demand and supply. It is this quality of the market that makes it a powerful institution to settle all aberrations in the market. Neo-classical economists in general rely on the efficiency of automatic free market mechanism to ward off all sorts of economic ills without the assistance of the government. The government in such a system is accorded a minimal role to regulate the economy.

The most important aspect of a market is that it automatically works for creating an ideal situation by eliminating undesirable differences. How does it achieve this outcome? It is mainly through free and fair competition. For instance, if a cardiologist's income is high in the market but a urologist's pay is low, then there would be a move on the part of would-be doctors to specialize in cardiology and after some time, there would be a larger supply of cardiologists, and through competition, the pay difference would be more or less eliminated, if all other things remain unchanged. This does not mean that a more skilled or qualified doctor will not receive higher pay according to the market system, but it simply shows that the average pay differences can still be there and would be equivalent to the average cost differences of obtaining the necessary qualifications.

However, it must be mentioned that for the automatic working of the market mechanism, some conditions are necessary. The market must work freely and fairly without interference from any quarters. Also, the exclusion principle must apply: if a person is not willing to pay for the goods demanded, then the person can be excluded from consuming them. Obviously, preferences and choices can be revealed in a market through demand, supply and prices. It is possible for individuals to make independent decisions in a market without being coerced by others. To work properly a market must give full freedom to its participants and must be highly competitive. A market should be open and ready for competition; that is, it must have contestability. A market should be complete and adequate without any missing component and a good market is characterized by a free flow of costless and asymmetric information. The transaction cost, information cost, contracting cost and enforcement cost in a perfect market is very low or zero. Finally, the knowledge and information system should be complete and easily accessible.

'Market failure' refers to those situations in which the market cannot work efficiently and automatically solve problems like unemployment, inflation and income inequality that would otherwise be solved by a normally functioning market. In the case of market failure, the rules of efficiency cannot be fully applied. The two most important rules of efficiency are that: (i) marginal cost (i.e., the cost of the last unit of the item) must be equal to the revenue from the last unit of the item (marginal revenue); and (ii) the social benefits at the margin (MSB) must be equal to the social cost at the margin (MSC) so that society's benefit is the maximum. The first rule suggests that if marginal cost (MC) is equal to marginal revenue (MR) from any project or enterprise, the price would be as low as possible and the output would as high as possible in the circumstances.

However, if competition is imperfect and restricted, MR will not be equal to MC. Such a situation is possible in the presence of monopoly power and restrictive trade practices. In the case of monopoly (one seller), there will be less production and more wastage. In the case of market imperfection and asymmetric information (where the participants do not have an equal stock of information), there may be either more or less production than that justified by an efficient market. In such a case, the ruling price level fails to clear the market; there may be either excess demand or excess supply. Market failure is characterized by different symptoms such as unemployment, recession, inequalities, inflation and stagflation (excessive price rise not accompanied by economic growth).

The main reasons for market failure can now be explained with reference to the HCS of a typical developing economy. It should be noted that the HCS includes many institutions, many types of services and products. The HCS can be a type of public good which could be enjoyed by all or many without having to make payments more often at the point of need. For example, spraying to kill mosquitoes or the chlorination of water by the health department are examples of public goods. Booklets or advertisements circulated freely by health authorities about the early symptoms of AIDS or cancer, are typical public goods. Public goods are those goods which can be simultaneously consumed by all people without harming the interest of any particular consumer. In the case of public goods in the realm of the HCS, it is often difficult to know the exact demand of the society; the demand is not revealed by the people because they think that they can enjoy the benefits of the commodity or services without making any payment – the so-called free rider problem. Thus, public goods cannot be produced in optimum amount, and generally, the actual production remains lower than the necessary production, and social efficiency cannot be attained in the matter of production of these goods. The market fails precisely because: first, it cannot prevent people from consuming the good even without payments (the exclusion principle, as discussed earlier, does not apply); second, the market has no way to know the total demand for the public goods, as some people will not reveal their demand for the fear of making payment; third, under these circumstances, the market cannot apply any rule or principle to allocate resources for the optimum supply of these goods. The market does not know what should be the optimal supply. Moreover, since these goods are not priced in usual way, the price mechanism becomes irrelevant.

Another main cause of market failure in the domain of the HCS is the prevalence of externalities. Externalities are costs or benefits thrust on other individuals by the actions of some individuals or firms (e.g., water pollution by a riverside drug factory). Externalities may be positive (beneficial) or negative (harmful). The damage caused by a drug factory or a chemical factory is a type of social cost that currently is not taken into account in the pricing and output decisions of the drug (or chemical) firms. Hence, social cost does not become equal to social benefits in such cases, and actual production of those goods is often higher than what would justified by a normal market system. The market tends to fail if there are considerable negative externalities in the HCS which cannot be internalized by the market prices; the social damage caused by wrong products or services is not reflected in the price mechanism. Externalities are not communicated through the market. Hence, the market mechanism does not address them.

Healthy persons can benefit the society in many ways. Like education, health has many types of positive externalities (or spill over effects). For instance, a healthy person is less contagious than a sick one. The spill over effect is responsible for market failure because the market cannot be expected to deliver the socially efficient level of health system (Todaro and Smith, 2003: 368). In the cases where the health care product market is imperfect (not many sellers or competitors), monopoly comes into existence and the allocation of resources cannot be done efficiently because cost does not become equal to revenue at the margin. Since under monopoly, output is generally lower and price is often higher, the society is deprived of the benefits of extra output which could have been produced had the HCS been allowed to work under a more competitive environment. Under such a system, the market fails for three reasons. First, under monopoly, the actual market price becomes higher than the competitive price. Second, actual output is lower than the competitive output. Third, the social benefit does not become equal to social cost at the margin. Moreover, in the case of natural monopolies like hospitals and hospital-based services (provided by very expensive equipment including ultrasound scanning and haemodialysis), the average cost decreases as the number of patients increases. Thus, as cost comes down, the price should come down but a private monopolist (for instance, a private hospital) will charge the same or a much higher price to the patients. If there is only a special private hospital offering a particular services or expertise, the right price cannot be determined by the market mechanism. The market fails. Hospitals can be called natural monopolies because their construction, infrastructures and services are so expensive that no competitive market may be expected to provide them in abundance especially in a developing country.

However, many writers from the Chicago-Virginia School argue that market dominance may not be a problem so long as there is potential competition or contestability (Posner, 1992). If any firm charges prices higher than average cost, other firms will enter the market and will take away the customers of the monopolist firm. The classic example is airlines. If any airline charges prices higher than the average cost, other airlines flying nearby will change the route and pick up the passengers by charging prices which are equal to average cost. However, such a line of argument is not applicable to health care systems. Hospitals are not mobile institutions. Also, many types of specialists may form a cartel which may be composed of, for example, highly specialized surgeons' or physicians' services. These are unique in many senses in a developing country where the supply of such specialists is highly limited in a particular region and the cost of transfer of patients in terms of inconvenience, time and money is extremely high.

Market failure may also arise out of information failure or, imperfect and incomplete information. There are many problems with the information system: the available stock of information may be incomplete, distorted and even wrong. Information asymmetry occurs when the two transacting parties (say doctor and patient) do not have an equal stock of information about the relevant problem (say disease). The uneven information between the two parties may make the cost different from the benefit at the margin. Therefore, the rules of efficiency cannot be properly applied. The market fails.

Information asymmetry may involve moral hazard when information about the actual action to be taken is not disclosed by one party. For instance, a doctor, who is posted with better information and knowledge than the patient regarding the disease and the medicines, may not disclose to the patient the line of treatment, its duration and the severity of the disease. Moral hazard is also present when the patient depends too much on the mercy of the doctor. In the case of moral hazard between the doctor and the patient, the social cost may be higher than the social benefit in the sense that the doctor gets an opportunity to play ducks and drakes with the life of a patient. Adverse selection (somewhat undesirable selection) occurs when information on which the transaction is to take place is hidden by one party from the other. For instance, a health insurance company always wants to insure a person of normal health without disease ('cream scheming'), but some persons sometimes hide information about their congenital bad health and get themselves insured. This is an example of adverse selection by the health insurance company. Agency problems are also associated with asymmetric information. The agents, for instance bureaucrats may not part with all the relevant information to the principal (may be the minister). In such a case, because of information asymmetry, there may be a divergence between social benefits and social cost at the margin, and there may not be any compromise (competitive equilibrium) between the two involved parties having unequal knowledge (say doctor and patient). The market often fails to remove the distortions contrived by a party for maximizing his personal gains. The allocation of resources cannot be efficient under such circumstances, as the risk and uncertainties are not properly evaluated on the basis of available stock of information. The market fails to alleviate the situation.

Market Failure in the Health Care System

Having understood the theoretical basis of market failure, it is now appropriate to discuss this problem with reference to the HCS. To appreciate the situation of market failure in the HCS, it is necessary to discuss first the major problems involved in this system. Basically, as discussed in the next two sections, there are three sets of associated problems concerning doctors, patients and insurance agents.

Demand Side Problems

A basic problem is the rising cost (expenditure) of public health services and products. In many developing countries, the rate of growth of the per capita cost of health services has outstripped the growth of real income per capita over time from the point of view of patients. The billing is too high. The information on the treatment between the doctor and the patient is asymmetric and something very secret; the patient cannot question the billing. There is no bargaining power of the patient who is generally a poor person in a developing country. Thus, there is an element of exploitation either potential or actual, implicit in the system and an in-built institutional discrimination against the patient.

As against the rising cost of private health expenditure, the real public expenditure on health is gradually going down even in most of the higher-income developing countries, including Malaysia (see Gomez, 1998) and the Organization for Economic Cooperation and Development (OECD) countries (see Table 1). Conceivably, the situation in poor developing countries is more bleak. As Table 1 shows, in all the countries for which data are available, the percentage of public health expenditure has shown a declining trend between 1980 and 2002. Interestingly, the fall in public health expenditure in these countries has occurred during the period when their governments had been aiming at higher rates of economic growth. One may suspect that public health expenditure is competing with expenditures that lead to quantitative growth of output in these countries. Evidently, globalization has not contributed to the betterment of public health in these countries. The initial years of globalization in the 1980s witnessed higher percentage of public expenditure on health but as the tempo of globalization increased, expenditure on health showed a declining trend: a comparison of 1980 and 2002 figures makes the point clear.

Table 1
Public Expenditure on Health (% of Total Expenditure)

Country	*1980*	*1990*	*2000*	*2002*
Belgium	—	78.5*	75.8	75.0
Canada	75.6	74.5	70.3	69.6
Czech Republic	96.8	97.4	90.5	89.7
Denmark	87.8	82.7	82.4	82.9
Germany	78.7	76.2	78.6	78.6
Hungary	—	89.1	70.7	70.2
Iceland	88.2	86.6	82.6	83.2
Netherlands	69.4	67.1	63.1	62.5
New Zealand	88.0	82.4	78.0	77.9
Norway	85.1	82.8	82.5	83.5
Slovak Republic	—	91.7*	89.4	89.1
Spain	79.9	78.7	71.6	71.3
Sweden	92.5	89.9	84.9	85.1
United Kingdom	89.4	83.6	80.9	83.4

Note: *Data for 1995.

Source: OECD Health Data (2006).

Apart from the constrained health expenditure, a patient's choice about the use of health care goods is extremely limited in less developed countries (LDCs), and there is low responsiveness of the market to consumers' demand. It is more the supply that creates demand, and not the other way round. This is so because of structural rigidity, supply constraints, limited technology and low effective demand for health products. For instance, a patient suffering from benign prostate enlargement (prostatitis) can ameliorate symptoms by taking a few herbal medicines including *Saw Palmetto* and *Pygeum Africanum*, but such herbal medicines are not available in many developing countries. There are indeed either incomplete or missing markets or both in developing countries for health care products or services. Moreover, the health care services market is less competitive, and the use of brand drugs rather than generic drugs escalates the cost of treatment. It is a popular perception that branded drugs are more expensive but of better quality. This may be true, as many poor hypertensive patients in developing countries generally use locally manufactured beta-blockers such as amlodipin or enalapril maleate, but their blood pressure does not often stabilize and continues fluctuating. Generic drugs are very cheap but the patients do not know their names and are not sure of their quality. The branded drugs produced by multinational firms are extremely expensive compared to generic drugs. For instance, the price of a branded anti-rheumatic drug like Voltaren (diclofenac Na. 25 mg tablet) is 900 per cent higher than the generic equivalent drug in Malaysia (Ghosh, 2000: 51). Likewise, the price of amoxycillin oral suspension (125mg/5ml) is 1,044 per cent higher in Malaysia compared to its generic substitute. There may be similar cases in many other developing countries.

There is unfortunately no incentive in the HCS for cost efficiency in LDCs. In the reimbursement system that prevails in many countries, neither the patients nor the doctors have any incentive to minimize the cost of treatment when the patients get their medical expenditure reimbursed. However, the poor patients not covered by the protective umbrella of reimbursement, do not have equal access to treatment. There are both vertical and horizontal equity problems. That is to say, there are inequalities among the equals (horizontal inequality) and also inequalities among unequals (vertical inequality). Such inequalities are created by distribution policies and undesirable delivery systems.

Distributional inequalities in the HCS encompass many dimensions that include inter-state disparities, group inequalities and rural-urban inequalities. For instance, like in many other developing countries, in the case of Mexico, public spending on health remained extremely urban biased between 1960 and 1980, in the sense that most of the advantages of such expenditure accrued only to the urban population. To take one example, in 1970, the ratio of inhabitants for paramedical personnel was 231 in the Federal District and 3, 432 in the state of Oaxaca (Aspe, 1993; Aspe and Sigmud, 1984). Many other health-related data confirm that the rural sector has been discriminated against.

As a matter of fact, in many cases, absolute income or even per capita income in a country does not become a true measure of the health level of its people. As A.K. Sen (1981) observes, it is not really the absolute income but the relative income as determined by the income distribution pattern of the country which is a more important determinant of effective entitlement for health services. Sen has found that despite low income, China, Sri Lanka and Kerala in South India have achieved a life expectancy of more than 70 years as compared to countries like Brazil, South Africa and Gabon which have lower life expectancy at birth in spite of their higher resources (Sen, 1999: 104). These countries have more inequitable distribution of health care facilities than those in many low income countries. Sometimes, through health subsidies and additional expenditure on health, governments try to mitigate the situation; but even in that case, the achievement remains far from the ideal in the sense that public expenditure as a percentage of total expenditure on health is low in many countries; it is lower than the private expenditure on health (see Table 2).

Table 2

*Private vs Public Expenditure (%) on Health (2000)**

Country	*Public*	*Private*	*Country*	*Public*	*Private*
Afghanistan	40.6	59.4	Mali	45.8	54.2
Armenia	41.5	58.5	Mauritania	30.3	69.7
Bangladesh	46.0	54.0	Mexico	41.0	59.0
Benin	47.2	52.8	Morocco	40.7	59.3
Bhutan	46.2	53.8	Myanmar	12.6	87.4
Brazil	48.7	51.3	Nepal	26.0	74.0
Brunei	40.6	59.4	Nigeria	28.2	71.8
Cambodia	9.4	91.6	Pakistan	22.9	77.1
Cameroon	20.1	79.9	Peru	39.7	60.3
China	24.0	76.0	Philippines	48.5	51.5
Congo	36.6	63.4	Korea (Rep.)	37.8	62.2
Côte d'Ivoire	38.4	61.6	Sierra Leone	09.7	90.3
Cyprus	38.8	61.2	Singapore	35.8	64.2
D.R. Congo	0.9	90.1	South Africa	46.5	53.5
Dominican R	38.5	61.5	Zimbabwe	43.4	56.6
Egypt	27.0	73.0	Sri Lanka	45.4	54.6
El Salvador	37.2	62.8	Sudan	20.9	79.1
Ethiopia	36.2	63.8	Suriname	34.0	66.0
Gambia	45.9	54.1	Syria	33.6	66.4
Georgia	08.6	91.4	Thailand	33.0	67.0
Ghana	47.0	53.0	Togo	42.8	57.2
Grenada	46.6	53.4	Tonga	46.0	54.0
Haiti	33.6	66.4	Uganda	35.1	64.9
Honduras	36.0	64.0	UAE	35.4	64.6
India	13.0	87.0	USA	44.1	55.9
Indonesia	36.8	63.2	Vietnam	20.0	80.0
Iran	42.8	57.2	Yemen	37.9	62.1
Lebanon	29.6	70.4	Zambia	38.2	61.8

*Estimates for 1997.

Source: World Health Report (2000: 192–5).

Studies by Pradhan (1996), and Jimenez (1995) have brought home the fact that the bottom 40 per cent of the population in many countries including Indonesia, Philippines and Malaysia received relatively lower health subsidies. In some cases, they find that the bottom 40 per cent of the population get a bit higher subsidies.

However, these studies do not give the breakdown of the exact share of the bottom 20 per cent of population. As Alesina (1998: 304) presumes, these people receive fewer benefits as compared to the higher quintiles. Greater subsidies to the poor do not mean that some sort of favour is shown to the poor. In the case of the poorest quintile, infant (or even adult) mortality may be much higher, indicating the case for a need-based subsidy. It is quite possible that while the lowest 20 per cent is getting the lowest subsidy, the upper 20 per cent in the same category of people get more of it. In fact, absolute poverty does become a constraint for the availability of health care facilities to the poor people in the developing world. To take but one example, Angell and Graham's (1995) study shows that the health system in Venezuela is extremely expensive and beyond the reach of the poor. The HCS is not only expensive but also inefficient, regressive and offers poor services. The situation is not substantially different in other LDCs.

Supply Side Problems

In the health care market, doctors are profit-maximizing monopolists, and in many cases, specialists do form a collusive cartel or what may be called a syndicate to protect their interest and raise their fees. It is a well-known fact that physicians have discretionary power over their fees and they are the price-makers and not simply price takers (Feldstein, 1970). They set their fees in such a way that excess demand for their services is created and sustained in the market. Fortunately or unfortunately, the importance of medical specialists in the HCS in future is going to be much higher in developing countries. This is because of higher future demand for those specialists in the context of larger population, and also because of possible higher per capita income in these countries. Such oligopolistic group practices contribute to higher prices of health care services. In a bid to maximize profits, there is a tendency to overtreat the patient. This is possible, under two situations: first, the patient's level of ignorance about his disease is absolutely very high; and second, the patient is completely dependent on the doctor. In many countries, iatrogenic illness arising out of the medical care process itself is a major problem and there is a widespread perception that many of the operations should not have been performed (Fuchs, 1981: 25). Too much dependency on the part of the patient is indeed a necessary evil. The patient has no right to know about the medicine used, its quality and also the quality of the care being taken by the doctor. The cost and quality of care vary from doctor to doctor, and also from hospital to hospital. But the poor patient has no way to determine all these crucial issues in detail before beginning the treatment protocol. It is also difficult within the system of bounded rationality for the patients to make proper choices before or during the period of treatment, and more often than not, things are forced on to patients. The doctor can compel the patient to buy more medicine than which is necessary and advise him to come more frequently for a check up. All this creates a supply-induced demand. In order to recover the heavy overhead costs of private hospitals, the innocent patients are often asked to undergo tests which are not really warranted but whose cost for the patients is extremely high. For instance, in North Cyprus patients whose PSA test showed normal (2.91 total PSA) are asked to undergo a biopsy test which is unnecessary. Unquestioned dependency on doctors in many cases leads to exploitation of patients in many ways in LDCs.

In the health care market in LDCs, doctors' perceptions, prescriptions and the time duration of treatment are never the same even for the same disease. This creates enormous difficulties to the patients in many ways. The doctor-patient relation is like the one that we encounter in a market having a single seller and a single buyer (often called bilateral monopoly). That is, both are unique in their own ways. A doctor, particularly a specialist, is a monopolist of his own trade in a specific geographical region, and therefore, can dictate his own terms and conditions, and will have many opportunities to exploit the patient mainly because of two reasons. First, the patient has no knowledge about the pathological genesis and the severity of his own disease. Second, different types of fees charged by the doctor are either institutionalized or fixed arbitrarily by the doctor in his favour. As for the consultation fees charged by the doctor, there is an element of rent-seeking behaviour in the sense that the doctor is getting a payment over and above his regular salary from the government hospitals or clinic where he is employed. Very often, doctors in government hospitals pester patients to see them in their private clinics. The hidden motive is obvious. Every patient with his disease along with his idiosyncrasies is a new world to a doctor who can convince the patient in a way he wants. The doctor can withhold his motive and information from the patient. The patient in such a system has no bargaining power. The patient, though the monopolist of all his troubles, has no control over his disease and has to completely submit to the doctor. One of the things the consumers are buying is the physician's knowledge and information, and the buyer has to rely extensively on the seller's judgement about the value of his money (Stiglitz, 1998: 37). The monopolistic behaviour of doctors in LDCs may be due to a shorter supply of specialists and also because of the very nature of the profession. For instance, a study by Baker and Perlman (1967: 186) shows that health professional workforce imbalances were very acute in Taiwan and the situation could continue for a few decades.

One of the reasons for the shortage of specialists in the medical profession in many developing countries is the continuous migration of doctors on a regular basis from developing to developed countries, commonly known as the problem of brain drain, which I have discussed in detail elsewhere (Ghosh and Ghosh, 1985). In addition, there is a more serious problem of efficiency in the allocation of resources for the development of the HCS. The problem is dualistic in nature. First, it involves the optimum allocation of available resources among different types of health care services, and second, it also involves the problem of relative allocation of national resources among many competing programmes such as education, public health, defence and so on. A decision on both these matters will have to consider the definition of health and health care services. In this context, the definition of 'health' by the WHO and by the World Bank may appear to be rather contradictory in the first instance. The WHO, in a 2000 report, observed that since health is a public good, the ultimate responsibility of a country's HCS lies in its government. However, health care is regarded by the World Bank as a type of private good, and therefore, the primary responsibility for health care lies basically with private individuals (see *Medical Tribune*, 1 May 1998: 15) and in such a case, the poor people especially in LDCs are very much adversely affected (see Nuruzzaman, 2007: 70). Although these contradictory definitions have enormous implications for investment in the HCS in developing economies, the opposing ideas can be reconciled by appreciating the fact that whilst health is a private good in individual micro-perspective, it becomes a public good in macro or social perspective. Body capital is an individual wealth, but from the collective perspective, social capital or collective human capital is national wealth. When considered as a public good, it is indeed the inability of the market to know the exact demand for different health care products and services that makes the market a failure to fix up prices and supply. This is one of the reasons why the supply of such services is often inadequate in the market. Given the nature of the HCS as a public good, Kenneth Arrow (1963), therefore, argues for subsidies for these types of goods.

Consequences of Market Failure

Market failure in the HCS leads to a number of unwanted consequences. A free and fair market stands for mitigating or correcting many undesirable evils in a neutral way. However, if the market mechanism fails to operate successfully, the consequences would be the proliferation of socio-economic problems. In the case of market failure in the HCS, it would be almost impossible to get the supply of these goods equal to their demand. For example, the demand for health infrastructure which is a public good benefiting all, cannot be correctly determined because all the citizens will not reveal their preference at the first instance for such a good when an estimate is being made through survey or contingent valuation technique. This happens because of two reasons. First, all people do not disclose their demand as they are afraid that if they do, they may have to pay for such benefits for national health goods like a pollution-free local health environment, better local sanitation and so forth. Second, some citizens think that when the government is providing such public good for the local people, they can enjoy the benefits of provisions even without making any payments. However, the point remains that in such a case, since the preferences of all people are not known, there would be over- or under-supply of those critical health goods.

Health goods often have positive externalities in the sense that they benefit many people even without their asking for it. So their benefits in the long run are always greater than costs. For instance, persons vaccinated against (say) AIDS are not only protected but also give protection to others with whom they have contact. However, health goods with positive externalities such as vaccines cannot be produced in abundance and their total inter-generational benefits cannot be precisely estimated for all citizens. Positive externalities cannot also be evaluated and incorporated in the pricing of health goods. Thus, market price remains an imperfect measure of the benefits of such goods, and the market produces too few of these goods. In case of a regrettable necessity like smoking, producing negative or harmful externalities, there has to be some provision about compensation. For instance, a smoker in a non-smoking zone can be compelled to pay for the health damages of non-smokers, and non-smokers in smoking zones may be asked to compensate for the loss of utility if a smoker is asked to stop smoking. This will, however, necessitate the enforcement of property rights and determination of the amount of payments in such cases.

The question of prices and payments for the HCS is partly related to the extent of competition in that market. The less the competition, the higher is the price and the lower the volume of products. So less competition or the growth of a monopoly which is the source of market failure can be harmful for the consumers of heath care products and services. Stiglitz (1981: 184–9) argues that the maintenance of monopoly position in the market may lead to wastage of valuable national resources. In fact, even if the actual competition is absent, there should be the presence of potential competition. This is the basic idea of contestability theory. Market imperfection may, however, be caused by imperfect and incomplete information. In the health care market in LDCs, many consumers suffer more in terms of excess expenditure simply because they have no complete information about either the disease or health care products, or market fees, or all these. Consumers' welfare cannot also be maximized in the cases of missing or incomplete markets in the health care system.

Market failure due to missing market and incomplete market can lead to consumers' dissatisfaction because of reduction in welfare. In such a case, the right medicine or health facilities may not be available in spite of the presence of adequate purchasing power. This speaks of the underdeveloped nature of the HCS and, may also be a reflection of improper distribution systems. For instance, some health care facilities like 'telemedicines' are not available to the rural people in developing countries, and demand does not create the supply. This leads to more and more inequality in the HCS. The inequality in the distribution of the HCS is not only a reflection of its failure, but also leads to further deterioration in the overall socio-economic and human capital (body capital) inequalities. The society then has to face a bigger problem of resource endowment and empowerment for the less fortunate people who are deprived of the basic health facilities. So, following the Rawlsian theory of justice, it can be said that the principle of difference is violated if the poor people cannot be provided with the minimum necessary medical facilities at affordable cost (Rawls, 1971).

Distributional inequality may aggravate political instability. Albanesi (2001) finds a relationship between political instability and inequality. As a matter of fact, political instability, distributional inequality and economic growth are mutually correlated. Venieris and Gupta (1986) observe that instability has a negative impact on growth. In fact, poor countries are more unstable because they cannot properly manage to be rich, and they cannot manage to be rich because they are not politically stable (Alesina and Perotti, 1994: 359). So, for the unstable poor countries, the vicious circle continues unabated and its impact is also felt in the health care system. Economic growth is also adversely affected by income inequality (Alesina 1988). A high degree of distributional inequality is associated with illegal activities, social instability and unrest. The model presented by Alesina and Rodrik (1994) comes out with the conclusion that there is an inverse relation between distributional inequality and growth. It is indeed true that inequality in the matter of health care services does produce more capability failures and less productivity and growth.

Market Failure, Policy Implications and Government

Market failures in the HCS have important policy implications for developing countries. When market principles cannot work, greater reliance has to be placed on the government for correcting the distortions that have been caused by market failure. The government will have its role in five distinct areas of the HCS, namely, production, distribution, cost and price, health care structure, and regulation and control. Government should clear out market bottlenecks and constraints and, ensure increased competition. In fact, the introduction of increased competition in the market can bring down the prices and increase the supply of health care products. It would also be necessary to de-monopolize specialists' cartels that aim at maximizing profits by increasing consultation fees and other medical cost for the patients. Although the system of group practice has done well in North Carolina (Scheffler, 1981: 478--88), the same is not true in LDCs. Even for the United States, as Scheffler cautions, without proper safeguards, the system of group practice by medical doctors will contribute to increasing cost of medical care. Any attempt to reduce the cost of health care services by the government in developing countries is sure to induce some additional demand: the price elasticity of demand for health services is less than one (Fuchs, 1981: 13). There are indeed many possibilities to reduce the medical cost in LDCs by prescribing generic drugs, by reducing the use of unnecessary clinical tests and expensive drugs. Simply by shifting to the use of generic drugs, health care cost can be reduced by at least 50 per cent in developing countries. In all these cases, governments do have positive roles to play. In order to help the consumers to know the cost of treatment, it would be imperative to introduce itemized billing by the private hospitals and clinics. This practice may be made obligatory so that the consumers are not exploited.

It is necessary on the part of the government to ensure that essential cheaper drugs are made available to the public in adequate amount. As in Malaysia, the national drug policy must ensure the availability, accessibility, affordability and rational use of drugs (Suleiman, 1997: 13). The drug policy, among other things, should pay attention to the safety aspect of each drug being used in the country. Although according to the list prepared by the World Health Assembly in 1978, only 200-plus preparations were considered adequate to meet the pharmaceutical health needs of developing countries, the actual number of branded drugs in these countries has exceeded several thousand preparations (Chetley, 1990). In many LDCs, drugs are not standardized on the basis of quality and toxicological tests. Moreover, health care products often do not mention the safety level, possible side effects and warnings for the consumers. In all such cases, government control is urgently needed. The public sector needs to be up-to-date in the method of drug formulation, drug listing, drug protocol and therapeutic guidelines. In this connection, it may be imperative to extend the regulatory activities to control the price mark-up of multinational drug industries operating in LDCs and also to control the prices of locally produced medicines. At the same time, there should be no compromise with the quality of products. Health being a public good, it is the responsibility of the government to make up for the missing or incomplete market by making available complementary, holistic and alternative medicines at the level justified by demand. In establishing new markets, the government has to perform the role of an innovating entrepreneur and undertake many types of risks which a private enterprise will generally try to shun.

As a pubic good, the supply of many of the health care services often remain sub-optimal, which the government needs to make up at the desired level. Government participation should be able to remove the supply side constraints in the market for health care services. However, in a bid to maximize the supply of health care products, healthy working conditions and health safety measures must not be overlooked. In many fast developing countries including China, Indonesia, Philippines and Thailand, workers have to work for long hours for low levels of pay in inhuman working conditions. *The Guardian* (3 December 1996) reports that in Jakarta, young women have to work in multinational factories under 30°C heat to earn only 16 pence an hour. The WHO estimates that more than a million workers in Latin America alone are poisoned every year and 10,000 die from exposure to toxic chemicals (cited in World Bank, 1995: 13). Bad health created under unhealthy environment may indeed lead to many negative externalities both inside and outside the affected families and commercial organizations.

In the case of positive externalities that health care services generate, some subsidies should be provided by the government to ensure their maximum possible supply while at the same time restricting the supply of those products, through taxes, that damage public health and environment (products with negative externalities). Since health generates externalities, intervention by the government becomes necessary to protect public health by reducing negative externalities. In order to settle the issues connected with negative externalities, the government has to legally fix up property rights. In many cases, if the property right is properly determined by the government, there may not be any need for corrective taxation (see Coase, 1960). The supply of necessary information about health, drugs and disease to the public is necessary to remove information asymmetry, which is one of the important causes of market failures.

Interactions between public and private sectors can help target public subsidies better if the higher income groups use privatized medical facilities (Griffin, 1992: 130). Since higher income groups generally prefer privatized medical facilities, a larger pool of resources can be created by privatization for the benefit of poor patients. A large part of the demand for public health services by the richer section consists of meta-needs, like attempts to slow down ageing, maintenance of a shipshape figure, cosmetic surgery and autonomous blood tests and so on. However, rampant privatization creates the unwanted possibility of diversion of limited resources towards a demand-based system to satisfy meta-needs at the cost of need-based priorities of the poor people (Chan, 1996: 345). Moreover, privatization of medical facilities involves allocative inefficiency in the sense that prices charged are much higher than the marginal cost. In fact, privatization may reduce the burden of the government but it generally increases the burden of the people as common people have to pay higher tariffs and higher prices for medical services (Ghosh, 1998: Ch. 20). Privatization of necessary medical services is unjust for the poor who need minimal entitlement for the medical services they need. The government should not really shy away from the basic responsibilities of providing the social reproductions of necessary merit goods like health and education in LDCs in the case of market failure. Even in a case where privatization creates private monopoly, there is enough justification for government intervention and control to increase production and reduce the price level of the product.

The issue of inequality in the distribution of health care services is a serious matter in less developed countries. There are indeed many types of inequalities in the distribution of medical care services in these countries. For instance, doctor-population ratio, numbers of hospitals and medical clinics per unit of population vary substantially from region to region. It is one of the duties of the government to make the distribution pattern more and more egalitarian as far as possible so that inequalities in many health indicators across the country such as the infant mortality rate and life expectancy can be eradicated in the long run. Good health is so fundamental to human life and existence that it cannot be left to the dictates of market forces (see Tobin, 1970). In fact, health has come to be regarded as a more fundamental responsibility of the government than even education, and hence health deserves more egalitarianism and equity considerations (see Stiglitz, 1998). The important responsibility of the government is to introduce many types of balancing in the HCS, for example, balancing between demand and supply of health care services, balancing between the demand for and supply of health manpower, rural-urban balance and so on. Although like any other macro policy, health policy is essentially a political matter, the governments in LDCs have to concentrate on the promotion of public health even at a higher cost when the trade-off between the allocation of resources for public health and that of economic growth has to be considered in favour of the latter. This is so because improvement of public health may ultimately benefit economic growth by increasing productive efficiency, capability and contestability.

Having pointed out the utmost importance of the role of government in the correction of market failure in LDCs, a note of caveat is in order. The introduction of government may not always automatically ensure market success because its role cannot be thought to be completely sacrosanct. It is likely that the government would be more vulnerable to temptation and rent-seeking behaviour, and bureaucracy may at times make things worse through procrastination, inefficiency and regulatory capture, and all these syndromes may lead to government failure in the HCS.

Concluding Observations

The health care policy of a developing country is now influenced by many deterministic external and internal factors and forces. These may be structural, economic, demographic and epidemiological in nature. An ageing population will mean more dependency load, higher medical expenses and higher gerentological investment. Having engaged in a capitalist method of industrialization buttressed by the philosophy of globalization, many of the LDCs are now moving towards predominantly 'capitalist diseases' such as hypertension, diabetes, coronary ailments, mental aberration, schizophrenia and so on. One can also observe in developing countries, the emergence of drug resistant pathogens and the resurgence of communicable diseases. All this will involve many challenges to keep the population in the wellness paradigm. Whilst health care cost is escalating rapidly, the allocation for the HCS is declining in many cases. In many countries, health care expenditure has to considerably depend on foreign aid which may be more than 50 per cent of all expenditures (World Bank, 1993). Walt (1994) has rightly observed that such an aid is more reflective of the interests of the donor rather than of the recipient country. These days, global processes have been shaping the development strategies of the LDCs and its impact is also being increasingly felt in the dynamics of the HCS (Larkin, 1998: 109). In the era of globalization, which experiences domestic political disintegration and weakening of the state power but increasing tempo of privatization and marketization, it is indeed difficult for any government to ensure a health care system, which is pro-poor, egalitarian and efficient.

Note

1. The author is aware of the works of many contributions to the *Journal of Contemporary Asia* that have considered this a peripheral debate in that the 'market failure' approach is too accepting of an ideological position that promotes the market and its supposed logic.

References

Albanesi, S. (2001) "Inflation and Inequality", Unpublished Paper, Northwestern University.

Alesina, A. (1988) "Macroeconomics and Politics", in S. Fischer (ed.), *NBER Macroeconomics Annual: Volume 3*, Cambridge: MIT Press, pp.13–52.

Alesina, A. (1998) "The Political Economy of Macroeconomic Stabilizations and Income Inequality: Myths and Reality", in Vito Tanzi and Ke-young Chu (eds.), *Income Distribution and High-quality Growth*, Cambridge: MIT Press, pp. 303–21.

Alesina, A. and D. Rodrik (1994) "Distributional Politics and Economic Growth", *Quarterly Journal of Economics*, 109, pp. 413–29.

Alesina, A. and R. Perotti (1994) "The Political Economy of Growth", *World Bank Economic Review*, 8, pp. 351–71.

Angell, Alan and C. Graham (1995) "Can Social Sector Reforms Make Adjustment Sustainable and Equitable?: Lessons from Chile and Venezuela", *Journal of Latin American Studies*, 13, pp. 625–40.

Arrow, Kenneth (1963) *Social Choice and Individual Values*, New Haven: Yale University Press.

Aspe, P. (1993) *Economic Transformation: The Mexican Way*, Cambridge: MIT Press.

Aspe, P. and P. Sigmud (1984) *The Political Economy of Income Distribution in Mexico*, New York: Holmes and Meir.

Baker, Timothy D. and M. Perlman (1967) *Health Manpower in a Developing Economy*, Baltimore: John Hopkins Press.

Chan, Chee Khoon (1996) "Health Care Financing", in K.S. Jomo and Ng Suew Kiat (eds.), *Malaysia's Economic Development*, Kuala Lumpur: Pelanduk Publications, pp. 329–47.

Chetley, A. (1990) *A Health Business: World Health and the Pharmaceutical Industry*, London: Zed Books.

Coase, R.H. (1960) "The Problem of Social Cost", *Journal of Law and Economics*, 3, pp. 373–95.

Cullis, J.G and P.A. West (1979) *The Economics of Health*, Oxford: Martin Robertson.

Feldstein, M. (1970) "The Rising Prices of Physicians' Services", *Review of Economics and Statistics*, 7, pp. 25–43.

Fuchs, Victor R. (1981) "Economics, Health and Post-Industrial Society", in John B. McKinlay (ed.), *Economics and Health Care*, Cambridge: MIT Press, pp. 12–27.

Ghosh B.N. (1998) *Malaysia: The Transformation Within*, Kuala Lumpur: Longman.

— (2000) *The Three Dimensional Man: Human Resource Development in Malaysia*, Kuala Lumpur: Utusan.

— (2001) *From Market Failure to Government Failure*, Leeds: Wisdom House.

Ghosh, B.N. and R. Ghosh (1985) *The Economics of Brain Migration*, New Delhi: Deep and Deep Publications.

Gomez, M. (1998) "Financing Malaysia's Health Care System", *Medical Tribune*, 15, pp. 23–8.

Government of Malaysia (2001) *Eighth Malaysia Plan*, Kuala Lumpur: Government of Malaysia.

Griffin, Charles C. (1992) *Health Care in Asia*, Washington DC: World Bank.

Jimenez, E. (1995) "Human and Physical Infrastructure: Public Investment and Pricing Policies in Developing Countries", in Hollis Chenery and T.N. Srinivasan (eds.), *Handbook of Development Economics*, 3, New York: North Holland, pp. 423–35.

Larkin, M. (1998) "Globalization Aspects of Health and Health Policy in Third World Countries", in Ray Kiely and Phil Marfleet (eds.), *Globalization and the Third World*, London: Routledge, pp. 107–22.

MONEE Database: International Child Development Center, Florence, Italy, http://www.unicef-icdc.org

Nuruzzaman, M. (2007) "The World Bank Health Policy Reforms and the Poor", *Journal of Contemporary Asia*, 37, pp. 59–72.

Organization of Economic Cooparation and Development (2006) OECD Health Data 2006: A Comparative Analysis of 30 Countries, www,aihw.gov.au

Posner, Richard A. (1992) "The Chicago School of Antitrust Analysis", in G.H. Burgess, Jr. (ed.), *Antitrust and Regulation*, Aldershot: Edward Elgar, pp. 73–89.

Pradhan, S. (1996) "Evaluating Public Spending: A Framework for Public Expenditure Reviews", Discussion Paper No. 323, Washington DC: World Bank.

Rawls, John (1971) *A Theory of Justice*, Cambridge: Cambridge University Press.

Scheffler, Richard M. (1981) "The Pricing Behaviour Group", in John B. McKinlay (ed.), *Economics and Health Care*, Cambridge: MIT Press, pp. 473–85

Sen, A.K. (1981) *Poverty and Famine: An Essay on Entitlement and Deprivation*, Oxford: Oxford University Press.

— (1999) *Development as Freedom*, New York: Alfred Knopf.

Sifford, D. (1977) "Medical Advice: Get Used to Plain", *Philadelphia Inquirer*, 28 August.

Stiglitz, J. (1981) "Potential Competition May Reduce Welfare", *American Economic Review*, 71, pp. 175–91.

— (1998) "The Role of Government in the Contemporary World", in Vito Tanzi and Ke-young Chu (eds.), *Income Distribution and High-quality Growth*, Cambridge: MIT Press, pp. 34–50.

Suleiman, Abu B. (1997) "Essential Drugs Concept: An International Perspective", Keynote Address to the Opening Ceremony of the Seminar, Essential Drugs Concept: An International Perspective, Penang, Malaysia, 17–19 September.

Tobin, J. (1970) "On Limiting the Domain of Inequality", *Journal of Law and Economics*, 13, pp. 26–54.

Todaro, Michael P. and S.C. Smith (2003) *Economic Development*. Boston: Addison-Wesley.

Venieris, Yannis and D. Gupta (1986) "Income Distribution and Socio-Political Instability as Determinants of Savings", *Journal of Political Economy*, 96, pp. 374–96.

Walt, J. (1994) *Health Policy*, London: Zed Books.

World Bank (1993) World Development Report: Investing in Health, Oxford: Oxford University Press.

— (1995) World Development Report: Workers in an Integrating World, Oxford: Oxford University Press.

World Health Organization (2000), World Healht Report: Health System Improving Performance, Geneva: WHO.

2

Eleventh Five-Year Plan on Food Security

Estimates and Interpretations

M.H. SURYANARAYANA

Planning process and policy formulation in India is one area, which calls for some serious review and consideration. One can cite several instances, which tend to generate such an impression:

(i) The Sixth Five-Year Plan (1980–85) justified its choice of growth with redistribution strategy for poverty reduction with reference to estimates of inequality measures based on price-unadjusted size distribution of consumption data, which show a trend decline in inequality (Government of India, 1981: 81). This exercise is methodologically unsatisfactory and estimates with appropriate corrections for grouping bias and prices do not bear out any such conclusion and the chosen strategy (Suryanarayana, 1983).

(ii) Plan exercises are carried out imposing assumed values for distributional parameters rendering the entire exercise an academic illustration for a wrong approach rather than one of serious policy pursuits (see, for instance, Government of India, 1981: 233, Suryanarayana, 1991).

(iii) This tradition seems to persist, with the latest addition being the Eleventh Five-Year Plan Strategy "Towards Faster and More Inclusive Growth". The approach paper does not define explicitly the concept, measure and parameters, leaving a field day for experts to make their own interpretations and recommendations, of course, without any conceptual and methodological bounds.

To cite and illustrate one particular consequence of such an approach, India realized the Sixth Five-Year Plan target of 30 per cent for poverty not in five years but after pursuing planned pro-poor growth strategies for two and a half decades. Incidence of poverty has finally declined to 28.30 per cent in the rural sector and 25.70 per cent in the urban in 2004–05 (Government of India, 2007b) thanks largely to growth and not any significant reduction in inequality.

This form of policy making is a luxury, which a poor country like India can ill-afford. Another policy area in the Eleventh Five-Year Plan, which calls for a serious review pertains to issues related to food security, morbidity and health status of the population. This is an area, which has received wide attention in the wake of food inflation across countries in the world. Experts have drawn inferences and made policy recommendations based on empirical details on partial profiles, or inconsistent details when the profiles are comprehensive and integrated. Even the Indian Planning Commission is not an exception to this syndrome. One such issue pertains to inferences and policy recommendations based on objective estimates of food consumption and exogenous threshold norms. There is scope for a careful review of empirical details.

The paper is organized as follows: The following section presents the Eleventh Plan prespectives on food security and health status based on estimates of food grain consumption and calorie intake. This is followed by a review and related estimates. The final section concludes with a summary.

Eleventh Plan Perspective on Nutritional Status

The Eleventh Plan is quite aware of the importance of food security in order to improve what it calls "nutritional outcomes" for the poor and to facilitate quick recovery from illness (Government of India, 2008: 128–48). In other words, food security is quite important as an answer to morbidity. All the more so given the (i) observed decline in pre capita cereal production; and (ii) stagnant income levels of the poor. The plan cites enough empirical details on nutritional status measures like low birth weight of newborn babies, weights and heights of adults, which are explained, inter alia, in terms of deficit in energy intake. The document provides information on trends in consumption pattern and calorie intake since 1972–73, which is as follows:

(i) Cereals are a major source of energy intake for the Indian population. Per capita cereal consumption has declined in both rural and urban areas.

(ii) One important reason for this is the decline in the share of food in total expenditure. Between 1972–73, 1987–88 and 2004–05, food share declined from 73 per cent to 64 per cent and finally to 55 per cent in rural India and from 65 per cent to 56 and to 43 per cent in urban India (Government of India, 2008: 131).

(iii) In urban India, the share in expenditure of other food items like milk and milk products, edible oils and sugar have declined. In rural India, though the shares of other food items like milk and milk products, fish, egg and meat, and fruits and nuts increased, the increase has not been sufficient to make up for the loss in calories due to decline in cereal consumption.

(iv) As a result, average per capita calorie intake per diem decreased from 2,221 kcals (1983) to 2,153 (1993–94), 2,149 (1999–2000) and to 2,047 (2004–05) in rural India, that is, by eight per cent between 1983 and 2004–05; the corresponding estimates for urban India being 2,089, 2,071, 2,156 and 2,020 involving a reduction in calorie intake of 3.3 per cent.

(v) Average calorie intakes in both rural and urban areas have fallen increasingly short of the calorie norms for official, poverty lines for the rural (2,400 kcals) and urban (2,100 kcals) areas.

Using similar statistics, several other study groups and experts have concluded that food insecurity and malnutrition has increased in India. This has led many experts to advocate universalization of the public distribution system (PDS). Our estimates by the poverty-line-calorie norms show that incidence of calorie deficiency is 90 per cent in rural India and 70 per cent in urban India. The plan document also cites evidence to show that the rate of malnutrition as reflected in estimates of underweight children has not declined at all between 1998–99 and 2004–05 though the economy was growing at the rate of 6 per cent per annum. As regards policies, the plan goes on to evaluate the PDS and concludes "PDS seems to have failed in serving the second objective of making foograins available to the poor. If it had, the consumption levels of cereals should not have fallen on average – as it has consistently over the last two decades" (Government of India, 2008: 135). However, the Plan is cautious and states that issues related to food security should not be examined in isolation but should focus on improving nutritional outcomes for the majority of the poor.

Table 1

Estimates of Average Per Capita Intake of Calorie, Protein and Fat Per Diem: Major States

State	Per capita per diem intake of														
	Calorie (kcal) according to					Protein (gm) according to					Fat (gm) according to				
	27th round (1972–1973)	38th round (1983)	50th round (1993–1994)	55th round (1999–2000)	61st round (2004–2005)	27th round (1972–1973)	38th round (1983)	50th round (1993–1994)	55th round (1999–2000)	61st round (2004–2005)	27th round (1972–1973)	38th round (1983)	50th round (1993–1994)	55th round (1999–2000)	61st round (2004–2005)
(1)	(2)	(3)	(4)	(5)	(6)	(7)	(8)	(9)	(10)	(11)	(12)	(13)	(14)	(15)	(16)
Rural															
Andhra Pradesh	2103	2204	2052	2021	1995	53.0	56.0	50.8	49.4	49.8	21.0	24.0	27.2	29.5	33.5
Assam	2074	2056	1983	1915	2067	53.0	52.0	49.5	47.7	52.7	15.0	18.0	21.0	22.3	26.7
Bihar	2225	2189	2115	2121	2049	65.0	65.0	60.2	58.7	57.8	17.0	20.0	23.0	26.5	28.4
Gujarat	2142	2113	1994	1986	1923	58.0	59.0	55.6	54.2	53.3	40.0	44.0	47.4	53.8	50.9
Haryana	3215	2554	2491	2455	2226	90.0	78.0	78.4	75.3	69.6	47.0	47.0	53.6	59.1	55.4
Karnataka	2202	2260	2073	2028	1845	57.0	60.0	55.1	54.2	48.8	23.0	26.0	28.6	36.6	33.9
Kerala	1559	1884	1965	1982	2014	38.0	47.0	50.8	52.4	55.4	19.0	32.0	32.7	38.8	40.8
Madhya Pradesh	2423	2323	2164	2062	1929	68.0	68.0	63.0	58.2	58.8	21.0	25.0	28.3	31.3	35.1
Maharashtra	1895	2144	1939	2012	1933	54.0	62.0	54.8	56.5	55.7	24.0	30.0	33.5	39.7	41.5
Orissa	1995	2103	2199	2119	2023	49.0	51.0	52.7	49.9	48.3	8.0	13.0	14.8	16.3	17.8
Punjab	3493	2677	2418	2381	2240	85.0	79.0	74.7	71.7	66.7	50.0	52.0	59.8	58.7	58.7

Cont'd…

Cont'd...

Rajasthan	2730	2433	2470	2425	2180	84.0	75.0	79.4	76.9	69.6	46.0	42.0	52.8	53.5	50.9
Tamil Nadu	1955	1861	1884	1826	1842	49.0	47.0	46.8	44.9	44.9	18.0	22.0	24.7	29.5	29.6
Uttar Pradesh	2575	2399	2307	2327	2200	76.0	73.0	70.4	69.7	65.9	28.0	29.0	35.5	37.6	37.5
West Bengal	1921	2027	2211	2095	2070	50.0	52.0	54.8	51.6	52.0	13.0	17.0	21.4	24.2	26.5
All-India	2266	2221	2153	2149	2047	62.0	62.0	60.2	59.1	57.0	24.0	27.0	31.4	36.1	35.5
Urban															
Andhra Pradesh	2143	2009	1992	2052	2000	51.0	50.0	49.6	50.8	50.9	31.0	32.0	34.9	41.5	43.2
Assam	2135	2043	2108	2174	2143	56.0	52.0	53.5	56.5	55.9	25.0	25.0	30.8	38.7	36.8
Bihar	2167	2131	2188	2171	2190	61.0	61.0	61.4	61.0	62.2	25.0	26.0	32.7	34.2	40.4
Gujarat	2172	2000	2027	2058	1991	57.0	55.0	54.9	54.7	57.3	58.0	53.0	57.9	67.0	63.5
Haryana	2404	2242	2140	2172	2033	67.0	67.0	63.6	62.5	60.5	42.0	49.0	49.4	56.3	54.4
Karnataka	1925	2124	2026	2046	1944	46.0	55.0	53.1	53.5	52.2	32.0	36.0	37.6	45.1	43.3
Kerala	1723	2049	1966	1995	1996	44.0	51.0	52.4	55.2	56.7	27.0	38.0	37.0	42.9	44.9
Madhya Pradesh	2229	2137	2082	2132	1954	61.0	62.0	59.8	60.6	58.2	34.0	36.0	40.3	43.5	43.4
Maharashtra	1971	2028	1989	2039	1847	55.0	56.0	55.5	55.9	52.1	41.0	45.0	47.9	52.6	50.1
Orissa	2276	2219	2261	2298	2139	55.0	56.0	57.2	57.8	55.2	23.0	24.0	28.1	27.4	28.3
Punjab	2783	2100	2089	2197	2150	70.0	63.0	61.8	64.8	63.4	52.0	49.0	53.7	57.9	61.0
Rajasthan	2357	2255	2184	2335	2116	70.0	69.0	66.5	70.4	64.0	47.0	47.0	51.6	61.5	56.4
Tamil Nadu	1841	2140	1922	2030	1935	44.0	45.0	48.7	51.7	49.2	23.0	29.0	33.9	43.2	41.1
Uttar Pradesh	2161	2043	2114	2131	2124	62.0	62.0	63.2	62.0	65.1	35.0	34.0	41.2	45.5	46.1
West Bengal	2080	2048	2131	2134	2011	58.0	55.0	56.6	55.5	55.1	31.0	31.0	34.2	40.2	39.1
All-India	2107	2089	2071	2156	2020	56.0	57.0	57.2	58.5	57.0	36.0	37.0	42.0	49.6	47.5

Source: Government of India (2007c; p. 54).

Table 2

Estimates of Per Capita Cereal Consumption: Rural and Urban All-India

(kg per 30 days)

Decile group	*Rural All-India*					*Urban All-India*				
	1972/73	1983	1993/94	1999/2000	2004/05	1972/73	1983	1993/94	1999/2000	2004/05
0–10	9.08	10.35	10.53	10.49	10.16	8.75	9.19	9.53	9.57	9.66
11–20	12.03	12.45	12.09	11.65	11.08	10.52	10.46	10.64	10.30	10.11
21–30	13.32	13.38	12.65	12.30	11.44	11.23	10.98	10.80	10.80	10.26
31–40	14.35	13.94	13.22	12.59	11.71	11.46	11.34	10.93	10.67	10.16
41–50	15.15	14.78	13.40	12.92	11.89	11.84	11.49	11.03	10.87	10.28
51–60	15.60	15.29	13.77	13.09	12.11	11.90	11.88	10.96	10.78	10.13
61–70	17.07	15.66	14.12	13.43	12.34	12.15	12.12	11.02	10.74	10.13
71–80	17.75	16.34	14.46	13.54	12.50	12.09	12.12	10.80	10.60	10.03
81–90	18.96	17.41	14.65	13.81	12.45	11.84	12.08	10.77	10.62	9.69
91–100	21.26	19.40	15.52	14.18	15.81	11.43	12.16	10.31	10.06	9.37
All	15.46	14.90	13.44	12.80	12.15	11.32	11.38	10.68	10.50	9.98

Source: Based on various NSS reports.

Table 3

Estimates of Energy Intake: Rural and Urban All-India
(Kilocalories per capita per diem)

Decile group	*Rural All-India*					*Urban All-India*				
	1972/73	1983	1993/94	1999/2000	2004/05	1972/73	1983	1993/94	1999/2000	2004/05
0–10	1192.09	1356.31	1460.12	1491.48	1480.52	1298.70	1331.76	1443.50	1520.88	1510.50
11–20	1591.90	1681.80	1731.32	1730.52	1681.42	1575.94	1588.29	1702.40	1731.16	1687.67
21–30	1783.40	1847.86	1850.00	1865.30	1800.00	1745.94	1724.00	1803.48	1912.56	1833.00
31–40	1944.00	1952.00	1971.66	1955.22	1882.45	1802.18	1861.19	1896.79	1970.46	1856.41
41–50	2115.04	2111.53	2056.48	2049.15	1958.95	1980.00	1912.41	1992.81	2092.92	1944.62
51–60	2210.00	2229.56	2156.34	2170.62	2044.32	2035.48	2046.00	2074.64	2189.89	2024.00
61–70	2451.41	2322.00	2275.17	2287.78	2158.00	2266.00	2221.13	2186.00	2297.00	2111.12
71–80	2581.40	2506.92	2410.00	2403.00	2290.00	2382.13	2294.20	2296.74	2467.69	2209.00
81–90	2929.00	2779.53	2584.72	2582.54	2376.40	2658.75	2500.71	2470.50	2536.00	2343.04
91–100	3861.77	3422.49	3034.19	2954.39	2797.94	3324.88	3410.30	2843.14	2841.53	2680.64
All	2266.00	2221.00	2153.00	2149.00	2047.00	2107.00	2089.00	2071.00	2156.00	2020.00

Source: Based on various NSS reports.

Table 4

Percentage Distribution of Households by Food Availability Status

Sector/round	Percentage of households				
	Getting enough food everyday throughout the year	Not getting enough food everyday		Not recorded	All
		Some months of the year	All months of the year		
Rural Sector					
NSS 61st round (July 2004–June 2005)	97.4	2.0	0.4	0.2	100
NSS 55th round (July 1999–June 2000)	96.2	2.6	0.7	0.5	100
NSS 50th round (July 1993–June 1994)	94.5	4.2	0.9	0.4	100
NSS 38th round (Jan–Dec 1983)	81.1	16.2	2.4	0.3	100
Urban Sector					
NSS 61st round (July 2004–June 2005)	99.4	0.4	0.1	0.1	100
NSS 55th round (July 1999-June 2000)	98.6	0.6	0.3	0.4	100
NSS 50th round (July 1993-June 1994)	98.1	1.1	0.5	0.3	100
NSS 38th round (Jan-Dec 1983)	93.3	5.6	0.8	0.3	100

Source: Government of India (2001, p.16 and 2007b; p. 22)

Table 5

Food Availability Status: Statewise Profile (2004–05)

State	No. per 1000 of households						
	Adequate food throughout the year			Getting inadequate food some months of the year	Getting inadequate food all months	Not recorded	All
	As ascertained by a direct question	As judged by the investi-gator	All				
Rural India							
Andhra Pradesh	526	467	993	6	0	1	1000
Assam	562	378	940	17	36	6	1000

Cont'd...

Cont'd...

Bihar	579	388	967	20	8	6	1000
Chhattisgarh	534	440	974	26	0	0	1000
Gujarat	498	500	998	3	0	0	1000
Haryana	265	735	1000	0	0	0	1000
Jharkhand	433	560	993	6	1	0	1000
Karnataka	619	378	997	3	0	0	1000
Kerala	420	555	975	22	3	1	1000
Madhya Pradesh	400	579	979	15	5	0	1000
Maharashtra	388	602	990	10	0	0	1000
Orissa	725	209	934	48	13	5	1000
Punjab	396	595	991	8	1	0	1000
Rajasthan	234	765	999	0	0	0	1000
Tamil Nadu	599	399	998	1	1	0	1000
Uttar Pradesh	328	653	981	14	3	3	1000
West Bengal	582	298	880	106	13	2	1000
			Urban India				
Andhra Pradesh	373	626	999	1	0	0	1000
Assam	435	538	973	3	21	3	1000
Bihar	408	567	975	8	11	7	1000
Chhattisgarh	342	657	999	1	0	0	1000
Gujarat	238	762	1000	0	0	0	1000
Haryana	197	801	998	0	2	0	1000
Jharkhand	330	670	1000	0	0	0	1000
Karnataka	398	600	998	1	0	0	1000
Kerala	359	623	982	17	1	0	1000
Madhya Pradesh	204	792	996	4	0	0	1000
Maharashtra	241	753	994	5	0	0	1000
Orissa	522	472	994	4	2	1	1000
Punjab	361	637	998	2	0	0	1000
Rajasthan	149	851	1000	0	0	0	1000
Tamil Nadu	358	639	997	4	0	0	1000
Uttar Pradesh	242	748	990	7	1	1	1000
West Bengal	366	618	984	7	6	4	1000

Source: Government of India (2007b; p. 20).

Table 6 (a)

Measures of Nutritional Status across States: 2004–2005

State	Rural Sector							
	% expenditure on		*per capita per day intake of*			*per consumer unit per day intake of*		
	Food	*Cereals*	*Calorie (kcal)*	*Protein (gm)*	*Fat (gm)*	*Calorie (kcal)*	*Protein (gm)*	*Fat (gm)*
Andhra Pradesh	55.2	19.4	1995	49.8	33.5	2475	61.8	41.6
Assam	66	24.8	2067	52.7	26.7	2515	64.1	32.4
Bihar	64.8	27.1	2049	57.8	28.4	2560	72.3	35.5
Chhattisgarh	56.2	27.2	1942	47.4	19.9	2424	59.2	24.8
Gujarat	58	13.3	1923	53.3	50.9	2380	65.9	63
Haryana	48.6	8.6	2226	69.6	55.4	2738	85.6	68.1
Jharkhand	61.9	27.2	1961	51.2	22.8	2440	63.8	28.4
Karnataka	55.7	16.5	1845	48.8	33.9	2276	60.2	41.8
Kerala	45	11	2014	55.4	40.8	2549	70.1	51.6
Madhya Pradesh	52.9	18.1	1929	58.8	35.1	2386	72.7	43.4
Maharashtra	51.7	14.5	1933	55.7	41.5	2405	69.3	51.6
Orissa	61.6	28.3	2023	48.3	17.8	2512	59.9	22.1
Punjab	49.2	8.8	2240	66.7	58.7	2763	82.3	72.5
Rajasthan	54.8	14.5	2180	69.6	50.9	2714	86.7	63.3
Tamil Nadu	52.4	15.5	1842	44.9	29.6	2294	55.9	36.9
Uttar Pradesh	53.6	17.6	2200	65.9	37.5	2743	82.1	46.8
West Bengal	58.7	23.4	2070	52	26.5	2545	64	32.6
All	55	18	2047	57	35.5	2540	70.8	44
Upper quartile	—	—	2070	58.8	41.5	2560	72.7	51.6

Source: Government of India (2007a; p. 44).

Table 6 (b)

Measures of Nutritional Status across States: 2004–2005

State	**Urban Sector**							
	% expenditure on		*per capita per day intake of*			*per consumer unit per day intake of*		
	Food	*Cereals*	*Calorie (kcal)*	*Protein (gm)*	*Fat (gm)*	*Calorie (kcal)*	*Protein (gm)*	*Fat (gm)*
Andhra Pradesh	41.6	12.2	2000	50.9	43.2	2449	62.4	52.9
Assam	49.5	13.6	2143	55.9	36.8	2593	67.6	44.5

Cont'd...

Cont'd...

Bihar	51.1	17.2	2190	62.2	40.4	2683	76.1	49.5
Chhattisgarh	39	12.1	2087	53.9	37.2	2550	65.9	45.4
Gujarat	44.9	8	1991	57.3	63.5	2436	70.1	77.7
Haryana	41.4	6.9	2033	60.5	54.4	2487	74	66.6
Jharkhand	46.9	13.4	2458	69.5	53.8	3013	85.2	65.9
Karnataka	43.2	11.1	1944	52.2	43.3	2385	64	53.1
Kerala	40	8.4	1996	56.7	44.9	2534	72	57.1
Madhya Pradesh	38.9	9.8	1954	58.2	43.4	2397	71.4	53.2
Maharashtra	40.4	8.4	1847	52.1	50.1	2261	63.8	61.3
Orissa	49.9	16.8	2139	55.2	28.3	2596	67	34.4
Punjab	37.6	6.4	2150	63.4	61	2614	77	74.2
Rajasthan	41.6	9.6	2116	64	56.4	2586	78.2	69
Tamil Nadu	42.7	10.3	1935	49.2	41.1	2394	60.8	50.8
Uttar Pradesh	45	11.4	2124	65.1	46.1	2598	79.7	56.4
West Bengal	43.4	11.3	2011	55.1	39.1	2467	67.6	48
All	42.5	10.1	2020	57	47.5	2475	69.9	58.2
Upper quartile			2139	62.2	53.8	2596	76.1	65.9

Source: Government of India (2007a; p. 44).

Table 7

Incidence of Calorie Deficiency with Reference to Alternative Norms: 2004–05

State	**Rural sector**		**Urban sector**	
	Incidence of calorie deficiency with respect to norm (per capita per diem) of		*Incidence of calorie deficiency with respect to norm (per capita per diem) of*	
	2100 kcals	*2400 kcals*	*2030 kcals*	*2100 kcals*
Andhra Pradesh	73.92	93.14	60.77	64.66
Assam	61.28	93.60	47.23	55.42
Bihar	62.06	87.74	43.39	47.44
Gujarat	82.22	93.17	53.94	72.20
Haryana	51.37	71.50	63.35	70.66
Karnataka	84.50	97.06	67.08	76.99
Kerala	71.15	84.89	60.45	64.90
Madhya Pradesh	76.25	82.43	66.38	71.24
Maharashtra	70.51	78.36	83.18	89.39
Orissa	64.94	85.55	45.70	52.42

Cont'd...

Cont'd...

Punjab	51.54	75.45	51.83	56.00
Rajasthan	57.36	80.41	48.27	60.73
Tamil Nadu	84.62	95.75	71.29	75.94
Uttar Pradesh	52.9	76.55	38.84	41.18
West Bengal	62.65	87.22	56.43	72.98
All-India	64.9	90.73	60.78	68.67

Source: Author's estimates (without any normalization for age-gender-activity parameters) based on Government of India (2006b and 2007c)

Table 8

Morbidity Profile across States

Major States	**Rural**			**Urban**		
	PAP	*PPC*	*IMR*	*PAP*	*PPC*	*IMR*
Andhra Pradesh	90	36	71	114	47	35
Assam	82	58	73	83	48	38
Bihar	53	32	62	63	30	50
Chhattisgarh	69	38	—	72	31	—
Delhi	—	—	—	—	—	—
Gujarat	69	29	68	78	29	37
Haryana	95	48	65	87	43	51
Himachal Pradesh	87	26	—	59	19	—
Jammu & Kashmir	70	30	—	78	34	—
Jharkhand	33	21	—	50	21	—
Karnataka	64	32	65	57	20	25
Kerala	255	103	11	240	100	8
Madhya Pradesh	61	32	90	65	36	56
Maharashtra	93	44	52	118	50	34
Orissa	77	49	91	54	30	56
Punjab	136	61	55	107	44	35
Rajasthan	57	23	81	72	27	55
Tamil Nadu	95	54	50	96	49	32
Uttaranchal	52	31	—	65	25	—
Uttar Pradesh	100	55	83	108	55	58
West Bengal	114	56	52	157	62	36
India	88	45	69*	99	44	40*

Notes: (i) PAP: Number (per 1000) of persons reporting ailment for 2004–05
(ii) PPC: Number (per 1000) of persons reporting commencement of any ailment during the last 15 days for 2004–05
(iii) IMR: Infant mortality rate estimated for 2002 through the Sample Registration Scheme of the Office of the Registrar General of India

Source: Government of India (2006a)

Table 9

Correlation Matrix: Rural and Urban Sectors (2004–05)

Rural Sector

Variables	*Per capita calorie intake*	*Cal. HCR_ 2100*	*Cal. HCR_ 2400*	*Food avail. status*	*PAP*	*PPC*	*IMR*
Per capita calorie intake	1.00	(–) 0.98 (0.0000)	(–) 0.70 (0.0039)	(–) 0.51 (0.0517)	(–) 0.14	0.09	(–) 0.10
Cal. HCR_ 2100	(–) 0.98 (0.0000)	1.00	0.72 (0.0026)	0.56 (0.0297)	(–) 0.23	(–) 0.30	(–) 0. 18
Cal. HCR_ 2400	(–) 0.70 (0.0039)	0.72 (0.0026)	1.00	0.79 (0.0004)	(–) 0.34	(–) 0.18	(–) 0.09
Food. Avail. Status	(–) 0.51 (0.0517)	0.56 (0.0297)	0.79 (0.0004)	1.00	(–) 0.14	0.09	(–) 0.10

Urban Sector

Variables	*Per capita calorie intake*	*Cal. HCR_ 2030*	*Cal. HCR_ 2100*	*Food avail. status*	*PAP*	*PPC*	*IMR*
Per capita calorie intake	1.00	(–) 0.88 (0.0000)	(–) 0.89	0.39	(–) 0.21	(–) 0.11	0.50 (0.0562)
Cal. HCR_ 2030	(–) 0.88 (0.0000)	1.00	0.90 (0.0000)	(–) 0.33	0.23	0.10	(–) 0.60 (0.0174)
Cal. HCR_ 2100	(–) 0.89	0.90 (0.0000)	1.00	(–) 0.32	0.21	0.04	(–) 0.61 (0.0165)
Food. Avail. Status	0.39	(–) 0.33	(–) 0.32	1.00	(–) 0.18	0.04	(–) 0.19

Notes: (i) Cal. HCR_2030 denotes percentage of population with per capita calorie intake per diem less than 2030 kcals

(ii) Cal. HCR_2100 denotes percentage of population with per capita calorie intake per diem less than 2100 kcals

(iii) Cal. HCR_2400 denotes percentage of population with per capita calorie intake per diem less than 2400 kcals

(iv) Food availability status refers to percentage number of households reporting adequate food consumption throughout the year.

(v) Figures in parentheses are p-values, which are reported only for estimates, which are significant at least at a 10 per cent level.

Source: Author's estimates based on the NSS data.

This kind of interpretations and policy recommendations raises several issues. How stagnant are the real incomes of the poor during the sample period under review? How meaningful are the interpretations of estimates of budget shares at current prices? How valid are the interpretations of such estimates for the total population? What do the estimates of quantities for different population groups suggest? How valid are the exogenous norms for threshold levels of calorie intake worked out in the 1950s and 1960s, that is, almost half a century ago since when the economy has experienced structural and technological change and improvements? What have been the temporal changes in calorie intake across different decile groups? What do they mean? How far perception of the population with reference to adequacy of food consumption corroborates such findings? The following section examines these issues based on past studies.

Review

Real Incomes and Budget Share Estimates

One important explanation put forward by the Eleventh Plan for the decline in average cereal consumption and hence, calorie intake of the population is stagnant real incomes. However, there have been studies, which have gone into these details using different deflators (see, for instance, Suryanarayana, 1995). Among them the results obtained using representative price indices for rural and urban India have brought out the following: In rural India, the poorest three decile groups experienced higher (in percentage terms) increases in consumer expenditure than the whole population during the period 1970–71 and 1988–89. The consumption expenditure (at constant prices) for the rural population as a whole increased by 18.88 per cent; it increased by 32.02 per cent for the poorest and by 28.05 per cent for the second poorest decile group. As regards the urban sector, the corresponding increases for different decile groups were broadly the same, between 16.50 and 20.25 per cent.

The plan provides regressive changes in consumption patterns involving a decline in budget shares for cereals and other essential food items as an important factor contributing to the decline in calorie intake. The estimates of budget shares are for the total population by sector at current prices. Needless to say, the observed changes in consumption patterns based on such estimates would also reflect changes in relative prices rather than consumption patterns. In addition, the plan has made little attempt to examine the structural changes underlying the estimates of budget shares on different broad groups of consumption. It is important to examine the changes in consumption patterns by population sub-groups in order to bring out differential behavioural changes. One such attempt (Suryanarayana, 1995) based on commodity-wise monthly per capita consumer expenditures at current as well as at constant prices for the period 1972–73 to 1988–89 has brought out the following:

(i) The budget share of the rural poorest decile group on cereals decreased from 62 per cent in 1972–73 to 43 per cent in 1988–89; a difference of 19 points. When the same is examined at constant prices, the decline is much less, that is from 59 per cent in 1972–73 to 51 per cent in 1988–89; a difference of only 8 points. Thus, changing relative prices have exaggerated the observed decline in the proportion of consumer expenditure on cereals.

(ii) Budget shares both at current and constant prices increased somewhat for the following commodity groups: (a) milk and milk products, (b) edible oils, (c) fruits, vegetables and nuts, (d) sugar, and (e) durables and miscellaneous goods and services. There was a real increase in the consumption of all these commodity groups, including cereals, for the rural poorest decile group.

(iii) For commodity groups like (a) meat, fish and eggs, (b) pan, tobacco and intoxicants, (c) clothing and footwear, and (d) fuel and light, consumption shares at current prices increased but at constant prices decreased. Per capita monthly consumer expenditure at constant prices on these items by the rural poorest decile group actually fluctuated around a stationary level.

(iv) Total consumption at constant prices increased by 28 per cent between 1977–78 and 1988–89. The commodities which largely accounted for this increase are (i) cereals and cereal substitutes (6.82%), (ii) fruits, vegetables and nut (4.92%), (iii) durables and miscellaneous goods and services (3.25%) followed by (iv) edible oils (2.93%), (v) beverages and refreshments (2.30%), (vi) milk and milk products (1.76%), (vii) betal, tobacco and intoxicants (1.72%), (viii) fuel and light (1.37%), (ix) pulses (1.32%) and (x) sugar (1.04%). For items like (a) salt and spice, (b) meat, fish and eggs and (c) clothing and footwear, there was virtually no increase in consumer expenditure. In sum, the consumption basket of the poorest decile group seems to have improved in terms of quality and diversity.

(v) One finds a similar profile for other decile groups and also for the entire population in the rural sector but with a difference. Cereal consumer expenditure declined for all the decile groups except the poorest two. As regards the rural population as a whole, total consumption increased by 5.99 per cent. The commodities which accounted for this increase are (i) fruits and vegetables (3.31%) followed by (ii) beverages and refreshments (2.07%), (iii) edible oils (1.40%) and (iv) milk and milk products (1.25%).

(vi) The story for the urban sector is no different. While the proportion of expenditure on cereals at current prices by the poorest decile group decreased from 49 per cent in 1970–71 to 34 per cent in 1988–89 involving a difference of 15 points, that at constant prices also declined but from 49 per cent in 1970–71 to 40 per cent in 1988–89 with a difference of 9 points. Total consumption at constant prices increased by 14.12 per cent for this decile group during the second period. This was largely accounted for by (i) durables and miscellaneous goods and services whose consumption increased by 4.16 per cent followed by (ii) milk and milk products (2.56%), (iii) edible oils (2.51%) and (iv) fruits, vegetables and nuts (1.45%). These four commodity groups accounted for bulk of the increases in total real consumption for other decile groups and also for the whole urban population.

This would lead us to a review of changes in cereal consumption basket in India in the following section.

Cereal Consumption

Of course, per capita estimates of cereal quantities consumed declined during the entire post-independence era of India (Suryanarayana, 1995 and Government of India, 2008). It is important to note that the cereal consumption basket has undergone a change in its composition in favour of superior cereals like rice and wheat. The average monthly per capita consumption of rice increased from 2.59 kg to 5.27 kg between 1954–55 and 1989–90 for the rural poorest decile group. Similar increases, though not of the same magnitude, occurred for the second poorest and third poorest but not for the middle decile groups in rural India. Shares of rice in the cereal basket increased from 25.00 to 48.10, 32.30 to 52.13 and 41.40 to 53.31 per cent, for the poorest three-decile groups respectively. Monthly per capita wheat consumption of the poorest decile group in rural India increased from 210 grams in 1954–55 to 1.57 kg in 1977–78 and to 2.84 kg by 1983; the corresponding share in total cereal consumption of wheat increased from 2.00 to 16.10 per cent and then to 27.41 per cent in the same years. Coarse cereals consumption by the rural poorest decile group declined from 7.57 kg per capita per month in 1954–55 to 4.44 kg in 1977–78 and then to 4.28 kg in 1983 and 2.82 kg in 1986–87; the corresponding coarse cereal shares in total cereal consumption decreased from 73.00 per cent in 1954–55 to 45.64 per cent in 1977–78, 41.37 per cent in 1983 and to 28.26 per cent in 1986–87. Similar changes occurred for other poor decile groups too.

The urban sector too experienced similar changes in the cereal consumption basket; but the pattern and magnitude of changes are not as striking as that for the rural sector. Both in the rural and urban sectors, the share of wheat in the cereal basket increased and that of coarse cereals decreased. In other words, it is important to emphasis the qualitative improvements in the diet habits of the population, though this has occurred at the cost of energy intake as shown below.

Such changes in the composition of the consumption basket could reflect partly changing tastes, consumer responses to changing relative prices and their substitution effects on consumer choices but largely changing production and supply conditions. Under the new agricultural growth strategy, benefiting largely wheat and rice, crop composition of food grains has changed considerably in favour of superior cereals. Between 1960–61 and 1989–90 per capita daily availability of rice increased from 201.10 grams to 212.60 grams (by 5.72%), that of wheat from 79.10 grams to 132.90 grams (by 68.02%) while that of other cereals decreased from 119.50 grams to 87.10 grams (by 27.12%) (Government of India, 1992:136).

Between 1960–61 and 1989–90, per capita physical consumption coarse cereals of the rural population declined by 62.60 per cent; as regards wheat, it increased by 52.60 per cent for wheat. For the urban population, coarse cereal consumption declined by 65.67 per cent and wheat consumption increased by 13.88 per cent. Structural changes in the rural economy involving a decline in coarse cereal availability and changes in labour markets could have accounted for some decline in total cereal consumption of the rural poorer decile groups.[1]

Calorie Intake

With the decline in average cereal consumption, a decline in average calorie intake would follow. The story based on averages would conceal rather than reveal any insight about the dynamics of the development process. Of course, the estimates for the total population would tell us that nearly 80 per cent of the Indian population is energy deficient with reference to the calorie norms underlying the official definition of poverty line. How did this come about? This has happened because of (i) a decline (by choice) in cereal consumption and hence, calorie intake of the richer decile groups; and (ii) an insufficient (relative to norm) increase in that of the poorer sections (Tables 2 and 3). The decline in the calorie intake of the richer sections could be explained in terms of changing consumption patterns in favour of non-calorie food and non-food items at the expense of calorie intake. The poor too seem to have opted for some diversification in consumption providing a more nutritious diet though not adequate energy (Suryanarayana, 1995).

What is important to note is that the calorie norms cited above have been worked out in the 1950s/60s and hence, may be outdated and irrelevant with improvements in modes of production and standard of living. This could be the reason for voluntary reductions in cereal consumption and calorie intake of the richer decile groups. Hence, it would not make sense to verify issues related to food security with reference to outdated exogenous norms. Instead, it is high time we revise the cereal and calorie norms for defining food security. However, it is important to examine how valid is the case for revising the norms for food security. One option could be to verify in terms of self-perception regarding adequacy of food consumption, which is done in the following section.

Perceptions on Food Adequacy

Since its 38th round (1983), the National Sample Survey Organization has periodically asked what are called probing questions like whether the household gets two square meals a day throughout the year. Such questions were asked during the 38th (1983), 50th (1993–94) and the 61st (2004–05) rounds. Till the 55th round, the investigator asked direct question to the household. In 1983, 81 per cent of the rural households reported adequate food consumption (two square meals a day); this percentage increased to 95 in 1993–94, 96 in 1999–2000 and to 97 in 2004–2005 (Table 4). In the urban sector, corresponding number increased from 93 per cent in 1983 to 99 per cent in 1999–2000 and 2004–05. In sum, this piece of evidence corroborates the perception that the population is well fed.

The NSS findings presented in the preceding paragraph would raise the question as to whether cereal/calorie shortfall is a question of voluntary choice or involuntary. As the preceding findings show, cereal consumption and calorie intakes of the richer decile groups have declined by choice. If the corresponding limits were to be the norm, then, after appropriate normalization, only about 30 per cent of the rural and 40 per cent of the urban population were food insecure and these macro estimates of food insecurity fell well in the neighbourhood of the poverty estimates (Suryanarayana and Silva, 2005). Therefore, it would be interesting to examine how far the objective measures of nutritional adequacy and subjective perceptions on food adequacy co-vary with estimates of morbidity and provide some base for policy choice.

Perceptions on Food Security and Morbidity

The preceding discussion would raise a number of issues: What would be the appropriate measure of food security? Should one consider objective estimates of food consumption relative to exogenous outdated norms? Could one base one's judgment on subjective perceptions of adequacy of food consumption? How do we verify these two questions? How far measures of association would validate these measures? What is the evidence?

The estimates of association as measured rank correlation coefficients are presented in Table 9. The estimates of association do not make much sense. For instance, cross-sectional evidence on household perceptions on adequate food consumption vary inversely with estimates of per capita calorie intake across states while the association is observed to be positive for the urban sector. Consistent with this finding, household perception on food adequacy bears significant positive association with incidence of calorie deficiency (with reference to alternative norms) in the rural sector and simple negative association in the urban sector. Only sensible estimate of association pertains to the ones between calorie intake and incidence of calorie deficiency in both rural and urban sectors. Other measures of association between subjective and objective measures of food security and alternative measure of morbidity/health consciousness are insignificant for the rural sector. As regards the urban sector, either they are insignificant or do not makes any sense. For instance, association between incidence of calorie efficiency and infant mortality is significant and inverse implying that higher the incidence of calorie deprivation lower is incidence of infant mortality, which is absurd.

Conclusion

Quite often one comes across studies or policy documents dealing with issues from a partial perspective. As a result, one finds misplaced interpretations and emphasis on policy choices and instruments. For instance, current advocacy for universalization of the public distribution system is based on the perception that about 90 per cent of the population is food insecure. This study illustrates this problem with reference to the Government of India Eleventh Five-Year Plan on Food Security and raises some methodological issues.

Recognizing the role of food security in ensuring sustained and effective response to morbidity, the Eleventh Plan makes a case to address issues related to food security. As per the plan, food security in India has worsened as measured by estimates of cereal consumption and calorie intake due to stagnant incomes of the poor and perverse changes in consumption patterns. This study reviews the basis for such assessments in terms of disaggregate analysis of changes in consumption patterns by decile groups in rural and urban India.

The assessment is carried out after appropriate consumption basket specific price adjustments for estimates of nominal consumption and in times of changes in physical quantities with reference to the observed structural changes in the economy. The study brings out that current price estimates of budget shares, as is well known, exaggerate changes in consumption pattern and analysis based on averages for the population could be misleading. It also shows that real consumption expenditures of all the decile groups, the bottom three decile groups in particular, increased since the mid-1970s. Per capita cereal expenditures of the bottom decile groups in rural India increased. However, this was not accompanied by corresponding increases in quantities of cereal consumption because of structural changes in the economy.

With casualization and hence, monetization of the labour market, there has been a progressive increase in the dependence of the poor households, landless labour in particular, on the commodity market. With changes in cereal production patterns and hence availability in favour of superior cereals, these households had to shift their consumption in favour of superior but costlier rice and wheat, which are inferior to coarse cereals in terms of calorie content. As a result, cereal consumption and hence, calorie intake has not increased to a commensurate extent. On the other hand, with changes in infrastructure and technology, average energy requirements seem to have declined calling for reduced calorie intake. This could be one major reason for the observed trend decline in average calorie intake of the richer decile groups in rural and urban India. Estimates of incidence of calorie deficiency with reference to outdated norms, hence, show a trend increase. Hence, there is a need for revising downward the calorie norms consistent with the converging pattern of changes in calorie intake across decile groups in rural and urban India.

The case for such an approach is validated by the survey findings which show that the percentage number of rural and urban households reporting adequate food consumption throughout the year has increased since 1983 and has reached almost 98 per cent. This would raise the question regarding an appropriate measure of food security. Should one measure it in terms of objective estimates of calorie intake with reference to and exogenous norm or subjective perceptions on adequate food consumption? The limited evidence in terms of bivariate correlations between subjective and objective estimates of food consumption, and measures of health status do not provide any unambiguous answer. The estimates are either weak or perverse which could be because of the simultaneous interaction of a host of variables in determining these outcomes.

Note

1. For further empirical details, see Suryanarayana (1995).

References

Government of India (1981): A Technical Note on the Sixth Plan of India (1980–85), Perspective Planning Division, Planning Commission, New Delhi.

—— (1992): Bulletin on Food Statistics: 1991, Ministry of Agriculture, New Delhi.

—— (2001): Reported Adequacy of Food Intake in India 1999–2000 NSS 55th Round (July 1999–June 2000), Report No. 466 (55/1.0/7), National Sample Survey Organisation, New Delhi.

—— (2006a): Morbidity, Health Care and the Condition of the Aged NSS 60th Round (January–June 2004), Report No. 507 (60/25.0/1), National Sample Survey Organisation, New Delhi.

—— (2006b): Level and Pattern of Consumer Expenditure, 2004 –2005, NSS 61st Round (July 2004–June 2005), NSS Report No. 508 (61/1.0)/1), National Sample Survey Organisation, New Delhi.

—— (2007a): Perceived Adequacy of Food Consumption In Indian Households 2004–2005 NSS 61st Round (July 2004–June 2005), Report No. 512 (61/1.0/5), National Sample Survey Organisation, New Delhi.

Government of India (2007b): Poverty Estimates for 2004–05, Press Information Bureau, New Delhi, India.

—— (2007c), Nutritional Intake in India 2004–2005 NSS 61st Round (July 2004–June 2005), Report No. 513 (61/1.0/6), National Sample Survey Organisation, New Delhi.

—— (2008): Eleventh Five-Year Plan 2007–12, Volume II, Social Sector, Planning Commission, Oxford University Press, New Delhi.

Suryanarayana, M.H. (1983): "Treatment of Poverty in the Sixth Plan", *Artha Vijnana*, Vol. XXV, No. 4, pp. 419–425.

—— (1991): "Distributional Assumptions and Their Implications for Plan Projections", *Artha Vijnana,* Vol. XXXIII, No. 2, pp. 142–50.

—— (1995): "Growth, Poverty and Levels of Living: Hypotheses, Methods and Policies", *Journal of Indian School of Political Economy*, Vol. 7, No. 2, pp. 203–55.

—— (2008): "Inclusive Growth. What is so Exclusive about it?", *Economic and Political Weekly*, Vol. 43, No. 43.

Suryanarayana, M.H. and Dimitri Silva (2005): "Is Targeting the Poor a Penalty on the Food Insecure? Poverty and Food Insecurity in India", *Journal of Human Development*, Vol. 8, No. 1, pp. 89–107.

3

Policy Reforms and Health Care System in Kerala

Constraints and Options

K. GANGADHARAN

Economic growth and development affect the health of the people by increasing their level of income, and hence the consumption-increasing goods and services. It means, there is a positive relationship between health and stages of economic growth and development but it is not always true. In this connection, it is useful to note two important consequences of the improvement of health: demographic transition and epidemiological transition. As populations become healthier, they also live long which is known as demographic transition. It occurs due to two reasons. First, when the health status of the individual improves, they live longer. Assuming a given birth rate, the net addition to the population each year increases, increasing the share of older people in the total population. Second, the fertility rate may tend to decline due to better health and greater economic security. As development proceeds, the pattern of diseases change which is known as epidemiological transition. This has also two effects. First, when some diseases and good health are controlled or eliminated, the relative importance of other diseases increases as a matter of arithmetic. Second, as individual live longer, diseases that only affect older individuals increase in absolute term. Similarly, reduction in maternal mortality leads to larger number of older women and also a greater prevalence of post-menopausal health problems.

Kerala, one of the socially advanced states in India, is now experiencing these two consequences of improvement in health, mainly demographical and epidemiological. This has culminated in the problem of ageing on the one side and increase in the morbidity load on the other. The present paper is an attempt to evaluate these changes that occurred in Kerala and also the consequences faced by the economy as part of the impact of policy reforms carried out by the country from 1991 onwards which ultimately pushed the state into a stage of health crisis.

The 40 years of planned development of the Indian economy ultimately culminated in a crisis in 1991. An impartial analysis of the situation of the crisis in 1991 definitely reveals that it was not a crisis of solvency but of mainly the liquidity crunch. The short-term market borrowing from global financial market, particularly from Euro-currency market at high commercial rates of interest, landed India into a crisis of liquidity. To solve this crisis, India opted to follow the IMF/World Bank prescriptions of Structural Adjustment Programme (SAP). The health care system in an open economy, which falls within the ambit of globalization, has to reckon with impact on health of the people of the country. Derek Yach and Douglas Bettecher (1998) identified certain global changes which have impact on health status (see Table 1).

Table 1

Global Changes vs Health Status

Global Transnational Factors	*Consequence and Probable Impact on Health Status*
Macro-economic prescriptions – . Structural adjustment policies and downsizing.	Marginalization, poverty, inadequate decreased social security nets, structural and chronic unemployment, higher morbidity and mortality rates.
Trade – tobacco, alcohol and psychoactive drugs.	Increased marketing availability and use.
Trade – dumping of unsafe or ineffective pharmaceuticals.	Ineffective or harmful therapy.
Travel – more than one million people crossing border per day.	Infectious diseases transmission and export of harmful lifestyles (high risk sexual behaviour).
Migration	Increases refugees population and rapid population growth – ethnic and civil conflict and environment degradation.
Environment degradation and unsustainable consumption patterns. Resource depletion especially access to fresh water – water pollution.	Global and local environment health impact. Epidemics and potential violence within and between countries (water wars).

Cont'd...

Cont'd...

Trade – trade of contaminated food stuffs/feeds.	Spread of infectious diseases across borders.
Ozone depletion and increased ultraviolet radiation – accumulation of green house gases and global warming.	Immuno-suppression skin cancers – major shifts in infectious disease patterns and vector distribution (chicken guinea) death from heat waves, increases trauma due to floods and storms and worsening food shortages and malnutrition in many regions of the world.
Foreign policies – based in national self interest, xenophobia and protectionism.	Threat to malnutrition and global cooperation required to address shared transnational health concerns.
Technology – patent protection of new technologies under the trade related aspects of intellectual property rights agreement.	Benefits of new technologies developed in the global market are unaffordable to the poor.

Health Care Sector in Kerala: The Post-Reform Scenario

The typical feature of the post-reform health scenario of India is that a shift occurred from health care to medical care. Social sector expenditure declined considerably during the post-reform period. During the First Plan 3.33 per cent of total plan expenditure (state and union government) was for health sector, while during the Eight Plan it was 1.75 per cent and it declined to further to 0.6 per cent in the Ninth plan and to 0.4 per cent during the Tenth Plan. The proportion of health expenditure in major states was in the range of 6–7 per cent during 1980s but came down to about 5 per cent during 1990s. A larger portion of public expenditure went towards salaries. Major portion was allocated towards tertiary level care. This results in a squeeze of resource for primary health care services in the country.

The health scenario in Kerala was hunky-dory during the pre-liberalization days. However, during the post-liberalization period many a problem cropped up in the health care system, and unfortunately, the health indicators gradually started showing an unfavorable trend, and in many cases, they are getting worse than the average all-India indicators over time. The morbidity rate is now all-time high, malnutrition and undernourishment alarming, various types of capitalist diseases are predominant, calorie intake going down and infant mortality has started rising up. In the meantime, the state expenditure has been declining, the government-run institutions stand outdated due to lack of modern health infrastructure and shortage of properly skilled manpower. There is perceptible decapitalization in the health sector. The globalization game has reduced the health sector into shambles and prepared a stage for the victory of the private sector, which now demarcates the configuration of a new history. There is a perceptible change in public expenditure on health care in Kerala. If the present trend continues, Kerala's percentile position is likely to fall further in the foreseeable future unless some checks and balances are placed in order, and Kerala will no longer hold its title as the best state in India as a health care provider.

The marketing strategies of medical care providers created growing health scarce, instead of health awareness. The increase in morbidity rate may be attributed to this phenomenon. Failure of government facilities to meet demand had led to the mushrooming of private sector and escalation in private health care expenditure. Also during the post-reform period more emphasis was laid on curative medicine and less on preventive medicine. The increase in heath care expenditure during the period is unprecedented. A hospitalized Indian spends more than half of his annual expenditure on buying health care. More than 40 per cent of hospitalized people borrow money or sell assets to cover hospital expenses. Among them, 35 per cent falls below poverty line (World Bank, 1993). Out-of-pocket expenses alone are estimated to push 2.2 per cent of the population below poverty line annually. Efforts are made and to an extent achieved to convert India into a hub of health tourism industry. However the negative impact of tourism industry in general and health tourism in particular are not addressed properly. Health care hitherto a sacrosanct area of public good is now converted into market-driven, profit-driven enterprise. Instead of competitive market we witnessed the emergence of an oligopolistic market with price leader. Often the prominent hospital, invariably the private hospital emerges as the price leader in this oligopolistic market.

The Structural Adjustment Programme, macro-economic prescriptions, trade, travel, migration, environmental and resource depletion etc., affected the Kerala's health care system. Failure of government—facilities to meet demand—led to the development of private sector. Large increase in private health care expenditure, privatization of medical education, reduction in public spending and health care and neglect of PHCs, hitherto sacrosanct area of public good converting health care into market-driven, profit-driven enterprise.

Decline in the quality of public sector because of financial restriction, shortage of supplies including medicines were other dominant influence of policy reforms on the health care segment of Kerala.

Table 2
Infant Mortality in Kerala and India

Period	*Kerala (K)*	*India (I)*	*K as of I*
1941–1950	153	192	80
1951–1960	128	140	91
1961–1970	66	114	58
1971	61	129	47
1981	37	110	34
1991	16	80	20
2001	11	66	17
2006	13	57	22
2007	14	58	24

Sources: 1. Kannan, KP., Thankappan, K.R. et al., 1991. Health and Development in Rural Kerala, KSSP.
2. Registrar General of India, Sample Registration System.

The movement of infant mortality indicated in Table 2 and Figure 1 reveals that Kerala is in the reverse trend of improvement in child health status. In the period after 2001 the infant mortality rate is steadily increasing year after year though the national figure is improving.

Figure 1
Infant Mortality in Kerala and India

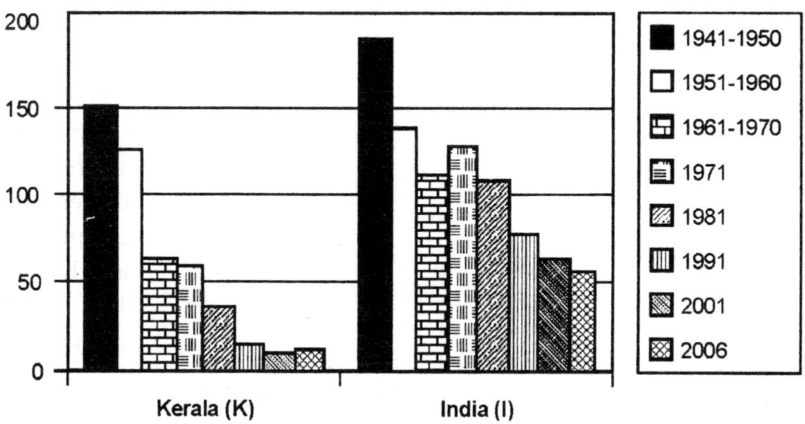

Table 3

Kerala's Health Indicators in Comparison to India as a Whole and to Some Other Countries

Countries	*IMR*	*Under 5 Mortality*	*Life Expectancy*	*TFR*	*Health Expenditure (as % of GDP)*	
					Total	%
Kerala	14	19	73.5	1.8	6.2	1.4 (22)
India	60	87	62	3.0	6.1	1.3 (21)
China	27	37	71	1.8	5.8	2.0 (34)
Sri Lanka	11	15	71	2.0	3.7	1.8 (49)
USA	5	8	77	2.1	14.6	6.6 (45)
Canada	7	6	80	1.5	9.6	6.7 (70)

Source: Economic Review, 2007; World Health Report, 2005.

In Kerala, urban health care facilities often benefit only the affluent minority and access to health care is restricted to poor and economically deprived. Difficulty in access to health care, impoverishment of a sizeable segment of population owing to high out-of-pocket health expenditure, prevalence of environmental related diseases owing to problems of community hygiene and pollution are the major health care hurdles faced by the urban dwellers in Kerala.

Table 4

Incidence of Morbidity by Type of Urban Households Kerala vs India (2004)

(per cent)

Household Type	*Kerala*	*India*
Self-employed (non-agricultural)	21.91	9.31
Regular wage salary	25.95	9.86
Casual labour	22.59	9.58
Others	30.58	15.60
All-India	24.06	9.95

Source: NSS 60th round.

The morbidity profile of Kerala is also alarming in the sense that the NSS 60th round reveals high morbidity in both urban and rural Kerala (Tables 4 and 5). High morbidity is reported among casual labourers and other type of manual workers. This reveals that the working class is subject to the brunt of both environmental and infrastructural deprivation in the health care sector.

The gender dimension of morbidity also reveals (Table 6) that females are subject to more of the health problems and morbidity in Kerala. This is also alarming in the sense that compared to the national level, 26 per cent of females are subject to one or other type of morbidity in Kerala whereas at the national level it is only 9 per cent. This also indicates the problems associated with the females and negligence of their health aspect. Females are facing this morbidity load mainly due to the problems associated with the child birth and also due to the problem of ageing. In the 60 plus categories in Kerala the proportion of females are more dominating than the males and usually the 60 plus period is a stage for an array of illness.

Table 5

Incidence of Morbidity by Type of Rural Household Kerala vs India 2004

(per cent)

Household Type	*Kerala*	*India*
Self-employed (Non-agricultural)	26.06	9.16
Agricultural labour	22.94	7.67
Other labour	27.49	10.64
Self-employed (Agricultural)	26.08	8.14
Others	23.23	12.33
All Rural	25.54	8.33

Source: NSS 60th round.

Table 6

Incidence of Morbidity by Gender and Sector (%) Kerala and All-India (2004)

Gender	*Kerala*			*All-India*		
	Rural	*Urban*	*All*	*Rural*	*Urban*	*All*
Male	24.28	23.56	24.09	8.36	9.11	8.56
Female	26.66	24.51	26.10	9.30	10.86	9.69
Total	25.53	24.06	25.15	8.82	9.95	9.11

Source: NSS 60th round.

Table 7

Percentage of Spells of Ailments Treated (non-institutional) during 15 Days and Percentage Distribution of Treated Spells of Ailments by Source of Treatment in Major States

Major States	*Rural*			*Urban*		
	% spells of ailments treated	*Source of treatment*		*% spells of ailments treated*	*Source of treatment*	
		Govt.	*Private*		*Govt.*	*Private*
Andhra Pradesh	77	21	79	88	20	80
Bihar	81	5	95	88	11	89
West Bengal	80	19	81	83	20	80
Gujarat	84	21	79	93	18	82
Haryana	94	12	88	95	20	80
Himachal Pradesh	94	68	32	92	86	14
J&K	82	52	48	94	51	49
Karnataka	78	34	66	87	16	84
Kerala	**87**	**37**	**63**	**90**	**22**	**78**
Madhya Pradesh	87	23	77	95	23	77
Maharashtra	88	16	84	92	11	89
Orissa	76	51	49	86	54	46
Punjab	94	16	84	96	48	82
Rajasthan	90	44	56	90	53	47
Tamil Nadu	78	29	71	87	22	78
India	82	·22	78	89	19	81

Source: Health Information of India, 2005.

In Table 7, the data related to utilization of public health care facilities and the spells of ailments treated etc., reveals that the monopoly of the state in the public health care system is vanishing as part of the policy reform measures. In Kerala only 87 per cent of the illness cases are reported for a treatment whereas in Himachal Pradesh, Haryana and Punjab 94 per cent ailments are treated and out of this 68 per cent have secured treatment from government hospitals. The position of Kerala is in the reverse trend in the sense that only 37 per cent has secured treatment from public hospitals and, private and corporate hospitals are dominating in Kerala and they canvassed 63 per cent of the total treatment cases. The Table 8 reveals the domination of private health care expenditure in the overall health care expenditure of certain selected countries. It reveals that the share of private expenditure in Kerala is somewhat at par with the health care expenditure of Togo, Myanmar, Pakistan etc., where the per capita income is comparatively far better than Kerala. This shows that overdomination of private health care expenditure is adversely affecting the capacity of the people for better living and also leads to some sort of financial and economic deprivation among them, especially among the communities at the socially and economically bottom level. Table 9 specially reveals the burden of health care and its impact on socially and economically poor sections. The BPL categories are forced to spend 31.7 per cent of the total family expenditure on health, at the same time the better groups in the society are spending only 10.4 per cent of their total income as the health expenditure. Thus, derailment of public sector in the health care area as part of downsizing of the government budget definitely affects the poor section of the community and data reveals that in Kerala this has adversely affected the prospects of the poor section of the society (see Table 10).

Table 8

Private Health Expenditure as Proportion of Total Expenditure on Health, 2004

Country	*Proportion of private health expenditure*
Global	44
Myanmar	87.1
China	62
Pakistan	80.4
Togo	79.3
Singapore	66.0
Cuba	12.2
United Kingdom	13.7
India	82.7
Kerala	78

Source: http: #www global health facts.org

Table 9

Treatment Expenditure in Relation to Various Socio-economic Classes

Categories	*Morbidity rate per 1,000*	*One-time health expenditure*	*Per capita annual health expenditure*	*Health expenditure as % of total family expenditure*
BPL poor	85.1	701.9	1552.9	31.7
APL poor	82.1	613.5	1309.7	18.1
Lower middle class	78.1	886.9	1801.0	13.0
Upper middle class	73.9	1686.1	3238.5	10.4
Total	79.2	830.7	1722.0	13.9

Source: KSSP, 2006.

Table 10

Revenue Expenditure on Health as % of Total Government Revenue Expenditure: India and Selected States (1980–2001)

Selected States and India	*1980–81*	*1990–91*	*2000–01*
Kerala	8.6	7.5	5.7
Maharashtra	6.5	5.5	4.2
Bihar	5.7	5.5	6.0
Rajasthan	8.3	7.2	5.8
India	3.3	3.0	3.1

Source: Budget documents of states and Government of India.

Table 11 also reveals the negligence of the health sector by the state government in all the period from 1965 onwards. This negligence itself was responsible for declining health package for a state which has been considered as an apex state in India in terms of health care development and human development.

Table 11

Government Expenditure in the Health Budget, 1956–2005

Years	*Government's expenditure*	*% of government's expenditure*
1956	386	8.00
1960	541	8.24
1965	981	8.74
1970	943	8.02
1975	4627	7.71
1980	7879	6.82
1985	12681	6.56
1990	22199	5.01
1995	35590	4.02
2000	59800	1.20
2005	111387.5	1.37

Source: Budget documents, Government of Kerala, various years.

The public sector hospitals are converting as a scarecrow by not filling the genuine posts of doctors vacant in these hospitals. Table 12 reveals the vacancy position of doctors in different PHCs and government hospitals in various districts in Kerala. In most of the hilly and tribal belt areas public hospitals are running in an anarchy as doctors are not willing to work there and no individual and personal attention is paid to the patients and those who approach for health care services. Due to lack of acumen and essential health care personnel to treat the children and mothers and pregnant women the maternal and child health status of Kerala also deteriorated over the time period from 1996 to 2006.

Table 12

Vacancies of Government Doctors in Kerala in 2007

District	*Assistant Surgeon*	*Civil Surgeon*	*Total*
Kasargod	36	12	48
Kannur	98	4	102
Wayanad	21	12	33
Kozhikode	2	10	12
Malappuram	36	21	57
Palaghat	73	11	84
Trichur	39	29	68
Ernakulam	58	1	59
Idukki	41	9	50
Kottayam	43	7	50
Alappuzha	34	10	44
Pathanamthitta	50	0	50
Kollam	26	0	26
Trivandrum	0	12	12
Total	567	138	705

Source: Directorate of Health Services, Thiruvananthapuram.

Table 13

Nutrition Status and Anaemia among Children and Adults Variation over Period in Kerala

(per cent)

Particular	*NFHS I*	*NFHS II*	*NFHS–III*		
			All	*Urban*	*Rural*
Women whose Body Mass Index is below normal	NA	18.7	12.5	9.1	14.3
Women who are underweight	NA	20.6	34.0	40.1	30.9
Men who are underweight	NA	—	24.3	28.0	21.9
Children in the age of 6–35 months who are anaemic	NA	43.9	55.7	51.3	57.9
Married women in the age of 15–49 who are anaemic	—	22.7	32.3	32.3	32.4
Pregnant women in the age group 15–49 who are anaemic	—	20.3	33.1	27.7	35.8
Children under 3 years who are stunted.	25.2	21.9	21.1	21.3	21.1
Children under 3 years who are wasted	12.8	11.1	16.1	10.1	19.1
Children under 3 years who are underweight	27.0	26.9	28.8	22.5	31.9

Source: NFHS, IIPS Mumbai, 2007.

Table 13 reveals the increasing trend by the National Family Health Survey (NFHS) with regard to anaemia and underweight problem among the children in Kerala. Compared to Tamil Nadu the position of Kerala was far better in the 1990s, now the trend is in the reverse direction as Tamil Nadu has improved a lot in maternal and child health status especially in anaemia reduction and reduction in underweight problem and also the advancement secured in the coverage of childhood immunization. Figure 2 shows the varitaion in underweight problem as a vital issue of nutritional deprivation in Kerala and Tamil Nadu over the period from 1992-93 to 2005-2006 (NFHS–I: 1992; NFHS–II: 1998-1999, NFHS–III: 2005-2006)

Figure 2

Children under 3 Years Who are Underweight, Variation over Period

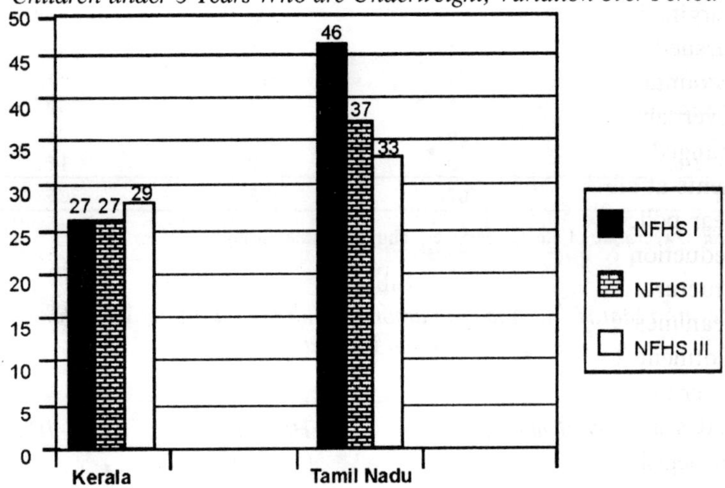

Constraints and Options Available

In both rural and urban areas, Kerala records the highest morbidity. Lack of basic infrastructural facilities in the slum and interior parts also pose a severe hurdle in the health care development in Kerala. Urbanization trends in Kerala adversely affected the health care for all. Fragile health budget and negligence of investment in health sector also play dominant role for the declining health status of Kerala. Decreasing allocation to public health sector, results in increasing privatization of health care. Public hospitals and PHCs are utilized mainly for maternal and child health care programmes and immunizations. Graying of Kerala due to hike in 60+ population and deteriorating environmental quality also leads to hike in morbidity. High provider induced demand for procedures and drugs, equipments but no acumen and supplies in government hospitals is also a severe hurdle in the health care advancement of the state. It is estimated that two-thirds of curative care is now in the private sector without government support. High level of mental distress, higher incidence of lifestyle diseases also makes Kerala a state with higher health distress than other states in India. Another major reason for the trailing of health care sector in Kerala is that in the public sector health budget salaries and allowances of the public health care persons form a major chunk of the health budget and the allocation for supplies and medicines is very meagre which has a direct effect on the needs and aspiration of the poor sections. This is the basic reason behind why public health care centres have become a scarecrow recently.

Improving quality of care and provision for accessibility of marginalized groups in the health care system is the basic policy to be pursued. Decision-making by local self-government and greater accountability for decision is essential under the era of decentralized governance in Kerala. All these are in papers alone and this must be changed. Equitable financing mechanism for proper health care requirements at all levels must be implemented. Technology upgradation with clear policy on technology diffusion at all levels must be implemented. Reduction of morbidity, both chronic and communicable, better infrastructure, drinking water, sanitation, drainage and environmental cleanliness must be maintained and provided at all levels. Hike in budget allotment for medicine supplies etc., in the health care budget of government in every year is indispensable to cater the supplies of the PHCs and government hospitals. Rehabilitation of private sector with due legislation and a monitoring cell to evaluate and check the working of PHCs is also essential. Protecting environmental quality and a check in ecological bankruptcy must also be followed as a supplementary tool to protect environment. Ensuring availability of doctors and para-medical staff in all PHCs and hospitals is the most important step to be undertaken by the government and public authorities. Targeted information, education and communication campaign for urban slums on family planning and RCH services, environmental and health awareness programme with NGO participation, better nutrition, environmental and preventive health care programmes, taxation of private health care for funding preventive health care services, and greater public investment in health sector etc., are the other important policy measures to be taken on a war footing level to bring back the derailed health care segment of Kerala.

Note

Private Health Expenditure: the sum of expenditures on health by prepaid plans and risk-pooling arrangements, firms' expenditure on health, non-profit institutions serving mainly households, and household out-of-pocket spending. Total Expenditure on Health: the sum of general government health expenditure and private health expenditure in a given year, calculated in national currency units in current prices.

References

Chakraborty, A. 2005. "Kerala's Changing Development Narratives", *Economic and Political Weekly*, February 5.

Chandrashekhar, C.P. and Jayanthi Ghosh. 2004. "Health Expenditure in India", *Business Line*, September 19, 2006

Gangadharan, K. 2006. "Morbidity in Kerala, Distributional Profile and Implications", *Indian Journal of Social Development,* New Delhi.

Government of India. 2001. Nutritional Intake in India: 1999–2000. National Sample Survey Organization, Ministry of Statistics and Programme Implementation.

——. 2005. "Health Information of India", Ministry of Health and Family Welfare, New Delhi.

Government of Kerala. 2007. Economic Review, State Planning Board, Thiruvanthapuram.

Kerala Sastra Sahithya Parishad. 2006. *How Kerala Thinks and Acts*. Sastra Sahitya Parisheth, Thiruvanathapuram.

Kurup, Gopalakrishna B. 1993. "Low Mortality and High Morbidity in Kerala, Reconsidered", *Population and Development Review,* Vol. 19, No.1.

National Family Health Survey. 1995. NFHS–I. International Institute of Population Sciences, Mumbai.

——. 2000. NFHS–II. International Institute of Population Sciences, Mumbai.

——. 2007. NFHS–III. International Institute of Population Sciences, Mumbai.

Thomaskutty, P.G. 2001. "Globalization and Its Impact on People's Health", *Social Science Abstract*, Vol. XXV, Indian Academy of Social Sciences.

Website: http: # www.global health facts.*org*

World Bank,1993. *World Development Report, 1993*. Investing in Health, Oxford University Press, New York.

Yach, Derek and Douglas, Bettecher, 1998. "The Globalization of Public Health, Threats and Opportunities", *American Journal of Public Health,* Vol. 88.

Section II

Health and Development: Issues and Strategies

4

Investing in Health

A Review of Measurement, Theory and Indian Evidence

MALATHY DURAISAMY AND P. DURAISAMY

Health is regarded as an important form of human capital formation and benefits of improving health status are far reaching (Sen, 1999). The health status of a population measures the quality of life of the people. It is both an end in itself and a means to achieve other ends. There are compelling arguments for accelerating investment in health. Good health is considered to be an integral part of development. Further it contributes to increasing the productivity of the economically active population which in turn enhances earnings. Health also accounts for longevity and well-being of children and the aged population. The benefits of good health both to the individual in whom it is embodied as well as to the society at large are so pervasive that health investments is accorded high priority everywhere.

There is growing research attention on several aspects of health and health care. Interestingly economists have made significant contributions to analysing health issues. The range of issues addressed include micro and macro concerns – from tracing the health effect on growth and poverty, the cost and financing of health care, public and private provisioning and utilization, demand for health care, burden of disease on households, specific disease impacts, disability measurement and adjustments, impact of technology on health, households health seeking behaviour, evaluating health and the like. The growing availability of data both at the aggregate as well as disaggregate levels has facilitated such analysis. India is a large country in terms of population and has made commendable achievements in several fronts. Yet its ranking in human development and several indicators of health status is rather low. Given the enormity of the health problems faced by the people, it is surprising that very little economic analysis has been conducted that can help formulate sound policies. It would be useful to throw light on some of the works in the area. The purpose of this paper is to provide insights into selected and frequently used indicators of health, review one of the popular and versatile theoretical frameworks to analyse health seeking behaviour and report some empirical evidence from Indian studies based on the reviewed theoretical framework.

The rest of the paper is organized as follows: Section II contains a discussion on health indicators focusing on their measurement and issues. Section III traces the trends in selected indicators of health status in India. Section IV presents the economic model. Some empirical evidence for India, based on the reviewed theoretical model, are given in Section V. The summary and conclusions are provided in Section VI.

II

Health Indicators: Measurement and Issues

Health status is multidimensional in nature and there is no consensus on how to summarily and precisely measure health status. It is captured through several outcome and input indicators. The outcome measures include mortality, morbidity and nutritional status. The health inputs are used to produce desired health outcomes and include availability of health infrastructure, expenditure on health etc. Each indicator serves a specific purpose and it may be worthwhile to consider the merits and demerits of some popularly used measures.

Mortality measures are perhaps the simplest ones and mortality data, to the extent available, are one of the most reliable data sets that provide a comprehensive picture of community health. Many different mortality measures are used and all are valid measures of the health of a community, but the information provided is from differing perspectives. These include, life expectancy at birth (which is a summary measurement of population health status based entirely on the mortality experience of a hypothetical cohort that is subjected throughout its lifetime to a set of age-specific death rates), crude death rates (calculated by dividing the total number of deaths from any cause in a given population by the number of individuals in that population which is expressed in terms of the number of events that occurred over a specified time period per unit of population per 1,000 or per 1,00,000 people), age-adjusted mortality rate (statistically removes the difference in age structure of a population), infant (under 1 year of age) and child mortality (children below 5 years) rates (number of infants and children reported dead per 1,000 live births) and years of potential life lost.

In contrast to mortality, *morbidity indicator* reflects severity of illness and is related to the pain and sufferings of the people unlike mortality which is a terminal event. Morbidity measures are of two types, namely, self-perceived and observed (Murray and Chen, 1992). Self-perceived morbidity measure is based on information about incidence or prevalence rate of illness, type of illness, functional disability and use of medical services collected through surveys. This measure however, critically depends upon a person's knowledge and perception of illness, and willingness to report the same. This is subjective and culturally conditioned, varies over space and time and renders comparisons difficult. Observed morbidity measure, on the other hand, is based on the illness pattern as assessed by an independent trained observer using specific methods that lend themselves for repetition with some degree of consistency. The methods include observing physical and vital signs, measuring physiological indicators by conducting laboratory tests, functional tests and making clinical diagnosis. Although clinically observed morbidity would yield more accurate data the method is seldom applied in practice due to the high cost involved in collecting the data. Hence, most large-scale morbidity surveys depend on the responses of individuals to structured questionnaires. The information is collected through a set of questions relating to illness symptoms, severity of illness, functional disability, the use of preventive and curative health services etc. The functional consequences of diseases like illness leading to bed-ridden days, work or school days or normal activities lost would yield more accurate measure of morbidity (Strauss and Thomas, 1998). More specific measures like disease patterns, reproductive, maternal and child health, health of elderly etc., are also used. Measures of morbidity are fraught with problems such as definition, choice of reference period, data collection methodology, recall bias and the perception and cultural influences which affect the reporting of morbidity etc. (see Duraisamy, 1995; 1998; 2000 and Duraisamy and Sukanya, 2002 for a discussion).

Nutritional indicators include anthropometric measures (body-mass index, height-for-age, weight-for-height, mid-arm circumference etc.) dietary and food intake assessment. Data on these are obtained through clinical examination, observation and measurement. Anthropometric measures as indicators of nutritional and health status are preferred as they reflect better the quality of life of the living and capture the combined past and present dietary intake, morbidity and health care.

The above indicators belong to the class of outcome indicators. The health input indicators that help generate desired levels of health include health infrastructure (hospitals/dispensaries, clinics, beds, drugs, materials) health manpower (doctors, nurses, staff). While these serve to indicate access to health, the health outcome depends importantly on utilization of services. In the event of illness or injury, most individuals and households seek treatment. Besides, several preventive measures like immunization are also used particularly for infants and children. Utilization of medical services is used as indicator of demand for health inputs that produce health outcomes. Related to utilization is type of provider (broadly public versus private) and system of medicine (allopathy versus indigenous systems). Another important and useful indicator is health expenditure.

Health expenditure (public/private expenditure) expressed as ratio of expenditure to income and variants of the same are widely used health indicators. Total expenditure on health measures the final consumption of health care goods and services (i.e., current health expenditure) plus capital investment in health care infrastructure. This includes spending by both public and private sources (including households) on medical services and goods, public health and prevention programmes and administration.

The above discussion provides a brief overview of health indicators that are widely used in health studies. Each has its own merits and demerits but largely the availability of data as well as the consistency and comparability of data act as constraints on which indicator is used by a researcher.

We now pass on to examine the trends in select indicators of health in India.

III

Health Status in India: Trends in Selected Indicators

The trends in infant mortality rate (IMR) and life expectancy at birth (LEB) are represented in the following figures. It may be noted that the

Figure 1

Infant Mortality Rate, 1971–2001, India

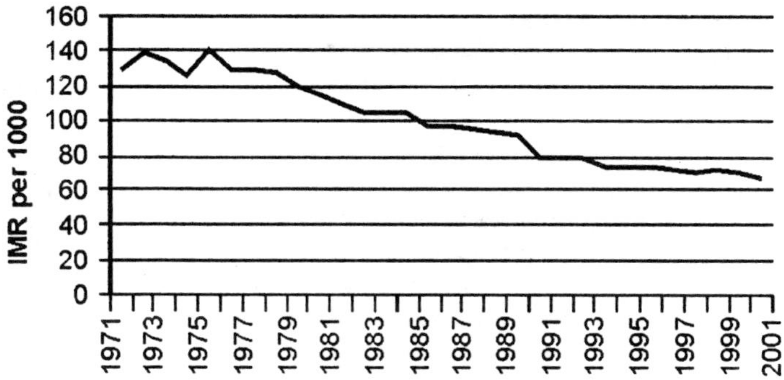

Figure 2

Trends in Life Expectancy at Birth, 1970–99, India

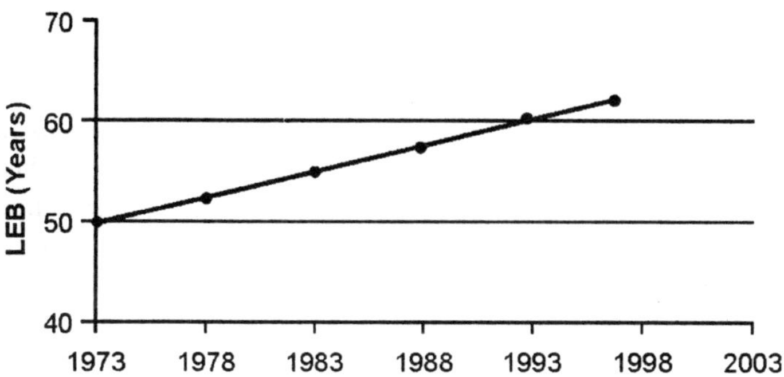

IMR has declined from 129 in 1971 to 68 in 2000 (Figure 1). Similarly, there is a remarkable improvement in LEB over this period, from 49.7 years during 1970–75 to 61.7 years during 1995/9 (Figure 2).

While the all-India figures are useful in themselves the vast differences across states call for a scrutiny of data at the state level. Data on IMR of the major states (shown in Figure 3) reveal that Kerala stands out with the lowest IMR of 14, per 1,000 live births, compared to 95 in Orissa, which has the highest IMR. Interestingly the second lowest IMR is 48 in Maharashtra, nearly three times higher than Kerala's IMR. This clearly shows that even states with better health status than all of India have a long way to go to 'catch up' with Kerala. Ten out of the fourteen states have IMRs lower than the all-India average.

Figure 3

Infant Mortality Rate by States, India, 2000

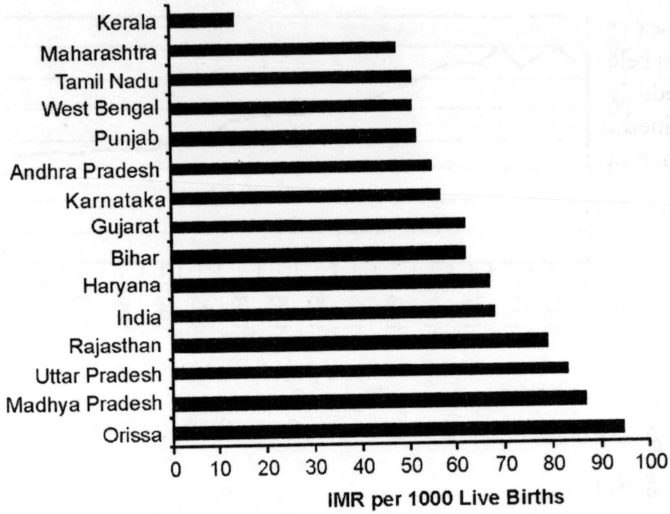

Similarly, life expectancy at birth (see Figure 4) is highest in Kerala (73.5 years) and lowest in Madhya Pradesh (56.4 years) which points to a difference of 17.1 years. Eight out of the fourteen states in our sample lie above the all-India average. Bihar which has the lowest per capita income seems to have fared better than Madhya Pradesh, Orissa (now Odissa) and Uttar Pradesh in this health status indicator.

Figure 4

Life Expectancy at Birth by States, India, 1995–99

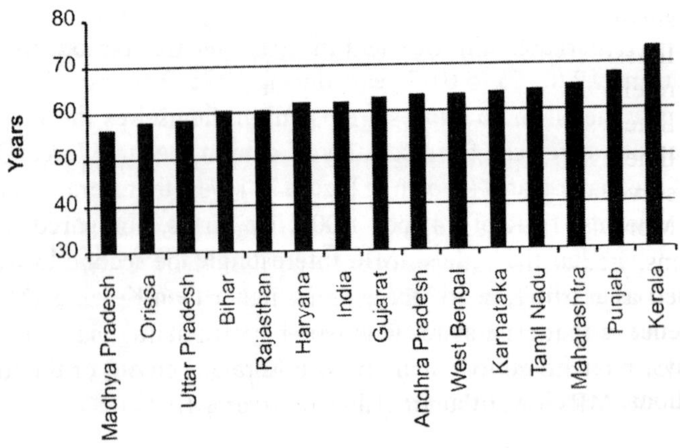

The IMR and LEB show considerable improvement in health status. It may be worthwhile to consider a related measure namely sex ratio, which is a reproductive health measure. Data shows a steady decline in the sex ratio from 972 females per 1,000 males in 1901 (see Figure 5 given below) to 933 in 2001 except for a slight increase over the previous decade in 1951, 1981 and 2001. On an average, the sex ratio has declined by 4 per thousand in a decade. This implies a disadvantage to women in the population. This is indeed a matter of concern.

Figure 5

Trends in Sex Ratio, India, 1901–2001

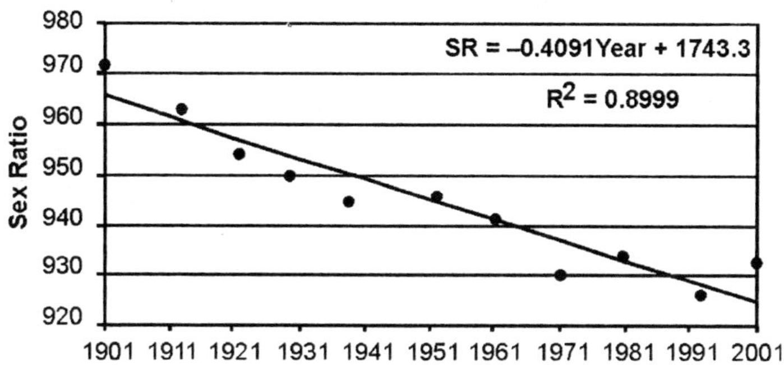

Next we present some estimates of morbidity in India. Morbidity measures are estimated based on number of illnesses in a specified period – 15 days, one month, one year etc., Morbidity can be divided into four categories

(i) Illness starting before reference period and continuing on date of survey
(ii) Illness starting before reference period and terminating within reference period
(iii) Illness starting and terminating within reference period
(iv) Illness starting within reference period and continuing on date of survey

Morbidity prevalence rate refers to the proportion of sick per 1,000 persons, irrespective of period of onset of disease. Incidence rate is defined as proportion of sick persons for whom illness started during reference period. Severity of illness is captured through number of ill-days, number of bedridden days, number of days of hospitalization, functional disability, number of school/work days affected.

The National Sample Survey Organization (NSSO), health and morbidity surveys, the National Family Health Surveys conducted by the International Institute for Population Studies and Surveys of the National Council of Applied Economic Research provide data on morbidity. The morbidity estimates from various studies are not comparable due to differences in definition and survey methodology. However, certain interesting patterns emerge from the data. First, morbidity was found to be higher among children and the aged thus exhibiting a U-shaped relationship between morbidity and age of the individuals. Second, females reported more sickness than males. Third, no clear pattern existed between morbidity and economic status measured by income or consumption expenditure. Last, education was negatively associated with morbidity.

Table 1 presents the available estimates on morbidity since 1961–62 based on various round of NSS data. Morbidity is measured as (i) number of ailing persons per 1,000 population (PAP) and (ii) prevalence rate (PR) in the reference period which refers to the proportion of sick per 1,000 persons, irrespective of period of onset of disease. The overall picture that emerges from the Table is that the morbidity rate has declined since 1961–62. The rural-urban difference in morbidity rates is large according to the recent survey. The reported morbidity rates of males are greater than for females in the earlier period but there is a reversal of this trend in the recent years.

Table 1

Trends in Morbidity Estimates in India, 1961–62 and 1995–96

Area	*Year*	*1961–62*	*1973–74*	*1986–87*	*1995–96*	*1995–96*	*2004**
	NSS	*17th Round*	*28th Round*	*42nd Round*	*52nd Round*	*52nd Round*	*60th Round*
	Definition Reference Period	*PAP 30 Days*	*PR 15 Days*	*PAP 30 Days*	*PAP 15 Days*	*PAP 30 Days*	*PAP 15 Days*
Rural	Male	139	47	64	54	84	83
	Female	123	40	63	57	89	93
	Total	132	43	64	55	86	88
Urban	Male	133	43	30	51	81	91
	Female	128	41	33	58	89	108
	Total	131	42	31	54	84	99

Note: PAP – Proportion of per 1,000 Ailing Persons, PR – Prevalence Rate.

Source: NSSO (1998), Table 4.6, p. 18, 1998, * NSSO (2006), Statement 9, p.15.

Illness prevalence rates are also influenced by non-medical factors like behaviour and habits such as smoking etc. The NCAER (1994) survey data contains data on smoking behaviour and the variation in the estimates of illness prevalence rates (IPR) by age group and smoking behaviour. It is observed that morbidity increases with age and is higher among the smokers compared to non-smokers.

IV

Economic Model of Demand for Health

The economic model of household decision-making, also known as household production model, due to Becker (1965) and Grossman (1972), is used to analyse several aspects of household decision-making including but not restricted to health. It is based on the premise that households are the main decision makers in choosing appropriate levels of final goods which contribute to their utility. Health is one such good produced within the household using inputs such as market goods and the time of members. This enters as an argument in the utility function and the usual constrained utility maximization framework applies. A detailed exposition of this approach and the relevant works are given in Duraisamy (2006) and Duraisamy and Sukanya (2002). Health can be thought of as a stock of human capital.

At a point in time, an individual's health stock depends upon the behavioural decisions concerning health such as food intake, tobacco or alcohol consumption habit, use of medical care, nature of work, physical exercise, besides the inherited genetic health endowments and the health environment in which the individual is placed. The change in the health status of a person, over a time period, is determined through a health production function.

$$H_t = H(H_{t-1}, X_t, M_t, E_t, \epsilon_t) \quad \ldots (1)$$

where H_t is the health at time t, X_t is a vector of health-related inputs such as nutritious diet, exercise, preventive care etc., M_t is curative care, E_t is a vector of individual, family and community characteristics and, ϵ_t is the unobserved initial endowments.

The household or family utility in any time period depends upon the stock of health of each member (H_t), leisure of family members (L_t) and a composite consumption commodity (C_t), given household environment (δ_t)

$$U_t = U(H_t, C_t, L_t; \delta_t) \quad \ldots (2)$$

The family is assumed to maximize a weakly time separable utility function (2) subject to the health production function (1), budget (3) and time (4) constraints:

$$Y_t = P_x X_t + PcC_{t =} wW_t + V \quad \text{... (3)}$$

$$T_t = L_t + W_t \quad \text{... (4)}$$

where: Y_t is real income in period t, V_t is the current annual household wealth or non-labour income, Pc and Px are relative prices of health inputs and consumption goods, w is the wage rate, T_t is the total available time, (such as 24 hours a day), L_t and W_t are leisure and work time respectively.

The constrained optimization process leads to a set of reduced-form demand functions for health demand (H_t) and health care (M_t) which can be specified as:

$$H_t = H\ (P_c, P_{x,}\ w, H_0, E; \varepsilon_t, \delta_t) \quad \text{... (5)}$$

$$M_t = H\ (P_c, P_{x,}\ w, H_0, E; \varepsilon_t, \delta_t) \quad \text{... (6)}$$

The subscript 0 in the above equations refers to the initial period.

Depending on the availability of data, one can estimate the health production function or the reduced form demand function or a mixture of both. Here we present empirical estimates of the reduced form health demand and health seeking behaviour functions.

V

Brief Review of Empirical Results

The available literature on health in Indian context has mainly focused on the levels and variations in health indicators. These studies are by and large based on aggregate data and are rather descriptive. Concrete and systematic evidence on the determinants of health status and health seeking behaviour is scarce (see Duraisamy 1995, 2006, 2007 for review of these studies). The available evidence using the above theoretical framework are synthesized here.

Demand for Health

The determinants of health, measured using morbidity, are examined using the NCAER (1994) survey data. The depended variable is defined as the probability of being ill, a dichotomous variable taking on values 0 (not ill) and 1 (ill), and is appropriately estimated using maximum likelihood probit method. Table 2 contains the estimates of the determinants of morbidity. As the estimates and the associated t values suggest, all the variables except some education level dummy variables and separate kitchen dummy in illness function are statistically significant at the 5 per cent level or better. The probability of being ill increases with age and is lower for women compared to men. Morbidity declines with education perhaps because the better educated take adequate preventive care. Household income exerts significant negative effect on morbidity. The estimated income elasticity is about –0.07 which indicates that a ten per cent increase in the income would result about 0.7 per cent decline in the illness prevalence rate. The coefficient of the dummy variables for caste and religion are positive and also statistically significant which indicates that the morbidity levels are higher in these population sub-groups than others. It is interesting to note that the two village level variables namely distance to doctor and good road exert significant effects in all the measures of morbidity. The results suggest that an increase in the distance to doctor (or health facility in general) increases morbidity levels and availability of good connecting road reduces the morbidity levels. This implies that access to health facility and good road contribute to improving health status and hence are important policy relevant variables to be taken into consideration. The second specification includes smoking and separate kitchen dummy variables. As expected the likelihood of being ill is higher among the smokers.

Determinants of Choice of Health Care

The NCAER data is also used to specify and estimate the conditional demand for curative care and is expressed as a trichotomous choice model involving no care, public service provider, private service provider) and is estimated using appropriate multinomial logit methods (MNL). The results, shown in Table 3, suggest that as age increases the chances of choosing public health care significantly increases. It is interesting to note that males are more likely than females to choose public and private care. The primary education has a positive and statistically significant effect on the choice of public and private care. A significant positive effect is observed for secondary level of education on the choice of private health care. In general, the better-educated persons show a preference for getting treated from private health facility than public or no care. As the household's income increases adults and elderly prefer to take treatment in a private facility rather than other providers. SCs and STs are less likely to choose public and private health care. Being a Hindu increases chances of using public care and reduces the likelihood of going to private care.

Table 2
Maximum Likelihood Estimates of the Determinants of Morbidity, Adults Aged 15–59, Rural India

Variables	*Illness dummy (Probit)*	
Age	0.00149 19.59)	0.00122 15.42)
Sex	–0.0227 (12.13)	–0.0333 15.87)
Education Dummy		
Primary	0.00198 (0.69)	–0.00200 (0.69)
Middle	–0.00495 (1.72)	–0.00404 (1.39)
Secondary	–0.0106 (3.63)	–0.00872 (2.92)
Graduate & above	–0.0196 (3.24)	–0.0178 (2.91)
Household income	–0.000186 (8.43)	–0.000178 (8.02)
Caste	0.00936 (4.84)	0.00723 (3.86)
Religion	0.00700 (2.84)	0.00735 (2.99)
Separate kitchen	—	0.000537 (0.29)
Smoking	—	0.0263 (11.51)
Distance to doctor	0.000242 (2.73)	0.000203 (2.28)
Good road	–0.00891 (4.73)	–0.00843 (4.48)
Constant term	–0.255	–0.249
Standard Error	—	—
Log-likelihood	–33943	–33,877
No. of observations	108 108	108,108

Note: 1. Asymptotic >t= values are in parentheses.
2. Marginal effects, not probit coefficients, are reported in Columns 2 and 3.

Source: Duraisamy (2007)

Table 3
Maximum Likelihood Estimation of Multinomial Logit Model of Choice of Curative Health Care, Adults and Elderly, Age 15 and Above, Rural India

Exogenous Variables	*Public*		*Private*	
	Coefficient	Asy. >t= value	Coefficient	Asy. >t= value
Age	0.00342	2.10	–0.00157	–1.12
Sex	0.147	2.76	0.0861	1.89
Education Dummy				
Primary	0.195	2.18	0.328	4.33
Middle	0.072	0.79	0.042	0.54
Secondary	0.142	1.38	0.243	2.82
Graduate & above	–0.250	–1.06	–0.00335	–0.02

Cont'd...

Cont'd...

Household income	0.0000441	0.05	0.00519	7.16
Caste	–0.122	–2.27	–0.222	–4.81
Religion	0.320	3.94	–0.152	–2.40
Distance to doctor	–0.00232	–0.98	–0.00283	–1.38
Good road	0.105	1.85	0.395	8.34
Constant term	–0.627	–5.56	0.529	5.78
Log-likelihood	–12758	—	—	—
No. of observations	12,470	—	—	—

Notes: 1. Base category is Self and No treatment.

Source: Duraisamy (2007)

Determinants of Child Morbidity in Rural Tamil Nadu

A study of child health was conducted in a rural district in Tamil Nadu based on a primary survey conducted during 1997–98. A host of morbidity measures like illness incidence and prevalence rates, (for short and long duration reference periods) severity of illness captured through duration of illness and functional consequences (number of days of restricted activity) were constructed. The overall morbidity prevalence rate was 204/1000 for a 30 days reference period. The variables included in the estimation of morbidity determinants were age and sex of the child, birth order, parent's education and occupation, religion, caste and family type, source of water, use of boiled water and availability of electricity. Key findings are: morbidity (illness prevalence) was found to be higher among earlier born children and higher in households where mothers were more educated. Source of water supply also played a significant role in affecting illness prevalence. (see Duraisamy and Sukanya, 2002 for more details)

Impact of Health on Wages and Labour Supply, Rural Tamil Nadu

It is well known that health status has far-reaching implications. One important effect of good health is the higher productivity as reflected through work and wages. Using primary data from rural farm households in Tamil Nadu, an attempt was made to measure the impact of health on labour supply and wages (Duraisamy and Sathiyavan, 1998), The major findings of the study are: Number of ill-days has a negative while body mass index (BMI) has a positive effect on wages and labour supply. A 10 per cent increase in BMI increased daily wages by 7 and 2 per cent respectively for males and females. The labour supply analysis demonstrated that a 10 per cent increase in ill-days reduced annual days worked by 0.6 per cent for both males and females while a 10 per cent increase in BMI increased male and female labour supply by 20 and 11 per cent respectively.

Intra-family Allocation of Resources to Child Health

A study based on primary survey of rural households in Tamil Nadu was undertaken to examine the determinants of gender difference in health investments using measure of child survival and preventive health care (immunization). Several household factors like parental education, assets, age, household caste and village level characteristics like distance to medical centre etc., were included as influencing factors. Notable findings are that mother's education (more than father's education) has a significant effect in increasing child survival and administration of preventive health care. There is also evidence of gender difference in these indicators with mother's education improving health outcomes of both boys and girls. (see Duraisamy and Duraisamy 1995 for more insights)

VI

Summary and Conclusion

Health status is multidimensional in nature and difficult to measure precisely. Various indicators like, mortality, morbidity, nutritional outcomes, health inputs etc., are used to measure the health status of a population. The available evidence on health indicators for India clearly point to the fact that there is a substantial improvement in the health status of the population. The most frequently used indicator of health namely infant mortality rate shows that it has almost halved during the last 30 years. Similarly, the life expectancy at birth has increased from 49.7 years in 1970–75 to 61.7 in 1995–1999. The available data on morbidity also show that morbidity rate has declined over a period of time. On utilization of health services, a majority of the population (80–81%) are found to choose private sector health facilities for out-patient care while 56–57 per cent uses the public health services.

The paper has reviewed a popular theoretical model used by economists to derive health demand functions for empirical estimation. Selected studies in Indian context based on this framework are also given. The factors that determine morbidity and choice of health provider in the event of illness are examined. There is a U-shaped relationship between age and illness prevalence rate, which indicates that the children and elderly face higher levels of morbidity than adults. Education (own education in case of adults and parents' education in the case of children) is an important determinant of morbidity, preventive health care, utilization and choice of health care. Household's income also exerts a significant effect on morbidity. Access to health care and source of water supply play major role in reducing morbidity. Good health has a positive influence on labour supply and wages. Importantly, boys are seen to score over girls in survival probability and immunization. Maternal education increases child survival and preventive health care utilization.

Policy decisions relating to health depends on reliable information on health status and health seeking behaviour of the population. Hence, the concepts and definitions of morbidity needs to be standardized in order to be able to compare the estimates over a period and the survey methodology needs to be improved to generate more reliable data. Moreover, analysing health within a household economics framework can shed light on household's responsiveness to factors. This will make way for informed policy making such as improving adult female literacy and awareness, improving access to health care etc.

References

Becker, G.S., (1965), "A Theory of the Allocation of Time", *Economic Journal*, Vol. 75: pp. 495–517.

Duraisamy, Malathy and S. Sukanya (2002), "Distribution and Determinants of Child Morbidity in Rural Tamil Nadu", *Asian-African Journal of Economics and Econometrics*, Vol. 2, No.1, pp. 67–90,

Duraisamy, P. (1994), "Do Parents Favour Boys Over Girls in Health Investments", in A. Ranga Reddy (ed.), *Health Care Services Management*, New Delhi: Delta Publishing House, 1994, pp. 20–36.

——. (1995), *Morbidity, Utilisation of and Expenditure on Medical Services in Tamil Nadu*, UNDP-Government of India Project Report, Studies on Human Development in India, CDS, Trivandrum (Thiruvananthapuram).

——. (1998), "Morbidity in Tamil Nadu: Levels, Differentials and Determinants", *Economic and Political Weekly*, Vol. XXXIII, No. 17: pp. 982–990.

——. (2000), *Health Status and Curative Health Care in India*, New Delhi: NCAER.

——. (2006), "Health Status and Choice of Health Care in India", in P. Duraisamy (ed.), *Studies on Human Development in India*, Chennai: University of Madras, pp. 07–36.

Duraisamy, P. (2007), "Health Status and Curative Health Care in India",, in A. Shariff and M. Krishnaraj (ed.), *State, Markets and Inequality*, New Delhi: Orient Longman, pp. 451–90.

Duraisamy, P. and A. Mahal (2005), "Health, Poverty and Economic Growth in India", in *Financing and Delivery of Health Care Service in India,* National Commission on Macro-economics and Health, Ministry of Health and Family Welfare, Government of India.

Duraisamy, P. and D. Sathiyavan (1998), "Impact of Health Status on Wages and Labour Supply of Men and Women: Evidence from a Rural Household Survey", *Indian Journal of Labour Economics,* Vol. 41, No. 1: pp. 67–84.

Duraisamy, P. and Malathy Duraisamy (1995), "Determinants of Investment in Health of Boys and Girls: Evidence from Rural Households of Tamil Nadu, India", *Indian Economic Review*, XXX (i): pp. 51–68.

Duraisamy, P., A.K. Ganesh et al. (2006), "Costs and Financial Burden of Care and Support Services of PLHA and Households in South India", *AIDS Care,* Vol.18, No. 2: pp. 121–132.

Grossman, M. (1972), "On the Concept of Human Capital and the Demand for Health", *Journal of Political Economy,* Vol. 80: pp. 223–55.

Murray, C.A. and L.C. Chen (1992), "Understanding Morbidity Changes", *Population and Development Review*, Vol. 18: pp. 493–503.

Sen, A.K. (1999), "Health in Development", *Bulletin of the World Health Organisation*, Vol. 77: pp. 619–23.

Strauss, J. and D. Thomas (1998), "Health, Nutrition and Economic Development", *Journal of Economic Literature,* Vol, 36: pp. 766–817.

5

Government Expenditure on Health Care Provision in India

K. GOVINDARAJALU

Good health is both the means and ends of development. It is identified that improved health contributes to economic growth in four ways. It reduces production losses, permits the use of natural resources, increases the enrolment of children and it frees for alterative uses of resources that would otherwise have to be spent on treating illness. Thus, improvement in health is an important factor for economic growth. Recent studies provide strong support for the notion of increasing government expenditure on health. Since India's level of government health expenditure is quite low in absolute terms as well as in comparison with other Asian countries, increase in government expenditure is advocated with this view. Despite the best efforts by the government to improve health status of the Indian population, health care provisions are far from satisfactory. The health infrastructure in India has a long way to go towards achieving health care delivery systems.

It is evident that health expenditure in India is dominated by private spending. To a large extent this is due to the inadequate public spending during the past fifty years. It is also evident that the financing pattern of the health care system in a country largely determines the volume of health care available to the population and also the extent and ease of access of the poor to health care. The total health expenditure of a country is classified under three major categories: (a) government expenditure on health, (b) non-household private expenditure, and (c) household expenditure. Among these three categories of expenditure, the roles of first two items are considered to be significant in reducing the burden of health care expenditure on the household sector. Hence, the present paper has examined the actual trend and pattern of government expenditure on health and also funding under National Rural Health Mission (NRHM).

Theoretical Support for Government Expenditure on Health

In line with the original economic perspective, which recognizes human capital as a determinant of investment and growth, several studies began to consider health not only as a good that individuals consume to enhance their personal satisfaction, but also as a capital stock that allows to increase the number of healthy days useful to work, to earn money and to consume other commodities to enjoy life, and have more opportunity to experience happiness. Health is considered to be both a consumption commodity and an outcome of a production process, which involves medical care and depends on individual behaviour and choices.

In the literature on health economics two alternative approaches are available to understand the decision-making processes on health. One is derived from neo-classical theory of demand for goods and services. This approach treats health care as only one of the several commodities over which economic agents have well-defined preferences. The other is based on human capital theory viz., health is a form of capital. There is a consensus among social scientists that health care is different from other goods and services, because of greater likelihood of "market failure". The two main characteristics of health care which lead to market failure are the presence of externalities and information asymmetries.

An externality results when an action of an agent has an effect not only upon the agent but also upon others. If a good or service not only benefits those who purchase these but others as well, then there is said to be a positive externality in its consumption. Conversely, a particular action of a producer may generate a negative externality, such as pollution. In the case of positive externalities, the operation of market forces alone would lead to sub-optimal consumption and production of the relevant good or service. This necessitates state intervention in order to ensure that sufficient resources are directed to the production of such goods or services, which in turn would result in an increase in the society's welfare.

The discussion on externalities reveals that it is less in the case of general health care services such as physician and hospital care and greater in the area broadly known as "public health". The latter relate to interventions targeted at overall conditions of nutrition and sanitation that determine health, as well as communicable diseases which are passed either directly among humans or indirectly through the physical environment. These positive externalities make government intervention essential. Asymmetric information reflects any situation in which one party to any contract or exchange has access to some information that is not known to the other party. Such information asymmetries, primarily between the service provider and patient, pervade the health sector and cause market failure in both health care and health care insurance markets.

For instance, in any society, patients know best how improvements in the health affects their own well-being, while providers have better information regarding both the causes of ill-health and the effectiveness of alternative health care services in restoring health or preventing the further deterioration of health. This background, stresses the need for government intervention in the form of regulation. Therefore, from both the efficiency and equity grounds, there is no alternative to the public provision of health care. Even for the success of insurance system based on private provision, increased public health spending and reforming of public health facilities are necessary. This is what makes the theoretical support for health expenditure by the government.

Pattern of Health Expenditure in India

The first systematic analysis of the distribution of health spending in India by source of funds, percentage of household spending, per capita spending etc., was published in the National Health Accounts of India, 2001–02. These analyses present the pattern of health expenditure in India in detail. In this section, the distribution of public and private health expenditure and selected indicators of health expenditure are presented.

Distribution of Public and Private Health Expenditure

The role of the public and non-household private sectors is considered to be important in reducing the burden of health care expenditure on households. It can easily be assessed that, in the absence of a well-developed non-household health care financing system, households are required to pay for the major part of health expenditure directly. The public health investments in the country over the years have been comparatively low, and as a percentage of GDP it has declined from 1.3 per cent in 1985 to 0.8 per cent in 2002. The share of public health expenditure varies from 17 to 21 per cent in health expenditure and balance being private health expenditure. Out-of-pocket payment in India is approximately 97 per cent of total private expenditure (WHO, 2003b). According to the WHO estimate, private pocket-expenditure as percentage of total health expenditure has been estimated at 80–81 per cent in India, which is much higher compared to many developing and most developed countries (WHO, 2005).

Figure 1

Percentage Distribution of Public and Private Health

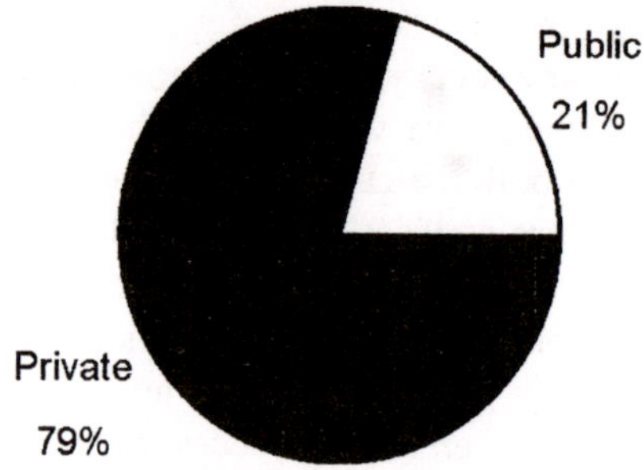

Source: World Health Organization (WHO) estimates (2005)

Selected Indicators of Health Expenditure

Health expenditure in India is around Rs 646, 055 million with more than 70 per cent consisting of private expenditure in the year 2002. Average per capita health expenditure is an indicator of how much public and household expenditure is made on health care, which comes to about Rs 617. However, average public per capita expenditure (Rs 163) is far less than household per capita expenditure (Rs 640). Share of public expenditure within plan and non-plan component of the budget stands in the ratio of 1:3 which shows that recurring expenditure like salary etc., constitutes an overwhelmingly large proportion of states expenditure. While the capital investment in total public expenditure is about 4.4 per cent the share of public expenditure on social and development expenditure of states are about 14.35 per cent and 7.94 per cent respectively. Share of total health expenditure to gross domestic product is about 3 per cent. It reveals that the pattern of government expenditure in health needs to be strengthened giving priority to government health expenditure (Table 1).

Table 1

Selected Indicators of Expenditure on Health in India, 2002

Selected indicators	*Value*
Public expenditure (million Rs) – on health	170,936
Private (household) (million Rs)	475,119
Total expenditure (million Rs)	646,055
Share (%) of public expenditure to total health expenditure	26.46
Share (%) of private expenditure to total health expenditure	73.54
Per capita average expenditure public (Rs)	163
Per capita average expenditure private (Rs)	473
Per capita average total health expenditure (Rs)	617
Public expenditure as percentage of GDP	0.8
Private expenditure as percentage of GDP	2.2
Total expenditure as percentage of GDP	3
Share percentage of OOPs in total consumption expenditure – All	6.39
Share percentage of OOPs in total consumption expenditure –Urban	5.82
Share percentage of OOPs in total consumption expenditure – Rural	6.15
Per capita public expenditure	579
Percentage of plan component to public health expenditure	30.45
Percentage of non-plan component to public health expenditure	69.55
Percentage of capital investment to public health expenditure	4.4
Percentage of public expenditure to social expenditure	14.35

Source: RBI report 2004–2005 and Consumer Expenditure Survey 1999–2000 NSSO.

Trends in Government Expenditure on Health

Total Health Expenditure

The public health systems in India has a diverse network of hospitals, primary health centres, community health centres, dispensaries and special facilities financed and managed by the central and state local government. Much of the funding for health facilities originates from the Union Ministry of Health and Welfare and is channelled to the state governments, which retain considerable authority for the expenditure decisions. Table 2 illustrates the total public expenditure on health. The public expenditures on health actually declined over the past decades. This declined from 3.12 per cent in 1992–93 to 2.99 per cent in 2003–04. Similarly, the combined expenditure (state and central government) on health as a percentage of GDP has also marginally declined from 1.01 per cent of GDP in 1992–93 to 0.99 per cent in 2003–04.

Table 2

Total Public Expenditure on Health (%)

Year	% GDP	% of Total Expenditure
1992–93	1.01	3.12
1993–94	1.05	3.28
1994–95	1.01	3.26
1995–96	1.00	3.39
1996–97	0.93	3.21
1997–98	0.95	3.32
1998–99	0.99	3.33
1999–00	1.04	3.34
2000–01	1.05	3.33
2001–02	1.03	3.25
2002–03	1.03	3.06
2003–04	0.99	2.99

Source: Public Finance Statistics, 2003–04.

Health Expenditure as Percentage of Total Expenditure – Statewise

The percentage of health expenditure incurred by the state governments and union territories from 1981 to 2005 is presented in the Table 3.

Table 3

Health Expenditure as Percentage of Total Expenditure (State and Union)

State	1981	1987	1991	1996	1998	2001	2003	2005
Andhra Pradesh	5.80	7.88	5.53	4.65	5.44	4.74	3.96	3.53
Arunachal Pradesh	5.91	9.77	4.89	4.66	5.04	NA	4.68	4.45
Assam	3.96	10.21	NA	5.84	5.87	4.66	3.69	3.06
Bihar	3.78	8.49	5.10	5.79	5.24	4.01	3.17	3.24
Chhattisgarh						4.13	3.99	3.74
Goa, Daman & Diu	7.19	13.45	8.70	5.39	4.89	3.90	4.02	3.27
Gujarat	4.38	9.58	5.03	4.70	4.57	3.38	3.21	3.05
Haryana	4.33	8.25	4.11	2.95	3.27	3.26	2.88	2.59
Himachal Pradesh	6.63	13.50	3.32	6.16	7.04	5.64	4.50	5.08
Jammu & Kashmir	3.79	12.50	5.56	5.50	4.97	4.89	5.30	4.78
Jharkhand						NA	4.18	3.65
Karnataka	3.79	8.23	5.40	5.28	5.85	5.11	4.17	3.49
Kerala	6.56	9.85	7.21	6.53	5.68	5.25	4.74	4.71

Cont'd...

Cont'd...

Madhya Pradesh	4.94	10.11	5.16	4.81	4.57	5.09	4.11	3.39
Maharashtra	4.85	9.38	5.13	4.56	4.29	3.87	3.71	3.51
Manipur	2.60	12.61	4.38	4.83	4.48	4.82	2.89	3.72
Meghalaya	6.25	13.25	6.26	6.19	6.86	5.65	5.88	5.23
Mizoram	7.89	11.85	3.50	4.18	NA	4.96	5.01	3.96
Nagaland	5.39	10.88	5.96	5.95	5.68	4.87	4.65	4.68
Orissa	5.17	8.50	5.13	5.16	4.82	4.15	3.75	3.90
Pondicherry	9.05	10.01	7.82	0.03	0.04	NA	NA	NA
Punjab	3.67	10.52	6.73	4.62	4.93	4.54	3.54	3.10
Rajasthan	4.85	14.48	6.50	5.70	7.97	5.16	4.24	3.94
Sikkim	4.49	6.44	7.89	2.72	1.92	3.67	2.03	2.56
Tamil Nadu	6.18	10.04	6.91	6.29	6.28	4.86	4.10	4.20
Tripura	2.51	7.37	5.18	14.74	4.79	4.04	3.79	3.79
Union Government	0.22	0.29	0.56	0.46	0.52	0.77	0.76	083
Uttar Pradesh	4.69	9.08	6.31	6.03	1.74	3.96	3.75	4.49
Uttaranchal						3.08	3.77	4.34
West Bengal	6.30	9.73	8.37	6.43	NA	5.63	4.94	0.93
All-India	1.52	3.95	2.93	2.01	1.75	2.77	2.41	2.42

Note: 2005 Budget Estimates; NA–not available; Data for Chhattisgarh, Jharkhand, Uttaranchal are located in their parent states.

Sources: Up to 1986 is combined. Finance and Revenue Accounts, Comptroller and Auditor General of India GOI, respective year. For year 2001 is State Finance: A Study of Budget of 2002–03, RBI. For year 2003 and 2005 is Public Finance, November 2004, CMIE.

The percentage of health expenditure was 1.52 per cent for all-India level during 1981 and it increased to 3.95 per cent during 1987 and declined to the lowest level of 1.75 per cent during 1998 and it was 2.42 per cent during 2005. The individual state percentage reveals that most of the states were having more than the national average. It was 5.80 per cent for Andhra Pradesh, 6.56 per cent for Kerala, 9.05 per cent for Pondicherry, 6.18 per cent for Tamil Nadu and 4.69 per cent for Uttar Pradesh and 3.67 per cent for Punjab during 1981. But, there was more than twofold increase in the percentage of health expenditure to total expenditure of most of the states during 1987. It was 3.95 per cent for all-India level during that period which was the highest level during the 25 years. During 1998, the figure was only 1.75 per cent for all-India level, which was the lowest level during the period. However, states like Andhra Pradesh, Himachal Pradesh, Karnataka, Kerala, Tamil Nadu have maintained the expenditure level almost equal or more than previous period. But, Pondicherry state has registered the lowest level of 0.03 per cent and 0.04 per cent during 1996 and 1998 respectively. After1998, the percentage has increased considerably during the period 2001, 2003 and 2005. It was 2.42 per cent for all-India level during 2005. Most of the states had maintained the percentage level during the past 5 years.

Health Expenditure as Percentage of GDP

One of the more obvious indicators of the inadequacy of public health spending in India is the very small amount of such spending relative to GDP. In developed countries, especially those with ageing populations, government health spending accounts for around 5 per cent of GDP or more. Even in Asian developing countries excluding India, the average is around 3 per cent of GDP. This makes it quite remarkable that India, which is currently seen internationally as an economic powerhouse and one of the success stories of global economic growth in the past decade, has government health expenditure amounting to less than 1 per cent of GDP. Further, this ratio is not only low internationally, but is even low compared to past experience.

Figure 2

Health Expenditure of Central and State Governments as per cent of GDP

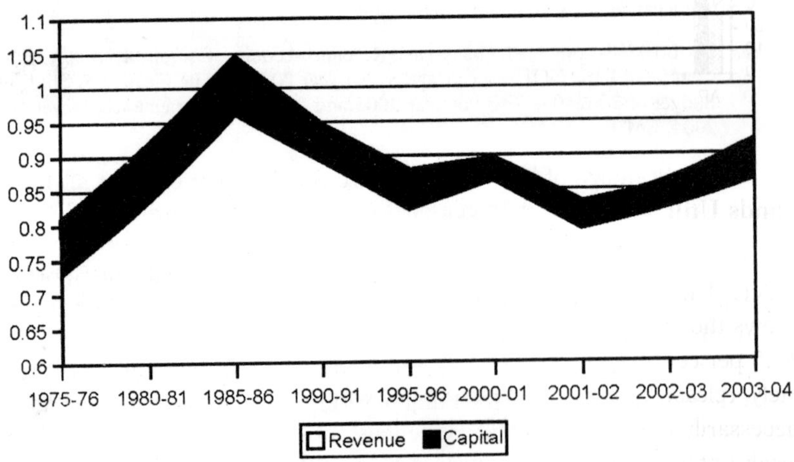

As the Figure 2 shows, even in the mid-1980s, health expenditure of central and state government taken together was more than 1 per cent of GDP, but now it is only around 0.9 per cent. Further, it has fallen as low as around 0.8 per cent in 2001–02 and 0.92 per cent during 2004. It is also significant that a greater proportion is taken up by revenue expenditure (essentially, the payment of salaries) rather than capital expenditure for creating much-needed basic physical infrastructure.

Share of Public and Private Expenditure to Total Health Expenditure

Public expenditure is more in less developed and middle developed states and on the contrary household expenditure is more in developed states barring a few exceptions (e.g., Uttar Pradesh). The share of household expenditure in less developed states is more than of some developed states because of direct intervention by NGOs (e.g., Tamil Nadu, Gujarat and Andhra Pradesh).

Figure 3

Share of Public and Private Expenditure to Total Health Expenditure (%)

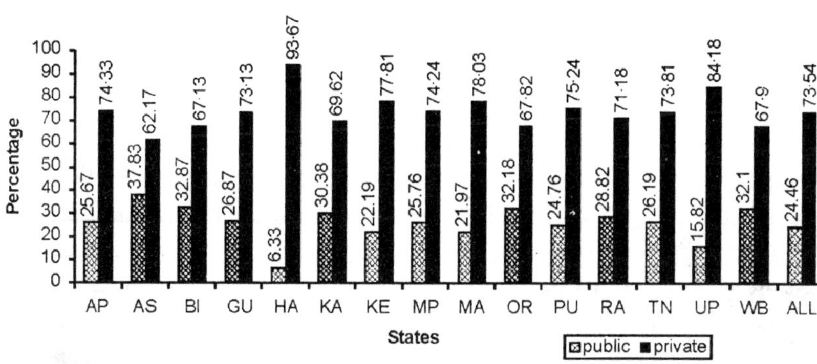

Funds Utilization under National Rural Health Mission (NRHM)

There is also a significant issue of utilization of NRHM funds by the states. The Government of India's expenditure statement for 2006–07 shows the budgetary provision for NRHM to be Rs 1,500 crore or about 17.5 per cent higher than what it could actually spend or more appropriately release as what appears as expenditure by the centre need not necessarily be what is actually spent by the states. Even then, there was a weak uptake under various NRHM sub-heads during 2006–07. Lack of uptake was nearly Rs 600 crore on account of rural family welfare services around Rs 250 crore on account of Reproductive and Child Health (RCH) programme, and Rs 130 crore on account of national disease control programmes – all these facts point towards capacity issues in spending increased resources under NRHM.

There are constraints faced by NRHM to be able to disburse fully its allocations. For example, the amount budgeted by the centre may be higher than what the centre can actually allocate, based on states project implementation plans (PIPS) and its own funds, and what the states are able to spend. In addition, the NRHM combines some funds tied to specific uses determined by the centre with little flexibility with others that are more flexible untied grants. In addition, there is little flexibility to move funds across sub-heads. The result is overspending under certain sub-heads and underspending in others, as it is recorded. Finally, NRHM emphasizes a new approach of need-based planning in a decentralized manner and offers some more flexible funds to support it. Managing this change at the state and district level requires a commitment from the states as well as new types of expertise which may take time to work effectively.

Conclusion

Even though India spends 6 per cent of its GDP on health care, more than 70 per cent of it comes from private sources out of which most of it is out-of-pocket expenditure in rural areas. From the viewpoint of public expenditure it has been found that even though both direct and indirect taxes are progressive in nature but in terms of government allocation of resources, rural areas have been neglected as most of the government expenditure have flowed to urban areas. Further, the government expenditure on preventive and curative services again tends to favour the urban and the richer groups. Allocation of government expenditure and provision between the centre and the state tend to be biased in favour of better-off states, which affects the poor in the poorer states adversely. Health care delivery has also been biased against the unorganized sector and particularly the urban poor.

Improved services and access to government facilities will have to continue as a major thrust area of the policy makers; the easy and unregulated expansion of the private sector health care market, and the continuous poor record of the government health facilities imply that the poor will have to rely on the private sector, despite the significant cost differences. This has been an area that has generated a lot of discussion including the possibility of public-private partnerships to enable the better use of existing government facilities.

References

Berman, Peter and Rajeev Ahuja (2008), "Government Health Spending in India", *Economic and Political Weekly*, June.

Economic Research Foundation (2006), "Government Health Expenditure in India: A Benchmark Study", New Delhi.

Government of India (2002), National Health Policy 2002, New Delhi.

—— (2005), Economic Survey 2004–2005, New Delhi: Economic Division, Ministry of Finance.

Mehta, Balwant Singh (2008), "Pattern of Health Care Expenditure in India", *The Indian Economic Journal*, Vol. 55, No. 4, January-March.

NCAER (2000), "Who Benefits from Public Health Spending in India?", New Delhi.

Planning Commission (2003), National Human Development Report, New Delhi: Government of India.

Reddy, K.N. and V. Selvaraju (1994), *Health Care Expenditure by Government of India 1974–75 to 1990–91*, New Delhi: Seven Hills Publications.

WHO (2003b), Shaping the Future: World Health Report 2003.

WHO (2005), Country Profile, http://whosea.org/cntryhealth/india/index.htm

6

Emerging Health Scenario in India

Present Challenges and Future Strategies

R. ANNAPOORANI

Health is an important aspect of human resource development and good health is considered as an integral element of development. As Gujarat proverb says, the first happiness is health, the second is a full stomach; one cannot enjoy food if one is not healthy. Viner (1953) observed, the first requirement of high labour productivity under modern conditions is that the masses of the population shall be healthy and sufficiently well fed to be strong and energetic.

The capability theory of living standard (Sen, 1987) holds that income, commodities and wealth do not ensure a decent living standard to their owners. It is the aggregate of certain capabilities like capability to live long, capability to be free from hunger and undernourishment and capability to enjoy personal liberty and freedom that provides a decent standard of living. Health is one of the important aspects that helps to develop capabilities, sustainability to work long and to contribute to economic growth. Similarly, World Development Report (1993) explained good health as crucial part of well-being. It focused on improving health, especially for women as a way to stabilize the growth of population. The International Conference on Population and Development (ICPD) goals for 2015 include reduction of infant mortality to below 35 and increase in life expectancy at birth to more than 75 years. According to Reddy (1995) improved health contributes to economic growth in four ways; it reduces production loss caused by workers' illness; it permits the use of natural resources that had been nearly inaccessible because of disease; it increases the enrolment of children in school and it frees for alternative use of resources that would otherwise have to be spent on treating illness. With increased urbanization and changing environment, deterioration of health resistance and the changing nature of health problems have become a great concern for the world today. Therefore out of ten millennium development goals, three goals emphasize on health. They are to reduce child mortality, improve maternal health and combat HIV/AIDS, malaria and other disease. The agreement adopted at the International Conference on Population and Development at Cairo in 1994 the use of natural resources that had been inaccessible because of disease; it increases the enrolment of children in school and it frees the alternative use of resources that would otherwise have to be spent on treating illness.

Health Scenario in India

The Directive Principles of State Policy in the Constitution of India provide that the state shall regard the level of nutrition and standard of living of the people and improvement of public health as among its primary duties. Several health committees such as Bohre (1946), Mudaliar (1962) and Mukherjee (1965) have made far reaching recommendations with a view to improve accumulation of services in both rural and urban area. However, India is still in the second stage of health transition characterized by high morbidity. According to Dr. C. Gopalan,

Table 1

Trends in Health Expenditure in India

Year	*Health Expenditure (in crores of rupees)*
1990–91	1040.8
1991–92	924.8
1992–93	1213.9
1993–94	1300.4
1994–95	1625.9
1995–96	1929.1
1996–97	2068.3
1997–98	2642.5
1998–99	5411.9
1999–2000	3568.7
2000–01	4348.8
2001–02	4411.0

we are only prolonging the lives of those who are in the sub-standard of health. It has been rightly pointed out by the World Health Organization (WHO) that health expectancy is more important and that life expectancy without health expectancy is an empty prize. The outcome of health scenario can be determined by the growth of health expenditure. Table 1 represents trends in health expenditure in India.

Health Performance Indicators in India

The population of India grew by one and half times in the first half of 20th century while in the later half it recorded almost a phenomenal threefold increase. Table 2 represents health performance indicators in India.

Table 2
Health Performance Indicators in India

Parameter	*1981*	*1991*	*2001*
Crude birth rate	33.9	25.5	26.1
Crude death rate	12.5	9.8	8.7
Total fertility rate	4.5	3.6	3.2
Maternal mortality rate	N.A.	437	407
Infant mortality rate	110	80	70

Source: Economic Survey, 2002–2003.

Between 1981 and 2001, crude birth rate declined from 33.9 to 26.1 and total fertility declined from 4.5 to 3.2. The crude death rate declined from 12.5 to 8.7 and infant mortality decreased from110 to 70. However, a comparative picture of India with other countries of the world indicates that India still has to intensify its health care effort in reducing death rate. Table 3 brings out India's global position in terms of socio-demographic parameters.

Table 3
India's Global Position in Terms of Socio-Demographic Parameters

Country	*Life expectancy*	*Under-five mortality rate (per 1,000 live births)*	*Infant mortality rate (per 1,000 live births)*	*Maternal mortality rate (per one lakh live birth)*
China	71	37	30	56
India	63	87	63	540
Pakistan	63	103	81	500
Sri Lanka	74	15	13	92
Bangladesh	63	69	46	380

In India infant mortality, under-five mortality rate and maternal mortality rate is higher than that China, Sri Lanka and Bangladesh. The prevalence of various diseases is an indicator of the poor health status of Indian population. Table 4 represents distribution of death by causes in India.

Table 4

Distribution of Death by Causes in India in 2000 (in %)

Disease	*Per cent*
Communicable disease	50.5
Tuberculosis	3.7
STD and HIV	2.7
Diarrhea	9.6
Childhood infections	6.7
Malaria	0.3
Worm infections	0.9
Respiratory infections	10.9
Prenatal causes	7.2
Others	7.1
Non-communicable diseases	49.5
Cancer	4.1
Nutritional deficiency	6.2
Ischemic heart disease	2.8
Others	27.3

It is estimated that by 2015, the number of HIV/AIDS cases would be three times more than the current level as would be the prevalence level of TB cases. Cardiovascular diseases and diabetes will more than double and cancer will rise by 25 per cent.

Disparity in Health Status among Major States

An attempt is made to assess performance of health indicators. Table 5 represents health indicators of major states in India.

A comparative analysis of various states reflects encouraging outcome of some of the middle income states. In contrast, some of the BIMARU states have to go a long way to meet the achievement level of better performing states. The estimated health index was the highest in Kerala while it was lowest in Madhya Pradesh. This might be due to differences in health expenditure among various states as evident from Table 6.

Table 5
Health Indicators of Major States in India

States	*CBR*	*CDR*	*TFR*	*IMR*	*MMR*	*Life expectancy*	*Estimated health index*
Andhra Pradesh	19.1	7.3	2.3	57	204	63.5	0.648
Assam	25.0	8.7	3.1	68	484	57.9	0.582
Bihar	30.4	8.1	4.3	61	436	60.8	0.670
Gujarat	23.7	7.1	2.9	54	137	63.4	0.643
Haryana	24.4	6.7	3.2	60	159	65.2	0.700
Karnataka	20.6	7.1	2.4	50	247	64.5	0.657
Kerala	15.0	6.4	1.8	14	136	73.5	0.805
Madhya Pradesh	29.4	9.0	4.0	76	411	56.9	0.560
Maharashtra	19.0	6.7	2.5	36	161	66.2	0.722
Orissa	22.3	9.5	2.7	75	377	58.5	0.582
Punjab	18.1	6.7	2.4	44	214	68.5	0.765
Rajasthan	28.6	7.0	4.1	68	484	61.1	0.625
Tamil Nadu	16.5	7.4	2.0	37	144	65.2	0.723
Uttar Pradesh	30.4	8.7	4.7	73	553	59.1	0.647
West Bengal	18.8	6.4	2.4	38	238	63.9	0.712

Source: Registrar General SRS Bulletin, various issues.

Table 6
State-wise Health Expenditure (2005–06)

State	*Real per capita health expenditure*	*Rank*	*Share of health expenditure to total expenditure*	*Share of health expenditure in gross state domestic product*
Andhra Pradesh	109.75	5	4.04	0.87
Bihar	61.23	14	4.27	1.53
Gujarat	87.36	11	3.22	0.67
Haryana	92.06	9	2.94	0.55
Karnataka	125.34	4	4.22	0.88
Kerala	145.89	1	5.01	1.03
Madhya Pradesh	69.74	13	3.85	0.92
Maharashtra	115.03	8	3.51	0.60
Orissa	74.60	10	3.82	1.08
Punjab	154.51	2	3.70	0.87
Rajasthan	106.69	7	4.67	1.10
Tamil Nadu	119.83	3	4.51	0.86
Uttar Pradesh	52.83	12	3.81	0.89
West Bengal	107.50	6	4.83	0.89

Rural-urban Disparity in Health

There is disparity in health indicators between rural and urban areas. This is evident from the following Table 7.

Table 7

Rural-Urban Disparity in Health Indicators, 2005–06

Indicators	*Rural*	*Urban*
TFR	3.0	2.1
Births delivered in hospitals (%)	31.1	69.4
Births assisted by health professionals (%)	39.1	75.2
Mothers who had at least three antenatal care visits for their last delivery (%)	42.8	73.8
Women whose body mass index is below normal (%)	38.8	19.8
Ever married women who are anaemic (%)	58.2	51.5
Children 12–23 months fully immunized (BCG, measles and 3 doses each of polio and DPT (%)	38.6	57.5
Children 12–23 months who have received 3 doses of DPT vaccine (%)	50.4	69.1
Children 12–23 months who have received 3 doses of polio vaccine (%)	76.5	83.1
Children with diarrhea in the last 2 weeks taken to a health facility (%)	55.6	65.3
Children with acute respiratory infection or fever in the last two weeks taken to a health facility (%)	59.9	78.1
Children aged 6–35 months who are anaemic (%)	81.2	72.7
Underweight children below 3 years age (%)	49.0	36.4
Infant death (per 1,000 live births)	62	51
Under-five mortality	103.5	63.1
CDR	10.4	7.4

Source: Compiled from National Family Health Survey reports.

There exists wide inequality in the distribution of health care infrastructure among rural and urban locations. In 2001, there were 0.54 hospitals, 1.49 dispensaries and 15.05 hospital beds per lakh population in rural India, while the corresponding figure in urban India were 0.80, 102.90 and 3.60 respectively. Access to water supply, drainage and sanitation contributed to good health in rural areas. However, in 2005 rural people fully covered with drinking water facilities were only 96.1

per cent. Lack of basic amenities of sanitation has posed a serious health hazard in rural areas.

National Rural Health Mission (NRHM) 2005–12 was formulated with the objective of improving the access to quality health care by rural people. It aims at integration of health concern with determinants of health, like sanitation and hygiene, nutrition and safe drinking water through a district plan for health. It tried to strengthen the primary health centres of which 8,756 have been 24 × 7. But it has focus only on 18 states–Arunachal Pradesh, Assam, Bihar, Chhattisgarh, Himachal Pradesh, Jharkhand, Jammu and Kashmir, Manipur, Mizoram, Meghalaya, Madhya Pradesh, Nagaland, Orissa, Rajasthan, Sikkim, Tripura, Uttaranchal and Uttar Pradesh. There are at present 1,46,026 sub health centres, 23,236 primary health centres and 3,346 community health centres in India. To meet 2001 population norm additional 19,269 SHCs, 4,337 PHCs and 3,206 CHCs are needed.

Infant and Child Health

The health of infants and children is determined by nutritional status and chronic illness is associated with poor nutrition among children. The proportion of children under three years of age who are underweight was 27 per cent and 25 per cent of the children are anaemic. Several studies showed that malnourished children are at a greater risk of dying than healthy children (Chan et al., 1990; Palletine et al., 1993; Rajaram, 2003 and Arnold, 2004).

Infant and child mortality rate reflect a country's level of socio-economic development and quality of life and are used for monitoring and evaluating population and health programmes and policies. The high infant mortality rate reflects the poor state of public health, inadequate medical attention during pregnancy and at birth and poor postnatal care.

The direct estimates of infant and child mortality are:

(a) *Neonatal mortality*: The probability of dying in first month of life
(b) *Post-neonatal mortality*: The probability of dying after the first month of life but before the first birthday
(c) *Infant mortality*: The probability of dying before the first birthday
(d) *Child mortality*: The probability of dying between the first and fifth birthdays
(e) *Under-five mortality*: The probability of dying before the fifth birthday

Table 8 shows direct estimate of infant and child mortality in India.

Table 8
Infant and Child Mortality

Years preceding the survey	*Neonatal mortality*	*Post-neonatal mortality rate*	*Infant mortality rate*	*Child mortality rate*	*Under-five mortality rate*
Rural 0–4	46.7	26.6	73.3	32.8	103.7
5–9	56.3	29.2	85.5	36.4	118.8
10–14	58.4	34.2	92.8	45.0	133.4
Urban 0–4	31.7	15.4	47.0	16.9	63.1
5–9	35.1	16.1	51.2	17.2	67.5
10–14	42.1	22.9	65.1	23.1	86.7
Combined 0–4	43.4	24.2	67.6	29.3	94.9
5–9	51.7	26.4	78.0	31.9	107.4
10–14	54.5	31.4	85.9	39.3	121.9

Source: National Family Health Survey, 1997–98.

Infant mortality in India declined from 86 deaths per 1,000 live births during 1984–88 to 68 deaths per 1,000 live births during 1994–98, an average rate of decline of nearly 2 infant death per 1,000 live births. Rural mortality rates are considerably higher than urban mortality rates. Child mortality is almost twice as high in rural areas as in urban areas. Neonatal mortality is 47 per cent higher in rural areas; post-neonatal mortality is 73 per cent higher in rural areas. The infant mortality is 56 per cent higher and under five mortality is 64 per cent higher in rural areas.

Table 9 represents a comparative picture of infant and child mortality in various states.

Infant mortality rate vary from 16 in Kerala to more than 86 in Uttar Pradesh, Madhya Pradesh and Meghalaya. Other states with infant mortality rate above the national average are Orissa (81), Rajasthan (80), Bihar (73) and Assam (70). The child mortality rate ranges from 3 in Kerala to 56 in Madhya Pradesh. Other states with child mortality above the national average are Uttar Pradesh, Rajasthan, Andhra Pradesh and Bihar. The major reasons for infant and child mortality are inadequate immunization, improper provision of clean drinking water and sanitation facilities to prevent infections and lack of professional attention among child birth.

Table 9
Infant and Child Mortality by States

State	*Neonatal mortality*	*Post-neonatal mortality*	*Infant mortality*	*Child mortality*	*Under-five mortality*
India	43.4	24.2	67.6	29.3	94.9
Delhi	29.5	17.4	46.8	9.0	55.4
Haryana	34.9	21.9	56.8	21.2	76.8
Himachal Pradesh	22.1	12.3	34.4	8.3	42.4
Jammu and Kashmir	40.3	24.7	65.0	16.1	80.1
Punjab	34.3	22.8	57.1	15.9	72.1
Rajasthan	49.5	30.9	80.4	37.6	114.9
Madhya Pradesh	54.9	31.2	86.1	56.4	137.6
Uttar Pradesh	53.6	33.1	86.7	39.2	122.5
Bihar	46.5	26.4	72.9	34.7	105.1
Orissa	48.6	32.3	81.0	25.5	104.4
West Bengal	31.9	16.8	48.7	19.9	67.6
Arunachal Pradesh	41.8	21.5	63.1	37.4	98.1
Assam	44.6	24.9	69.5	21.4	89.5
Manipur	18.6	18.4	37.0	19.9	56.1
Meghalaya	50.7	38.3	89.0	36.2	122.0
Mizoram	18.8	18.2	43.9	18.4	54.7
Nagaland	20.1	22.0	36.7	22.7	63.8
Sikkim	26.3	17.8	43.9	28.4	71.0
Goa	31.2	5.5	36.7	10.5	46.8
Gujarat	39.6	23.0	62.6	24.0	85.1
Maharashtra	32.0	11.7	43.7	15.0	58.1
Andhra Pradesh	43.8	22.1	65.8	21.0	85.5
Karnataka	37.1	14.4	51.5	19.3	69.8
Kerala	13.8	2.5	16.3	2.6	18.8
Tamil Nadu	34.8	13.3	48.2	15.9	63.3

Table 10 helps to analyse the source of high infant and child mortality.

Table 10

Source of High Infant and Child Mortality

(in per cent)

Children 12–23 months without immunization	
BCG	28.4
DPT	44.9
Polio	37.2
Measles	49.3
All	58.0
No access to drinking water	
Rural	7.5
Urban	9.8
No sanitation facilities	
Rural	91.9
Urban	50.7
Births not attended by medical professionals	
India	57.5
Kerala	5.1

Source: National Family Health Survey–II (2000).

Findings of the Research Study on Infant Mortality

A research study on "Differentials and Determinants of Infant Mortality in Coimbatore: A Micro Level Analysis" was formulated with the following objectives.

(i) To analyse the differentials in infant mortality as related to demographic characteristics, socio-economic characteristics, health care of infants and environmental condition, and

(ii) To identify the determinants of infant mortality.

The study covers 50 households in rural area and 50 households in urban area, in Coimbatore in Tamil Nadu. The required data relating to general information, family background, family property, family expenditure, savings and borrowings, fertility details, details of infant death, health care of infants, environmental conditions and measures recommended to reduce infant mortality rate etc., were collected by administering an interview schedule to the respondents chi-square analysis was used to find out the association between age at marriage of the respondents and infant mortality; educational level of the respondents and infant mortality and economic status and infant mortality.

The current study applied discriminant analysis to find out the significant factors causing differences in determinants of infant mortality in rural and urban area. In order to understand the effect of the selected variables on infant mortality, the samples were classified into two groups – (i) the respondents in rural area are termed as Group I, and (ii) the respondents in urban area are termed as Group II.

Using discriminant analysis, an attempt was made to find out the variables which significantly discriminated the determinants of infant mortality in two groups. The variables chosen for the analysis were age at marriage of the respondents (X_1), current age of the respondents (X_2), educational level of the respondents (X_3), occupational level of the respondents (X_4), income (X_5), socio-economic status (X_6), order of birth of children (X_7), place of delivery (X_8), number of children ever born (X_9), duration of rest after delivery (X_{10}) and special food taken during pregnancy (X_{11}).

When Group I was compared with Group II on the basis of measurement of several variables, a discriminant co-efficient function, which can discriminate between the two groups significantly was derived. To test whether there exists a significant difference between the two groups; the following 'F' tests were used.

$$F = \frac{N_1 + N_2 - (P - 1)}{P} \frac{N_1 + N_2}{(N_1 + N_2)(N_1 + N_2 - 2)} \times D^2$$

Where, N_1 – Number of cases in group I;
N_2 – Number of cases in group II;
V_1 – P x (the number of variables included);
V_2 – N_1 + N_2 – (P – 1) and
D^2 – Mahalanobis D square statistic.

In order to find out the relative importance of variables the discriminate between the two groups, the relative share of different variables has been calculated.

The relative share of each variable was calculated from DP^2 which can be expressed as

$$DP^2 = \lambda_1 d_1 + \lambda_2 d_2 + \lambda_3 d_3 + \lambda_4 d_4 + \lambda_1 d_1 + \ldots \lambda_P d_P$$

δ_1 is the coefficient of first variable in the discriminant function separating the two groups and d_1 is the difference in the mean value of the two groups for the first variable. In DP^2, δ_i, d_i gave the contribution of ith variable to the total distance. The percentage of each variable to the total distance has been calculated to bring out the relatively more important variables in discriminating the two groups. The study found that in rural area, eight per cent of the infant death were for illiterate women and 44 per cent of the infant death have occurred for respondents who have finished primary education.

However, in the urban area, 54.55 per cent of infant deaths have occurred for respondents who have completed secondary education and 27.27 per cent were for women who have completed collegiate education. In rural area, 16 per cent of the infant deaths have occurred in the families in which the respondents were coolies. In urban areas, 36.36 per cent of the infant deaths have occurred in the families, in which the respondents were industrial workers. In rural area, 56 per cent of the infant deaths occurred in the families of very low economic status, 20 per cent have occurred in the families of low economic status and 16 per cent have occurred in the families of medium socio-economic status. In urban area, only 18.18 per cent of the infant death were found in the families of very low economic status, 9.09 per cent of infant death have occurred in the families of low socio-economic status and 45.45 per cent of the infant death have occurred in the families of medium socio-economic status.

With the help of discriminant analysis, the current study tried to find out the variables, which significantly discriminated the determinants of infant mortality in rural and urban areas.

Table 11

Wilks Lambda and Relative Canonical Discriminating Function Power of the Selected Variables

Variable	*Wilks Lambda*	*Group I*	*Group II*	*Relative discriminating power*	*Contribution of the variables to discriminating power (%)*
X_1	0.996	5.14	5.30	0.382	19.10
X_2	1.000	1.27	1.31	0.130	6.50
X_3	0.996	2.83	2.31	0.038	1.40
X_4	1.000	1.57	1.20	0.071	2.15
X_5	0.961	1.04	1.60	0.653	20.00
X_6	0.963	0.45	0.95	0.473	17.20
X_7	0.998	2.50	2.38	0.098	3.30
X_8	0.991	0.44	0.52	0.241	8.34
X_9	0.959	0.29	0.386	0.109	5.15
X_{10}	0.991	3.58	3.80	0.323	16.10
X_{11}	0.997	1.94	1.95	0.011	0.76

The unit variate 'F' test indicates significant difference for 7 out of the 11 variables at 5 per cent or 1 per cent significant level. The mean of these variables – age at marriage of the respondent, current age of the respondents, educational level, occupation, monthly income, socio-economic status, order of birth of children, place of delivery, number of children ever born, duration of rest after delivery and special food during pregnancy were significantly different between Group I and Group II.

The canonical correlation, which is the measure of the degree of association between the discriminate score of the group, was 0.798. To test the significance of lambda, it was transformed to chi-square equivalent. The value of chi-square was 20.758 and it's significance level indicates that the two groups were different.

The estimated Fisher's discriminant function was as follows:

$$Y = 7.86 + 0.398\,X_1 + 0.000\,X_2 + 0.428\,X_3 + 0.007\,X_4 + 3.93\,X_5 + 3.80\,X_6 + 0.174\,X_7 + 0.921\,X_8 + 4.19\,X_9 + 0.93\,X_{10} + 0.28\,X_{11}$$

From the discriminant function, the relative contribution of individual variables to the total distance had been calculated. Discriminating power for X_1 was 19.1 per cent, X_2 was 6.5 per cent, X_3 was 1.40 per cent, X_4 was 2.15 per cent, X_5 was 20.00 per cent, X_6 was 17.20 per cent, X_7 was 3.30 per cent, X_8 was 8.34 per cent, X_9 was 5.15 per cent, X_{10} was 16.10 per cent and X_{11} was 0.76 per cent.

Women's Health

A primary way that parents discriminate against their girl children is through neglect during illness. A study in Punjab shows that medical expenditures for boys are 2.3 times higher than for girls, as adult women get less health care than men. They tend to be less likely to admit that they are sick and they will wait until their sickness has progressed before they seek help. Female life expectancy is an indicator of women's health. Table 12 provides a comparative picture of life expectancy of males and females in Indian states.

The top five states in respect of female life expectancy are: Kerala, Punjab, Karnataka, Maharashtra and Haryana. The lower five states are: Bihar, Assam, Orissa, Madhya Pradesh and Uttar Pradesh. There exist variations in maternal mortality rate between different states. The vital events survey revealed MMR of 130 per 1,00,000 live births in Tamil Nadu while it was only 30 in Kerala. With a view to promote maternal health in

Table 12
Life Expectancy of Males and Females in Indian States

State	*Male life expectancy*	*Female life expectancy*
Andhra Pradesh	63.40	65.93
Assam	61.14	61.18
Bihar	62.81	62.78
Gujarat	62.94	65.59
Haryana	66.21	65.94
Karnataka	65.55	66.55
Kerala	68.23	73.62
Madhya Pradesh	61.50	60.81
Maharashtra	65.45	66.31
Orissa	62.13	61.15
Punjab	67.61	67.80
Rajasthan	62.50	63.59
Tamil Nadu	64.85	65.20
Uttar Pradesh	60.09	56.09
West Bengal	63.95	64.19

1996, safe motherhood and child health service was integrated into the reproductive and child health programme. The programme includes:

(a) Provision of ante-natal care treatment of anaemia in mothers and management of high risk pregnancies
(b) Encouragement of institutional deliveries
(c) Provision of postnatal care
(d) Identification of sexually transmitted infections

Health Status of the Elderly Population

Ageing is described as depreciation of the individuals health capital. Health is a major concern in later life because it is the most important factor in predicting life satisfaction and well-being of the aged people. Hence care should be taken for monitoring the health status of the elderly. In India the elderly population increased from 5.6 to 7.9 per cent during1960–2005 and the growth rate of elderly was much higher of 3 per cent than the general population growth rate of 2 per cent during the period. This has serious implications in terms of how the elderly will survive and therefore is a subject of serious concern with policy implications.

Agenda for Action

The principal goal of development policy is to create sustainable improvement in the quality of life for all people. Besides enhancing per capita income and consumption, concentration must be on the objective of expanding access to health services (World Development Report 1999–2000).

A. Foster an enabling environment for the households to improve health. This calls for:
   1. Pursuing economic policies that benefit the poor.
   2. Expanding investment in female education.
   3. Promoting the rights and status of women through economic empowerment.

B. Improving government investment in health. This implies:
   1. Financing and ensuring delivery of essential clinical services especially to the poor.
   2. Financing and ensuring delivery of public health package including aids prevention.
   3. Improving the management of public health service.

C. Facilitate involvement by the private sector:
   1. Encouraging private finance and provision of insurance for all discretionary clinical services.
   2. Encourage private sector delivery of clinical services.
   3. Providing information on performance and cost.

D. Specifically to improve women health the following strategies may be adopted:
   1. Focused attention should be paid to meeting the nutrition needs of women at all stages of lifecycle.
   2 Special effort should be made to tackle the problem of nutrient deficiencies especially among pregnant and lactating women.
   3 Widespread use of nutrition education should be made to solve the issue of intra-household imbalance in nutrition.
   4. Steps should be taken to remove drudgery of women both at home and work place. Above all, community participation programme should be emphasized and this may increase access to local services and may also promote rapid transmission of health information.

To improve the health of infants and children there is need for regular monitoring of immunization programme, establishment of more primary health centres with child specialist and health awareness should be created among mothers about cleanliness and dietary habits of children.

Above all, public and private sector employees should be brought under health insurance scheme making mandatory for employees 50 per cent of the premium. The hospitals in private sector should be motivated to treat the poor at a subsidized cost and in government hospitals, the code of conduct has to be designed so as to encourage doctors, to stay at the place of work and attend to the work with commitment. With help of these measures it is possible to achieve first happiness in life, i.e., health.

"Health is not everything but everything is nothing without health"

References

Gopal, Rani (2003), "Health Implications of The Census of India-2001", in *Census 2001 and Human Development in India,* edited by G. Ramachandra Rao and M. Prasada Rao, Serials Publications, New Delhi, pp. 312–325.

Reddy, Ranga (1995), *Health Care Services Management for Underprivileged*, Delta Publishing House, New Delhi, pp. 135–141.

Sen, Amartya (1987),. *Commodities and Capabilities*, Oxford University Press, New Delhi, p. 42.

Viner, Jacob (1953), in Report of the Committee for Economic Development S.H. Ruttenberg, American Federation of Labour and Congress, p. 100.

Reports

National Family Health Survey–II (1998–99), International Institute for Population Science, Mumbai, pp. 178–195.

Reports of the National Committee on Health – (Bohre Committee, 1946, Mudaliar Committee 1962, Mukherjee Committee, 1965) – Published by National Institute of Health and Family Welfare, New Delhi.

State of the World (2002), 'A World Watch Institute Report on Progress Towards a Sustainable Society', Norton and Company, New York, pp. 127–148.

Tamil Nadu Development Report, Planning Commission, Government of India, New Delhi, pp. 170–171.

Tenth Five-Year Plan of India (2002). Vol. II, Planning Commission of India, New Delhi, p. 149.

World Development Report (1993), Oxford University Press, New Delhi, pp. 108–110

7

Cost of Treatment

A Study Based on Medical Pluralism

V. ANITHA

Economic development can be seen as a multidimensional process involving improvements in human well-being. Good health enables individuals to be active agents of change in the development process. The scope of health economics covers a wide range of issues such as interrelation between health and economic development, health planning, costs and benefits of medical care, choice of resource allocation, financing of health care services, demand and supply of health care services, economic efficiency and equity in medical care provisions, health as consumption versus investments, etc., (Panikar, 1993). In order to attain more effective financing, it is necessary to determine the cost, benefit and effectiveness of different health care services. The issues discussed by health economics are ever-widening. A concept that gained a great deal of attention in the gamut of health economics is 'medical pluralism'. In this context, it is useful to examine how various authors have sought to define medical pluralism.

Medical Pluralism: Meaning and Definition

The concept of 'medical pluralism' was used by Leslie (1980) as cosmopolitan medicine competing with numerous alternative therapies (local medical system). According to Lee (1982), the systems of medicine practised in China, Hong Kong and Taiwan reveals the presence of pluralistic system of medical practice. Bhardwaj and Paul (1986) used the term as different medical cultures in Bangladesh. The two formally structured systems of medicine, modern and traditional; existing side by side in Sri Lanka is considered as plural medicine by Waxler-Morrison (1988). The alternative systems of medicine practised in India are treated as medical pluralism by Minocha (1980). In Kerala, Boban (1990) used the concept of medical pluralism in the sense of more than one type of medical system that came into practice in the tribal world. In the present study, the concept is used to denote the alternative/different systems of medicine particularly allopathy, ayurveda and homoeopathy followed by the Keralites.

Relevance of Medical Pluralism

In the developing world there are two major systems of health care that coexist – the traditional and the modern. According to the report of WHO (1997), over 80 per cent of the world population depends on traditional systems of medicines, largely plant-based, to meet their primary health care needs. WHO strongly supports promotion and development of rational use of traditional medicine throughout the world. There is a growing realization all over the world that traditional systems of medicine offer cost-effective option. The world is witnessing a resurgence of traditional systems of medicine. In India, the different systems of medicine include allopathy, ayurveda, siddha, unani and naturopathy and yoga which were evolved as a part of the ancient civilizations of the subcontinent or assimilated from other civilizations. Homoeopathy is widely practised and officially recognized in India. Thus, there is the prevalence of more than one system of medicine, viz., medical pluralism in India.

Review of Literature

On the basis of the available literature related to comparative costs, including cost analysis of various types of services or programmes, an attempt has been made here to make a brief review of the important works among them. The main objective of the Babson's (1973) study is to derive a methodology for costing treatments. The study has outlined in considerable detail the methods of attributing hospital resources to treatments in the given disease categories. Market values are used to estimate costs. The author argues that the study justifies considerable optimism regarding the feasibility of disease costing.

The benefits and costs arising from the treatment of rheumatic diseases have been dealt in Brooks' (1969) analysis. The costs considered are the costs of providing hospital and other facilities for treatment. The benefits are those arising from the productive output gained from patients who are able to return to work. The study assumes that all the improvements in health are due to the treatment. The costs of treatment are estimated using market values. The value of the production of those in employment is valued at gross earnings. A wage is imputed for housewives using the wage of domestic helps. The study concludes that there is a prima facie case for the investment of resources in centres of rheumatic diseases. Carter et al. (1976) in their study, analyse the comparative costs of hospital and home treatment for adult haemophiliacs. Only changes in health service resources use were considered. Other costs, i.e., resulting from production loss were not considered. An attempt was made to identify precisely the changes in resource use arising from the out-patient element of hospital treatment. The in-patient estimate was based on average hospital costs and the cost was valued at market values. The result of the study is that cost of home treatment was found to be only 16 per cent of that of hospital treatment.

The costs and effectiveness of alternative health care programmes for the elderly are analysed by Doherty and Hicks. (1977). The alternatives are institutional care versus day care, versus home care. The costs considered were those resulting from health service and other community resource use. But the results did not lead to a definite ranking of the programmes. They showed that the day-care programme was the preferred choice on each of the effectiveness criteria, whereas home care was preferred on the overall cost criteria.

The main purpose of Cooper and Rice's (1976) study was to indicate the costs to society from different forms of illness. The economic cost of illness was considered to be due to the direct resource outlays for prevention, detection and treatment and the indirect costs or loss in output due to disability and premature death. The costs of pain and suffering were noted but not considered. Aggregate data from a number of sources were used for measurement. They found that the total cost of illness for 1972 was US $189 billion at a 4 per cent discount rate. About $40 billion was for persons suffering from diseases related to the circulatory system, $27 billion for accident victims and $17 billion each for cancer patients and victims of gastro diseases.

Krishnan (1994) has focused on the inter-state variations in the utilization of health services for in-patient care and has raised the important issue of the cost of treatment and the burden of treatment that fall on the lower strata of people. To him the discussion of health care financing and provision include access to health care and the quality of services, the importance of building stocks and capital formation in health services, cost effectiveness and the role of technology in determining cost of health care. Krishnaswami (2004) has made an attempt to measure the burden of disease in terms of the number of days lost due to illness and the costs incurred by the household, through cost of treatment and through loss of household income. The study concludes that allopathy is the preferred system of medicine, acute morbidity is the major cause in the total number of days of work lost and that the average cost of treatment of acute illness is high.

The Research Problem

In Kerala, there exist different systems of medicine like allopathy, ayurveda, siddha, naturopathy and homoeopathy. The whole medical care system including both the modern and traditional systems tries to safeguard the community from ill-health (preventive approach) and to provide effective care (curative approach) at lower costs. At present the general trend is the increasing influence of modern medicine on the one side and the disintegration of traditional systems of medicine on the other. It is often found that the government does not give due importance to the non-allopathic systems while allocating resources. In this context it is important for the government to understand the cost of treatment of systems of medicine in both rural and urban areas. It may enable the government to allocate resources more fruitfully among different systems of medicine.

Objective of the Study

The main objective of the present study is to analyse the cost differentials among different systems of medicine in Kerala.

Methodology

The study is primarily empirical. Both primary and secondary data are used for the study. Therefore, a sample household survey of both rural and urban population was conducted. The three different indicators usually used for analysing human development include the standard of living, level of literacy and the health of the population. In the case of variables such as per capita income, the proportion of people living in permanent type of houses, literacy rate, child mortality rate, the percentage of institutional deliveries, the percentage of old-age population, etc., the figures pertaining to Kollam district compares favourable with the all-Kerala average (*Economic Review*, 2002). Therefore, Kollam provides an appropriate case for the field survey related to the present study. Moreover, the district has rural and urban areas, both having access to different systems of medicines like allopathy, ayurveda and homoeopathy. Hence, Kollam district is selected purposively for the household survey. Altogether 200 households were covered in the field survey – 100 from the rural areas and 100 from the urban areas. Data have been collected through the interview method.

Purposive random sampling technique was also applied for the selection of the rural area for the field survey. The rural area for the study is Eroor panchayat, a typical rural one among 69 village panchayats of Kollam district. Kollam Corporation is selected as the urban area for the study as Kollam is the only corporation in the district. Systematic sampling is used for selecting the household units. Every 100th house is selected as a sample unit from each ward in the urban area, whereas in the rural area, every 25th house is selected. The number of household units selected in each ward depends on the size of the population. Assessment registers of the panchayat and corporation are used to identify the houses. A detailed questionnaire was prepared for collecting primary data. Selection of a proper reference period was one of the questions regarding the survey. A longer recall period increases the probability of memory lapse resulting in underreporting or over-reporting. Here a recall period of 30 days prior to the date of survey was selected. The household survey was conducted during the month of February-March 2002. The software – Statistical Package for Social Science (SPSS) – is used for processing the data. Average cost of each system is calculated for analysing the cost variation among different systems of medicine.

Limitations of the Study

The study mainly takes into account the curative aspects of different health care systems and deals with only a minor part of its clinical aspects. The cost of treatment is analysed on the basis of market prices during the period of the survey. No attempt has been made to value the benefits. It is a one-time survey and therefore does not reflect the seasonal variations in the disease pattern.

Health Care in Kerala

Kerala, the southern-most state of India has a unique position in the matter of health consciousness. The total area of the state is 38,863 sq.

kms and its population is 318.39 lakh (2001 census). The state is divided into 14 revenue districts and 63 taluks with Thiruvananthapuram as its capital. The rate of growth of population is 0.91 per cent per annum as against the Indian average of 1.93 per cent. The state has the highest density of population, 819 persons per sq. km, as against the national average 324. In Kerala, 74.04 per cent of the population lives in rural areas, which is almost the same as the national average. The economy is highly rooted in agriculture. However, the relative contribution of agriculture and allied sectors has been declining in recent years. Kerala has a long history of medical and health care systems. Health indicators of Kerala are comparable to those of developed countries. In Kerala the rural-urban differences is very low compared to the national average. However, most of the health development indicators are favourable to urban area. This may be due to the better health care facilities in the urban areas.

Though Kerala has achieved many of the health goals set for the year 2000 by 1991 itself, the state now faces problems like high morbidity rate, growing prevalence of lifestyle diseases and diseases of the elderly. Thus, the state is not free from epidemiological transition. This is one of the dominant second generation problem facing the economy. According to the available morbidity statistics, the morbidity rate in Kerala is much more than that of the all-India level, especially in the case of chronic diseases.

As mentioned earlier, Kerala has a well-established plural medical system. Majority of its health care systems consist of allopathy, ayurveda and homoeopathy. These three systems of medicine together have 2,706 institutions and 48,834 beds. Out of the total institutions, 47 per cent belong to allopathy, 32 per cent to ayurveda and 21 per cent to homoeopathy. Out of the total beds, 89 per cent belong to allopathy, 8 per cent to ayurveda and 3 per cent to homoeopathy (Economic Review, 2004). In the year 2003, altogether 18.84 lakh in-patients and 756.6 lakh out-patients were treated under these three systems. But this number has decreased by 2.6 per cent in the case of in-patients and 6.5 per cent in the case of out-patients. However, out-patients treated under allopathy have increased from 48 per cent in 2002 to 53 per cent in 2003. Thus, the health care facilities and utilization under the government sector also shows that allopathy ranks first followed by ayurveda and homoeopathy (*Economic Review*, 2004).

The Kollam District

Kollam district is located in southern Kerala with Arabian Sea in the West, Alappuzha and Pathanamthitta districts in the North, Ramnath district of Tamil Nadu in the east and Thiruvananthapuram district in the south as boundaries. This district has three geographical regions – the easternmost part consisting mainly of hills and forest area, known as 'malanadu', the western most part which forms coastal area which is even, and the middle portion, known as 'idanadu'. The people in general are engaged in different fields like agriculture industries, service sectors, etc. Cashew factories form the industrial base. The rural people of the district are primarily engaged in agriculture and animal husbandry. The level of urbanization is also high in the district (18%). Average rainfall in the district is 2,182 mm. It is hottest in March, April and May (temperature 32–33°C). The district gets monsoons from June to October. The minimum temperature is experienced in January (22°C). The district has a pleasant climate during September to February. Humidity rate is 63 per cent in January and 87 per cent in June-July.

Kollam Corporation

Kollam city is divided into 36 wards with a total area of 57.28 sq. km. The total population of the corporation is 3,61,560 and the sex ratio forms 1,035 according to 2001 census. The density of population is 6,309 per sq. km. The number of households in the corporation area is 78,182. People are mainly engaged in fishing, trade, business, communication, etc. Majority of them have regular work.

Health care facilities are one of the major factors that determine the health of the people. Information regarding health facilities available in the corporation area is shown in the Table 1. The health care system consists of allopathy, ayurveda and homoeopathy. But under the government sector, only two systems – allopathy and homoeopathy are available in the corporation area. The two systems of medicine together have 10 institutions in the government sector with 181 beds and 20 doctors. Out of the total institutions, five are under allopathy and homoeopathy. Out of the total beds available, 156 are under allopathy and 25 are under homoeopathy. In the private sector, the three systems of medicine together have 37 institutions with 699 beds and 110 doctors. Out of the total institutions, seven are in allopathy, 13 under ayurveda and 17 in homoeopathy. Out of the total beds available, 676 are under allopathy and 23 under ayurveda. Out of the total doctors, 74 belong to allopathy, 17 to ayurveda and 19 to homoeopathy.

Table 1
Government and Private Health Care Facilities in Kollam Corporation

Institutions	*Number*	*Beds*	*Doctors*
	Government		
PHC	4	12	5
Allopathic hospital	1	144	8
Homoeopathic hospital	1	25	3
Homoeopathic dispensary	4	—	4
Total	10	181	20
	Private		
Allopathic hospital	7	676	74
Ayurvedic hospital	3	23	6
Ayurvedic dispensary	10	—	11
Homoeopathic dispensary	17	—	19
Total	37	699	110

Source: Economics and Statistics Wing, Collectorate Office, Kollam, 2002.

Eroor Panchayat

Eroor panchayat is situated in Pathanapuram taluk in Kollam district. This panchayat has a total area of 44.74 sq km. According to 2001 census, the total population is 32,413 of which 15,693 are males and 16,720 are females. The density of population is 724 per sq km and the literacy rate is 91 per cent. The villagers are primarily engaged in agriculture. There are fifteen schools including 4 high schools in the village. Eroor panchayat consists of two villages – Eroor and Ayiranaloor, spread over 13 wards. Table 2 shows hospital facilities in Eroor panchayat. There are 9 institutions in the government sector with three doctors and no in-patient facilities. There are no government homoeopathic institutions in the panchayat. In the private sector, the three systems together have 5 institutions and 5 doctors. Out of the total institutions, 3 are under allopathy, one under ayurveda and one under homoeopathy. There is no in-patient facility in the government sector.

Table 2
Government and Private Health Care Facilities in Eroor Panchayat

Institutions	*No.*	*Doctors*
	Government	
PHC	1	1
Sub-centres	6	—
Allopathic hospital	1	1
Ayurvedic dispensary	1	1
Total	9	3
	Private	
Allopathic dispensary	3	3
Ayurvedic dispensary	1	1
Homoeopathic dispensary	1	1
Total	5	5

Source: Panchayat Office, Eroor, 2002.

General Characteristics of Sample Population

Some of the basic background information taken into account under demographic characteristics is age, sex, marital status, religion and caste. The total sample population was 967, of which 434 (45%) were from rural areas and 533 (55%) from urban areas. The sex ratio is higher in rural areas (1,087) than in urban areas (1,058). From the survey, it is clear that there is only a slight disparity in the age distribution of the population excepting the population above 60 years, which is higher in the urban areas. In the case of marital status the percentage of widows is higher than that of widowers in both rural and urban areas. This underlines the high female life expectancy in Kerala. The Hindu households formed 54.5 per cent, Christians 29.5 per cent and Muslims formed 32 per cent of the total samples. Of the total households, 14 per cent were SCs and 5.5 per cent STs.

Regarding average monthly income of the households, majority (59%) of the rural households come under the middle income group (Rs 2,501–4,500), while it is 22 per cent in the urban areas. The majority (69%) of the urban households come under the higher income group (Rs 4,501 and above), whereas it is 17.2 per cent in rural areas. This is mainly because the proportion of casual workers is higher (31%) in rural areas while it is only 20.2 per cent in urban areas. Unemployment is also high in rural areas.

Literacy rate is found to be high in both the regions (around 92%). Usually higher qualification of any one member in a family is reflected on the improved health status of the whole family. Fortunately there were no households in the survey area where all the members of the household were illiterate. Education always plays a vital role in the improvement of individual's health status.

Table 3

Distribution of Patients on the Basis of the Intensity of Disease

Classification of disease	*Number of people*		*Total*
	Rural	*Urban*	
Serious communicable disease	2 (0.97)	3(1.1)	5(1)
Acute illness	131(63.3)	146(53.7)	277(57.8)
Chronic illness	62(29.95)	119(43.75)	181(37.8)
Accident	12(5.8)	4(1.5)	16(3.3)
Total	207(100)	272(100)	479(100)

Note: Figures in the parentheses show percentage.

Source: Sample Survey.

Out of the total 967 total sample population, 479(49.5%) are found to have illness during the reference period. In rural areas, 48 per cent of people are found to have illness during the reference period while in urban areas it is 51 per cent. For the purpose of analysis, episodes of illness are classified into serious communicable disease, acute illness, chronic illness and accident (Table 3). Here, jaundice and tuberculosis are the two major serious communicable diseases reported. Acute diseases are those of short duration and sudden onset. Acute illness consists of diseases like respiratory infection, non-specific fever, skin disease, eye or ear problems, headache/body ache/back ache, stomach problems etc. Chronic diseases are those from which the patient was suffering before and during the reference period. Diseases like rheumatism, heart ailment, hypertension, diabetes, asthma, mental disorder, goiter, allergy etc., come under the category of chronic illness. Any injury suffered in the reference period of the survey is considered as accident. From the table, it is clear that the proportion of people suffering from acute illness is high in both areas. Compared to urban areas, instances of acute illness is higher in rural areas while chronic illness is higher in urban areas. Poor housing conditions in the rural areas often create respiratory problems. This may increase the incidence of acute illnesses. Changes in lifestyle form the major cause of high levels of chronic diseases in urban areas.

Treatment and Systems of Medicine

The number of people reporting clear preference to any one system is 444(92.7%). About 35(7.3%) people did not go for any kind of treatment on account of financial problems (For further analysis, such cases have been put under the classification 'others'). Some among them resorted to home remedies and few others depended on religious practices and rituals for healing. Distribution of patients on the basis of systems of medicine followed during illness is illustrated in Table 4 on the basis of their residential status. Here, a remarkable point is that the percentage of homoeopathic users is high in rural areas (18.35% as against 8.45% in urban area). In rural areas people generally prefer to avail cheaper treatment. Homoeopathy is found to be relatively cheaper than other systems of medicine. Again the category 'others' is also high in rural areas (10.6% as against 4.8% in urban areas). A few people in rural areas do not undergo any treatment because of financial problems. They mainly resort to home remedies or follow religious practices and rituals. However, urban people are more conscious of their health and of the harmful effects of sickness and they react more quickly in seeking treatment.

Table 4

Distribution of Patients on the Basis of Systems of Medicine Availed at the Time of Treatment: Rural-Urban

Systems of medicine	*Number of people*		*Total*
	Rural	*Urban*	
Allopathy	117(56.5)	185(68)	302(63)
Ayurveda	30(14.5)	51(18.75)	81(16.9)
Homoeopathy	38(18.35)	23(8.45)	61(12.7)
Others	22(10.6)	13(4.8)	35(7.3)
Total	207(100)	272(100)	479 (100)

Note: Figures in parentheses show percentage.

Source: Sample Survey.

The preference shown to any system of medicine by people belonging to both rural and urban areas is mainly based on reasons like absence of side-effects, economy, proximity or nature of disease

(Table 5). In rural areas about 2.4 per cent people prefer a particular system due to the absence of side-effects and 8.2 per cent due to proximity. People generally regard ayurveda and homoeopathy to have little side effects. About 45 per cent prefer a system for economic reasons and almost an equal proportion due to the nature of disease. In urban areas, slightly more than 50 per cent prefer a system of medicine owing to the nature of disease. About 5.9 per cent prefer a particular system due to the absence of side effects. The remaining prefer a particular system due to economy (39.7%) and proximity (22.1%). The category 'others' under the system of medicine is preferred mostly for economic reasons. The study revealed poor availability and limited accessibility of ayurvedic and homoeopathic systems of medicine, particularly in rural areas.

Table 5

Distribution of Patients on the Basis of the Reason for Availing Each System of Medicine: Rural-Urban

System of medicine	*No side-effect*	*Economic*	*Proximity*	*Nature of disease*	*Total*
		Rural			
Allopathy	0	24(20.5)	17(14.5)	76(65)	117(100.0)
Ayurveda	1(3.3	4(46.7)	0	15(50)	30(100.0)
Homoeopathy	4(10.5)	34(89.5)	0	0	38(100.0)
Others	0	21(95.5)	0	1(4.5)	22(100.0)
Total	5(2.4)	93(44.9)	17(8.2)	92(44.4)	207(100.0)
		Urban			
Allopathy	0	23(12.4)	53(28.6)	109(58.9)	185(100.0)
Ayurveda	6(11.76)	10(19.6)	4(7.8)	31(60.18)	51(100.0)
Homoeopathy	10(43.4)	2(8.7)	3(13.04)	8(34.8)	23(100.0)
Others	0	13(100)	0	0	13(100.0)
Total	16(5.9)	108(39.7)	60(22.1)	148(54.4)	272(100)

Note: Figures in parentheses show percentage.

Source: Sample Survey.

Cost of Treatment

The cost of treatment consists of doctor's fees, cost of medicine, hospital charges, laboratory charges, transport cost to access the medical facility, wages and income lost during the period of disease, etc. Here costs are classified into direct cost and indirect cost. Direct cost consists of consultation fee, cost of medicine, hospital rent, charges for lab tests etc.

On the other hand, indirect cost consists of travelling expenses of the patient and accompanying persons, food and accommodation of the companion, wages and income loss due to illness, etc.

The total health care expenditure of the patients in the sample population during the reference period was Rs 22,531 in the rural area and Rs 85,503 in the urban area. This works out to Rs 122 per capita expenditure per month in the rural area and Rs 330 in urban area. It is 11.03 per cent of the average per capita income in rural area and 20.7 per cent in urban area.

Table 6

Distribution of Patients on the Basis of the Distance Travelled for Availing a Particular System of Medicine: Rural-Urban

System of medicine	*Distance in kilometres*			
	0–3	*4–7*	*8 and above*	*Total*
		Rural		
Allopathy	34(29.1)	23(19.7)	60(51.3)	117(100.0)
Ayurveda	21(70)	2(6.7)	7(23.3)	30(100.0)
Homoeopathy	37(97.3)	0	1(2.6)	38(100.0)
Others	22(100)	0	0	22(100.0)
Total	114(55.1)	25(12.1)	68(32.9)	207(100.0)
		Urban		
Allopathy	111(60)	53(28.6)	21(11.35)	185(100)
Ayurveda	40(78.4)	4(7.84)	7(13.7)	51(100)
Homoeopathy	21(91.3)	1(4.3)	1(4.3)	23(100)
Others	13(100)	0	0	13(100)
Total	185(68)	58(21.3)	29(10.7)	272(100)

Note: Figures in parentheses show percentage.

Source: Sample Survey, February-March 2002.

The average direct costs in respect of allopathy, ayurveda and homoeopathy treatment in rural areas were Rs 140, Rs 36 and Rs 21 respectively and in urban areas Rs 356, Rs 261 and Rs 158 respectively (see Figure 1). The corresponding indirect costs in rural areas were Rs 30, Rs 13 and Rs.10 and in urban areas were Rs 40, Rs 20 and Rs 8 (see Figure 2). When the average costs were calculated, non-paying patients treated at the government hospitals were also included. As a result, the direct costs incurred by rural people who mainly depend on government hospitals were less than that of the urban people. Usually indirect cost is influenced by the transportation costs. The low indirect cost in rural area does not mean that there is easy access to medical facilities. Even if there is an easy access to medical facilities in urban areas, people spend money by using transport facilities like car, autoriksha, etc. In rural areas, the average distance the patient travels to get allopathic treatment was 8 kms while in urban areas it was 3 kms. The average distance travelled in the case of ayurveda and homoeopathy in rural areas was 6 kms and 5 kms respectively, while in urban areas it was 3 kms and 1.28 kms respectively. The detailed figures are shown in the Table 6.

The comparative cost analysis of serious communicable diseases and accidents are avoided here, as the majority of the people who come under these categories follow only allopathic treatment. The average direct cost of acute illness in rural areas is Rs 107, Rs 43 and Rs 20 for allopathy, ayurveda and homoeopathy respectively while in urban areas it is Rs 321 Rs 130 and Rs 48 respectively. The loss of earnings due to illness/disablement, was not included in the calculation of indirect cost. In rural areas, especially in the case of labourers, it is very difficult to calculate the wages and income loss due to the episodes of illness (because it needs guess work in the case of casual workers while in the case of regular workers there is no loss in income due to the availability of reimbursement and eligible leave). There are two such cases reported in rural areas and eleven cases in urban areas.

Figure 1

Average Direct Cost of Treatment on the Basis of Residential Status and the System of Medicine: Rural-Urban

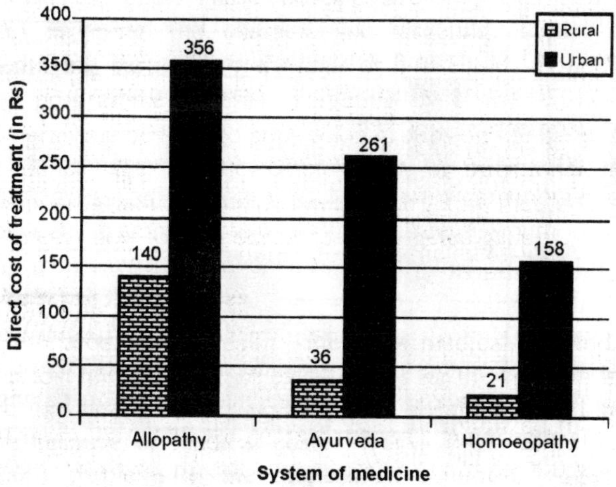

Source: Developed from sample data.

Average indirect costs of treatment for acute illness in rural areas are Rs 21, Rs 16 and Rs.10 for allopathy, ayurveda and homoeopathy respectively. The corresponding figures in urban areas are Rs 16, Rs 22 and Rs 8 respectively. The average direct cost of chronic illness in rural areas is Rs 41, Rs 122 and Rs 25 for allopathy, ayurveda and homoeopathy respectively, while in urban areas it is as high as Rs 406, Rs 190 and Rs 235 respectively. The average indirect costs of treatment for chronic illness in rural areas are Rs 7, Rs 10 and Rs 11, while the same cost in urban areas is Rs 66, Rs 17 and Rs 8 respectively. From this analysis it is evident that there are very high cost differences among the different systems of medicines like allopathy, ayurveda and homoeopathy. The cost is much higher in urban areas than in rural areas. The cost of allopathy treatment is generally greater than that of ayurveda. Like that the cost of ayurvedic treatment is higher than that of homoeopathy. But in the case of chronic illness in rural areas, the average direct cost of ayurveda is higher than that of the other two systems. As per the survey the direct cost of chronic illness with regard to homeopathic treatment is greater than that of ayurvedic treatment for the same in urban areas (Rs 235 for homoeopathy and Rs 190 for ayurveda).

Figure 2

Average Indirect Cost of Treatment on the Basis of Residential Status and the System of Medicine

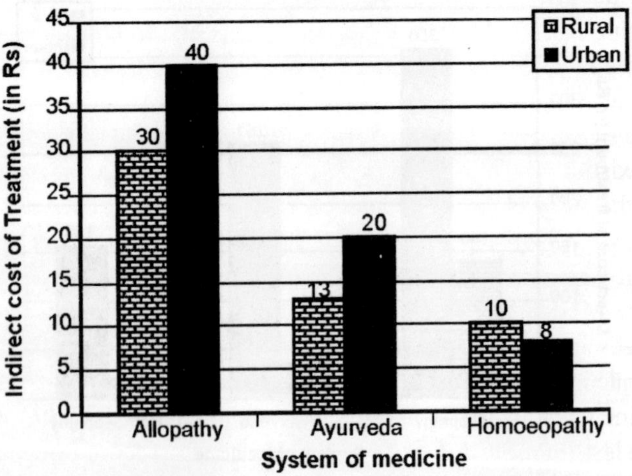

Source: Developed from sample data.

Table 7

Distribution of Patients on the Basis of Direct Cost of Treatment Under Different Systems of Medicine: Rural-Urban

Systems of medicine	*Direct cost of treatment (in Rs)*					
	<50	*51–100*	*101–300*	*301–500*	*501 and above*	*Total*
			Rural			
Allopathy	8(6.8)	40(34.2)	24(20.5)	31(26.5)	14(12.1)	117(100.0)
Ayurveda	17(56.7)	5(16.6)	2(6.7)	6(20)	0	30(100.0)
Homoeopathy	37(97.4)	1(2.6)	0	0	0	38(100.0)
Others	21(95.5)	0	1(4.5)	0	0	22(100.0)
Total	83(40)	46(22.2)	27(13)	37(17.9)	14(6.7)	207(100.0)
			Urban			
Allopathy	20(10.8)	41(22.2)	28(15.1)	48(25.9)	48(25.9)	185(100.0)
Ayurveda	24(47.1)	7(13.7)	9(17.6)	5(9.8)	6(11.7)	51(100.0)
Homoeopathy	12(52.2)	4(17.4)	2(8.7)	3(13)	2(8.6)	23(100.0)
Others	11(84.6)	2(15.4)	0	0	0	13(100.0)
Total	67(24.6)	54(19.9)	39(14.3)	56(20.6)	56(20.6)	272(100.0)

Note: Figures in parentheses show percentage

Source: Sample Survey, February-March 2002.

The detailed figures related to direct costs under different systems of medicine are shown in the Table 7. It can be seen that direct cost favours the rural areas. This is mainly because most of the patients in the rural areas use government hospitals and they avail themselves of Employees State Insurance benefits. At the same time, the price discrimination existing in the medical field, especially in the case of doctor's fee favours the people in the rural areas. About 40 per cent of the rural people have the direct cost less than 50, while in urban areas only 24.6 per cent come under this range during the survey period (February-March, 2002). The proportion of people who pay more than 500 rupees in rural areas was only 6.7 per cent among the allopathy users, while in urban areas it was 20.6 per cent. Moreover, in rural areas the cost incurred by ayurveda users is less than Rs 500 and homoeopathy users are less than Rs 100. But in urban areas, all of them range between less than Rs 50 to Rs 501 and above.

Table 8

Distribution of Patients on the Basis of Indirect Cost of Treatment Under Different Systems of Medicine: Rural-Urban

Systems of medicine	Indirect cost of treatment (in Rs)			
	<50	51–100	101 and above	Total
		Rural		
Allopathy	29(24.8)	76(65)	12(10.3)	117(100)
Ayurveda	20(66.7)	10(33.3)	0	30(100)
Homoeopathy	37(97.4)	1(2.6)	0	38(100)
Others	22(100)	0	0	22(100)
Total	108(52.2)	87(42)	12(5.75)	207(100)
		Urban		
Allopathy	99(53.5)	57(30.8)	29(16.1)	185(100)
Ayurveda	37(72.5)	12(23.5)	2(3.9)	51(100)
Homoeopathy	19(82.6)	4(17.4)	0	23(100)
Others	13(100)	0	0	13(100)
Total	168(61.8)	73(26.8)	31(11.4)	272(100)

Note: Figures in parentheses show percentage.

Source: Sample Survey, February-March 2002.

Almost the same pattern is prevailing in the case of indirect cost of treatment (Table 8). About 94.2 per cent (52.2% and 42%) of the rural people pay an indirect cost upto Rs 100, while in urban areas only 88.6 per cent (61.8% and 26.8%) come under this category. In the case of ayurveda and homoeopathy, most of the people come under this range in both rural and urban areas. In rural areas, about 10.3 per cent (6% + 3.4% + 0.9%) incur indirect costs greater than Rs.101 for allopathy, while in urban areas 16.1 per cent (8.1% + 5.4% + 2.6%) pay the same amount.

Major Findings

Following are the major finding of the study:

- It is noted that there exists large disparity in the cost of treatment in different systems of medicine. The cost of allopathy is the highest in both rural and urban areas followed by that of ayurveda and homoeopathy.
- In rural areas, both direct and indirect costs of different systems of medicine influence the people's preference for a particular system of medicine. This phenomena is found to be more pronounced in rural areas.

- The average direct cost of treatment regarding acute illness as well as chronic illness under all the systems of medicine in urban areas is greater than that in rural areas.
- In rural areas the average direct cost of treatment under allopathy for acute illness is greater than the average direct cost of chronic illness. However, the average direct cost of treatment under both ayurveda and homoeopathy for acute illness in rural areas is less than the same for chronic illness. But in urban areas, the average direct cost of acute illness under all the systems of medicine is less than the average direct cost for chronic illness.
- The average indirect cost of treatment under allopathy and ayurveda for chronic illness in urban areas is greater than that in rural areas while in the case of homoeopathy, the average indirect cost of acute illness as well as chronic illness in rural areas is greater than that in urban areas.
- There are variations in the preference pattern of the people for different systems of medicine in rural and urban areas. The preference for allopathy and ayurveda is greater in urban areas while the preference for homoeopathy is relatively more in rural areas. There is high rural-urban disparity in the availability of and accessibility to different systems of medicine.

Suggestions

The study offers the following suggestions for improving the efficiency and quality of health care in Kerala:

- Government policies should be oriented more towards the improvement of rural health care.
- A viable system of health care financing needs to be developed.
- An effective linkage between different systems of medicine needs to be established.
- The R&D and the supply of raw materials regarding traditional medicine have to be strengthened.
- The government should promote different cost-effective systems of medicine regarding chronic diseases.
- Effective implementation of National Rural Health Mission (NRHM) is required for the maximum utilization of the fund allocation by the central government particularly for the development of alternative systems of medicine and for the overall development of the health sector in the state.

Conclusion

It is evident from the present study that there is widespread prevalence of medical pluralism in Kerala. The major systems of medicine followed by the people are allopathy, ayurveda and homoeopathy. Of late, the disease pattern in Kerala has been changing dramatically. Communicable diseases continue to be the major cause of morbidity and mortality. However, changing lifestyles, urbanization, industrialization and ageing of the population as a result of increased life expectancy have resulted in the increase in non-communicable diseases like cardiovascular diseases, cancer, diabetes, etc., as the major cause for morbidity and mortality in recent times. This increasing burden of chronic and degenerative diseases demands drastic improvement in the present health care system which needs to be more effective and affordable to all the sections of the society. This requires the systematic expansion of medical pluralism in the state. Thus medical pluralism, which has the potential to provide cost-effectiveness, accessibility, availability and equity in the field of health care needs to be promoted further in the state of Kerala.

Select References

Andrews, S. (1973), Feasibility of Involving Indigenous Medicine Practitioners for Family Planning Service Delivery in Kerala, India, Ph.D. Thesis, Johns Hopkins University, School of Hygiene and Public Health, (Unpublished).

Anitha, V. (1997), Medical Pluralism in Rural Kerala: A Socio-economic Study of Chirakkara Village, M.Phil Thesis, Department of Economics, University College, Thiruvananthapuram (Unpublished).

Anitha, V. (2007). "Role of Medical Pluralism on India's Health Care", Seminar Proceedings, Economics of Human Rights and Health Care, Scott Publications, Nagercoil, pp. 130–35.

Antia, N.H. (1993), "World Bank and India's Health", *Economic and Political Weekly*, Vol. XXVIII, No. 52, December 25.

Babson, J.H. (1973), "Disease Costing, Studies in Social Administration", in *Studies in Economic Appraisal in Health Care*, ed. M.F. Drummond, (1981), Oxford University Press.

Banerji, D. (1979), "Place of the Indigenous and the Western Systems of Medicine in the Health Services of India", *International Journal of Health Services*, 9 (3): pp. 511–19.

Bannerman, R.H. (1982), "Traditional Medicine in Modern Health Care", *World Health Forum*, 3 (1): pp. 8–13.

Bhardwaj, S.M. and B.K. Paul (1986), "Medical Pluralism and Infant Mortality in a Rural Area of Bangladesh", *Social Science and Medicine*, 23 (10): pp.1003–10.

Boban, Jose K. (1990), Changing Medical and Related Ritual Practices among the Tribals: A Study among the Muthuvans and Mannans of Iduki Districts, Doctoral Thesis, Dept. of Sociology, University of Kerala.

Brooks, R.G. (1969), "Cost-Benefit Analysis of Patients Treated at a Rheumatism Centre", *Annuals of Rheumatic Disease*, 28, pp. 655–61.

C.S.O. (2001), Statistical Pocket Book, India 2001, Ministry of Statistics and Programme Implementation, Government of India, New Delhi.

Carter, F., C.D. Forbes, J.D. Mac, Farlane and C.R.M. Prentice, (1976), "Cost of Management of Patients with Haemophilia", *British Medical Journal*, ii, pp. 465–67.

Cooper, B.S. and D.P. Rice, (1976), "The Economic Cost of Illness Revisited", *Social Security Bulletin*, February, US Dept. of Health, Education and Welfare.

Doherty, N. and B. Hicks, (1977), "Cost-effectiveness and Alternative Health Care Programs for the Elderly" in *Studies in Economic Appraisal in Health Care* ed. M.F. Drummond, (1981), Oxford University Press.

Drumond, M.F. (1981), *Studies in Economic Appraisal in Health Care*, Oxford University Press.

Government of India (2001), Census Reports.

ICMR (1976–77), "Alternative Approaches to Health Care", New Delhi.

Krishnan, T.N. (1994), Access to Health and Burden of Treatment in India: An Inter-State Comparison, Studies on Human Development in India, Project of the UNDP. Discussion Paper Series, No. 2, CDS, Thiruvanthapuram.

Krishnaswami, P. (2004), Morbidity Study – Incidence, Prevalence, Consequences and Associates, Kerala Research Programme on Local Development, Discussion Paper No. 63, CDS, Thiruvanthapuram.

Lee, R.P. (1982), "Comparative Studies of Health Care Systems", *Social Science and Medicine*, 16 (16): pp. 629–42.

Leslie, C. (1980), "Medical Pluralism in World Perspective", *Social Science and Medicine*, November, 1413: pp. 191–95.

Ministry of Health and Family Welfare (1999), Indian Systems of Medicine and Homoeopathy in India 1998, Planning and Evaluation Cell, Dept. of ISM and Homoeopathy, Government of India, New Delhi.

Ministry of Health and Family Welfare (2001), Annual Report 2000–01, Department of Ayurveda, Yoga, Naturopathy, Unani, Siddha and Homoeopathy, Government of India, New Delhi.

Minocha, A. (1980), "Medical Pluralism and Health Services in India", *Social Science and Medicine,* November 14B (4): pp. 217–23.

Panikar, P.G.K. (1993), *Economics of Health and Nutrition*, Indian Council of Social Science Research, New Delhi.

Sankar, Deepa (2005), "The Role of Traditional and Alternative Health Systems in Providing Health Care Options: Evidence from Kerala", //www.Google.scholar.com//

Sharma, H.R. and J.C. Bhattia, (1971), "A Case Study of Rural Health Cooperatives", *Indian Cooperative Review*, VIII.

State Planning Board (2001, 2002, 2003, 2004, 2005, 2006 and 2007), Economic Review, Government of Kerala, Thiruvananthapuram, February.

Waxler-Morrison, N.E (1988), "Plural Medicine in Sri Lanka: Do Ayurvedic and Western Medical Practices Differ?", *Social Science and Medicine,* 27 (5): pp. 531–44.

World Bank (1993), "Investing in Health", World Development Report, Oxford University Press.

World Health Organization (1978), "Alma-Ata 1978: Primary Health Care", Geneva, WHO, p. 4.

World Health Organization (1997), "Conquering Suffering Enriching Humanity", World Health Report, Geneva.

8

Health-Related Millennium Development Goals in India

Realties and Challenges

K.P. VIPIN CHANDRAN

The world countries have started their new millennium with an ambitious development agenda planned in the Millennium Development Goals (MDGs). The MDGs assume strategic importance for governments and development agencies as they provide a focus and a way for the global development agenda. MDGs adopted by the United Nations in 2000, represent commitments by governments worldwide to do more to reduce poverty and hunger and to tackle ill-health, gender inequality, lack of education, lack of access to clean water, and environmental degradation and build development partnerships. The MDGs have gained widespread acceptance in rich and poor countries alike. They are seen to provide an overarching framework for development efforts, and benchmarks against which to judge success. With the MDG target date of 2015 not so far away, now is the time to review progress, take stock of achievements, and address challenges of health-related MDGs. Among all the goals, health assumes centre of the development agenda.

Study Setting and Methods

The present paper focuses on the specific issues related to the health-related MDGs and its realties and challenges in India. The study was carried out with three objectives in view. The first intention is to have an examination of the progress regarding health-related MDGs. Second, to examine the current trends of health-related MDGs in India and lastly to suggest the policy initiatives and strategic approaches to achieving health-related MDGs in India.

The study is based on secondary data; data from health-related MDGs and its facts and challenges in India are available from different sources like WHO, UNDP, World Bank and UNICEF publications, National Sample Survey Organization (NSSO) reports, various issues of National Family Health Survey (NFHS), National Nutrition Monitoring Bureau (NNMB) reports, reports of National Centre for Health Statistics (NCHS), Government of India publications, district level household survey on reproductive and Child Health, various articles and other publications are used for this study.

Millennium Development Goals and Health

In 2000, UN prepared, following the summit, established goals and targets to be reached by 2015. The eight MDGs are as follows: (1) eradicate extreme poverty and hunger; (2) achieve universal basic education; (3) promote gender equality and empower women; (4) reduce child mortality; (5) improve maternal health; (6) combat HIV/AIDS, malaria, and other diseases; (7) ensure environmental sustainability; and (8) develop a global partnership for development. The MDGs place health at the heart of development. Improvements in health are important in their own right, but better health is also a prerequisite and a major contributor to economic growth and social cohesion. Economic capabilities affect health, as low income constraints access to health care and health promoting opportunities. Equally significant is that the ill-health limits people's ability to earn higher incomes, and contributes to poverty. It is therefore important that the health-related MDGs are not seen in isolation as discrete programmes.

About 18 targets and 48 indicators have been adopted to monitor the Eight Millennium Development Goals. Of these, eight targets and 18 indicators are directly related to health. While many health indicators are "truly health indicators" such as prevalence and death rates associated with malaria and tuberculosis, some are related to critical factors for health such as access to improved water supply or dietary energy consumption (health-related indicators). India is committed to achieve the targets under the MDGs by 2015.

Progress Towards Health-Related MDGs in India

Health is at the heart of the MDGs – recognition that health is central to the global agenda of reducing poverty as well as an important measure of human well-being. Health is represented in four of the eight goals, and makes an acknowledged contribution to the achievement of all the other goals, in particular those related to the eradication of extreme poverty and hunger, education and gender equality. Importantly, the health goals also focus on problems which disproportionally affect the poor.

The reduction of proportion of people living below poverty line has been particularly sharp in the 1990s, when there has been a 10 percentage points decline between 1993–94 and 1999–2000. These trends indicate that India is on track with respect to the target of halving the proportion of people below poverty line. Global action for child survival is an ongoing challenge. The child mortality rate declined to 90 per 1,000 births in 2002 from 202 per 1,000 births in 1970. However, the rate of decline slowed in 1990s and with the current rate, achieving the MDGs target is impossible. In India, approximately 1.72 million children die every year before reaching their first birthday. Though the survival rate is much improved in recent years, the slow pace of reduction in infant mortality rate (IMR) hinders the reach of target of MDGs. The IMR has also come down from 80 per thousand live births in 1990 to 57 per thousand in 2005 and the proportion of one-year-old children immunized against measles has increased from 42.2 per cent in 1992–93 to 59 per cent in 2002–03. The principal causes of infant mortality in India are prematurity, diarrhoeal diseases, acute respiratory infections, vaccine-preventable diseases, inadequate maternal and newborn care; malnutrition contributes to over 50 per cent of child deaths, low birth weight and birth injury. However, the rural-urban disparity is still a prominent determinant of receiving basic health services (World Bank, 2004; Government of India, 2005; Gangadharan and Chandran, 2008). India must reduce maternal mortality rate from 437 deaths per 1,00,000 live births in 1990 to 109 by 2015. Adequate housing, water and sanitation are major issues in urban and rural development and empowerment of the poor. These issues are closely related to the quality of life, affecting multiple dimensions including psychological, sociological, cultural and economic factors.

Table 1

Progress Towards Achieving Health-Related MDGs in India

Indicator	*Year*	*Value*	*Year*	*Value*	*MDG target value*
Proportion of population BPL (%)	1990	37.5	1999–2000	26.1	18.75
Undernourished people as % of total population	1990	62.2	1999–2000	53	31.1
Proportion of undernourished children	1990	54.8	2005–06	46	27.4
Under-five mortality rate (per 1,000 live births)	1988–92	125	1998–2002	98	41
Infant mortality rate (per 1,000 live births)	1990	80	2006	57	27
Maternal mortality rate (per1,00,000 live births)	1991	437	2001–2003	301	109
Safe deliveries (%)	1990	34	2005	54	84
Population with sustainable access to an improved water source, rural (%)	1991	55.54	2005	90	80.5
Population with sustainable access to an improved water source, urban (%)	1991	81.38	2001	82.22	94
Population with access to sanitation, rural (%)	1991	9.48	2005	32.36	72
Population with access to sanitation, urban (%)	1991	47	2001	63	72
Death due to malaria per 1,00,000	1994	0.13	2004	0.09	—
Death due to TB per 1,00,000	1999	56	2003	33	—
Death due to HIV/AIDS	2000	471	2004	1114	—

Source: Millennium Development Goals: India Country Report, 2005.

Current Picture of Health-Related MDGs Goals

Eradicate Extreme Poverty and Hunger

The Planning Commission of India has always assigned poverty reduction as an important goal. Consequently, a number of anti-poverty programmes have been launched from time to time to reduce the incidence of poverty in the country. The reduction of proportion of people living below poverty line has been particularly sharp in the 1990s.

when there has been a sharp decline between 1993–94 and 1999–2000. Child malnutritionm – easured as poor child growth – is internationally recognized as an important public health indicator. South Asia, where the largest number of malnourished children resides, made substantial progress in reducing malnutrition by decreasing the share from well over 70 per cent to 46 per cent between 1970 and 2005. However, this cannot be a satisfactory performance (Table 2).

Table 2

Measures of Undernourishment of Children

Indicators	*1992–93*	*1998–99*	*2005–06*
Children (< 3years who are underweight (%)	51.5	47.0	45.9
Children (< 3years who are wasted (%)	NA	15.5	19.1
Children (< 3years who are stunted (%)	NA	45.5	38.4
Children aged 6–9 months receiving solid and semi-solid food and breast milk (%)	NA	NA	55.8

Source: Various Rounds of National Family Health Surveys.

With over 200 million people who are food insecure, India is home to the largest number of hungry people in the world. India has consistently ranked poorly on the Global Hunger Index (GHI). The Global Hunger Index 2008 (Von Grebmer et al., 2008) reveals India's continued lackluster performance at eradicating hunger; India ranks 66th out of the 88 developing countries. This is a serious problem throughout the country but with large disparities between states and groups (Table 3). There is no single state in India falls in the 'low hunger' or 'moderate hunger' categories defined by the GHI (2008). Instead, most states fall in the 'alarming' category, with one state – Madhya Pradesh – falling in the 'extremely alarming' category. Four states – Punjab, Kerala, Andhra Pradesh and Assam – fall in the 'serious' category (Menon et al., 2008).

The major causes of hunger and malnutrition are lack of public health services in remote and interior regions of the country, poor access to subsidized health care facilities, declining state expenditure on public health, and lack of awareness about preventive child health care. In December 2006, the Supreme Court of India passed an order, which requires the budget allocation of the central and state governments to increase funding for supplementary nutrition for severely malnourished children, pregnant women, nursing mothers and adolescent girls.

Furthermore, given the large share of underweight children and the high proportion of the population living on minimum consumption level, the Supreme Court of India reiterated the low prospect of India reaching the MDG target on hunger.

Table 3

Severity of Indian State Huger Index by States

< 4.5 (Low)		*<5.0–9.9 (Moderate)*		*10.0–19.9 (Serious)*		*20.0–29.9 (Alarming)*		*>30.0 (Extremely)*	
State	*ISHI*	*State*	*ISHI*	*State*	*ISHI*	*State*	*ISHI*	*State*	*ISHI*
None	....	None	....	Punjab	13.6	Haryana	20.0	M.P.	30.9
				Kerala	17.7	U.P.	20.9		
				A.P.	19.5	Tamil Nadu	21.0		
				Assam	19.8	Rajasthan	21.0		
						West Bengal	22.2		
						Karnataka	22.8		
						Orissa	23.7		
						Maharashtra	23.8		
						Gujarat	24.7		
						Chhattisgarh	26.6		
						Bihar	27.3		
						Jharkhand	28.7		

Source: NFHS–III (2005–06), NSSO 61st round (2004–05) and Menon et al. (2008)

Reduce Child Mortality

Infant mortality is a good indicator at how well nations are doing in protecting their most vulnerable members. Both infant and child mortality have continued their declining trend, but remain at high levels in India. Most of the under-five deaths in India result from diarrhoea, acute respiratory infections, and vaccine-preventable diseases. Malnutrition continues to be a major underlying cause of death. In India approximately 1.72 million children die each year before reaching their first birthday. Infant mortality has declined significantly in India from 129 in 1970 to 57 in the year 2006. While the expected fall in IMR is at 47 based on current rate, it is still above the millennium development goal of 28 per 1,000 live births by 2015. India's performance in reducing mortality rates, compared to similar Asian developing countries like China, Indonesia and Thailand, is poor. The level of IMR is much higher in India even compared to some of the South-East Asian countries like

Bangladesh and Sri Lanka. Though the long-term reduction in mortality rates is striking, the concern is the decline in slowing down during the recent decade. But, the tempo has not been sustained during the recent years (Table 4).

Table 4
Mortality Profile of India

Morality Indicators	*1995*	*2000*	*2005*
Crude death rate	9.0	8.5	7.6
Infant mortality rate	74.0	68.0	58.0
Neonatal mortality rate	48.1	44.0	37.0
Postnatal morality rate	25.9	23.0	22.0
Perinatal mortality rate	44.6	40.0	37.0
Still birth rate	9.2	8.0	9.0

Source: Statistical Report, Registrar General of India 2005.

There is urgent need for new approaches and priorities in the overall strategy to reduce mortality rates among children. There are wide inter-state disparities in infant mortality rates and under-five mortality rates. The IMR varies from as low as 14 (Kerala) to as high as 96 (Orissa) and weaker states like Uttar Pradesh, Rajasthan, Madhya Pradesh, Orissa and Assam have IMR higher than the national average. There are substantial differences not only in the IMR but also in the neonatal, and under-five mortality rates between states. The Ministry of Health and Family Welfare is implementing several programmes and schemes to address the issue of high infant and child mortality.

Improve Maternal Health

Ensuring safe motherhood is one of the biggest challenges faced in India. WHO estimates show that out of 5,29,000 maternal deaths globally each year 136,000 (25.7%) are contributed by India. This is the highest burden for any single country in the world. The National Population Policy (2000) seeks to reduce maternal mortality ratio to less than 100 per 1,00,000 live births by the year 2010. Women in the reproductive age group of 15–49 years are more vulnerable to maternal mortality and morbidity due to causes related to pregnancy and childbirth. Maternal mortality in India continues to be a major concern given the reduced social, cultural and economic status of Indian women that inhibits them from adequate access to health facilities.

The overall average rate of maternal mortality ratio (MMR) decline during the period 1997–2003 has been, of 16 points per year. At this rate of decline, both the NRHM goal of 109 by 2015 may be difficult to achieve. The SRS has published data on MMR for the years 1997–98, 1999–2001, and 2001–03. About two-thirds of maternal deaths occur in a handful of the states – Bihar, Jharkhand, Orissa, Madhya Pradesh, Chhattisgarh, Rajasthan, Uttar Pradesh, Uttaranchal and Assam. Though estimates are indicative, they reflect the relative neglect of women's health in India (Table 5).

Table 5

Statewise Trends of Maternal Mortality Ratio

Major State	*MMR (1997–98)*	*MMR (1999–01)*	*MMR (2001–03)*
India	398	327	301
Assam	568	398	490
Bihar/Jharkhand	531	400	371
Madhya Pradesh/ Chhattisgarh	441	407	379
Orissa	346	424	358
Rajasthan	508	501	445
Uttar Pradesh/Uttaranchal	606	539	517
Andhra Pradesh	197	220	195
Karnataka	245	266	228
Kerala	150	149	110
Tamil Nadu	131	167	134
Gujarat	46	202	172
Haryana	136	176	162
Maharashtra	166	169	149
Punjab	280	177	178
West Bengal	303	218	194
Others	—	276	235

Source: RGI, (SRS), 1997–98, 1999–2001, 2001–03.

The NFHS–III (2005–06) reveals that there has been improvement in provision of antenatal care, institutional and safe deliveries and postnatal care. There are several causes attributed to maternal deaths.

Some of the direct causes associated with maternal deaths such as haemorrhage, puerperal complications, obstructed labour, abortions and toxemia of pregnancy, anaemia, pregnancy with TB/malaria, viral hepatitis and others account for rest of the deaths (Table 6). The Government of India has introduced the "Janani Suraksha Yojana", which is a modification of the National Maternity Benefit Scheme, which provides comprehensive medical care during pregnancy, childbirth and postnatal care and thereby endeavours to improve the level of institutional deliveries in low performing states to reduce maternal mortality.

Table 6

Proportion of Antenatal Care and Safe Deliveries

Indicator	*NFHS–I 1992–93*	*NFHS–II 1998–99*	*NFHS–III 2005–06*
Antenatal care			
Any visit	62.3	65.4	—
Three visits	43.9	44.2	50.7
Deliveries			
Institutional	26.1	33.6	40.7
Safe deliveries	33.0	42.4	48.3
TT (pregnant women)	53.8	66.8	—

Source: Millennium Development Goals, India Country Report, 2007.

Combat HIV/AIDS, Malaria and Other Diseases

According to 2006 Report on Global AIDS Epidemic the number people living with HIV is 5.7 million, which is more than two-thirds of the total number living with AIDS in Asia. In 2004, of the estimates 55,000 children born with HIV every year due to parent to child transmission, infection was averted in about 2,150 children only. In India, the national prevalence rate is estimated at 0.9 per cent. However, there are considerable differences in the prevalence rates across different geographical regions. Nevertheless, HIV infection rates among people of nomadic tribes in Andhra Pradesh and pregnant women in some southern and western states of India are higher. The HIV prevalence is stabilizing and states like Tamil Nadu, Andhra Pradesh, Karnataka, Maharashtra, and Nagaland have started showing declining trends. Table 7 clearly indicates the status of various indicators under MDG: 6. The HIV prevalence has increased from 0.74 per hundred pregnant women aged 15--24 years in 2002 to 0.86 in 2003 and since then has been dropped to 0.68

by 2006. In the same way, the age group 25–49 has declined to 0.60 per hundred pregnant women by 2006. As per the Baseline BSS Report 2001–02, only 40.1 per cent of the population who had sex with non-regular partners used condom and 16.5 per cent people between ages 15–49 years have comprehensive correct knowledge about HIV/AIDS.

Table 7

Status of Various Indicators Under MDG: 6

Indicator/year	*2001*	*2002*	*2003*	*2004*	*2005*	*2006*	*Source*
HIV prevalence among pregnant women aged 15–24 years (%)	NA	0.74	0.86	0.80	0.80	0.68	Annual sentinel surveillance
HIV prevalence among pregnant women aged 25–49 years (%)	NA	0.80	0.88	0.98	1.00	0.6	
Condom use with non-regular sex partner during last sex	49.3%	—	—	—	66.1%	58.3%	Behavioural surveillance survey 2001-02 and 2006
Percentage of population aged 15–49 with comprehensive correct knowledge about HIV/AIDS	46.8%	—	—	—	57.2%	40.3%	

Source: Ministry of Health and Family Welfare.

As per DLHS (2002–04), 54 per cent of currently married women in India had heard about HIV/AIDS. Knowledge of HIV/AIDS is much lower among rural women, non-literate women, women from scheduled tribes, women from households with low standard of living, among young women and women from same religious groups. Around 78 per cent of urban women had heard of HIV/AIDS compared to only 42 per cent of rural women. Knowledge of HIV/AIDS steadily increased with an increase in educational status and standard of living. A total of 1,82,787 AIDS cases have been reported since 1986 till 31 July 2007. About 86.3 per cent of the infections were transmitted through the sexual route and perinatal transmission accounted for 4.34 per cent of infections. Comparatively, only 1.8 per cent and 1.9 per cent of infections were acquired through injecting drug use and contaminated blood and blood products respectively.

Table 8
AIDS Incidence by Categories of Risk/Transmission (as on 31 August, 2006)

Risk/transmission categories		*No. of cases*	*%*
Sexual		106669	85.34
Perinatal transmission		4755	3.80
Blood and blood products		2563	2.05
Injecting drug users		2930	2.34
Other (not specified)		8078	6.46
Total		124995	100.0
Age group	*Male*	*Female*	*Total*
0–14 years	3313	2283	5596
15–29 years	23905	15876	39781
30–49 years	54905	16701	70905
> 50 years	6843	1890	8713
Total	88245	36750	124995

Source: Millennium Development Goals, India Country Report, 2007.

Malaria is a public health problem in several parts of the country. About 95 per cent population in India resides in malaria endemic areas and 80 per cent of malaria reported in India is confined to areas consisting 20 per cent of population residing in tribal, hilly, difficult and inaccessible areas. The annual parasite incidence rate has consistently come down from 2.57 per thousand in 1990 to 1.54 per thousand in 2006 but confirmed death rates due to malaria have been fluctuating in this period between 0.04–0.14 deaths per 1,00,000 population. More than 80 per cent of malaria cases and deaths are reported from northeast states, Chhattisgarh, Jharkhand, Madhya Pradesh, Orissa, Andhra Pradesh, Maharashtra, Gujarat, Rajasthan, West Bengal, and Karnataka. Dengue fever and Chikungunya are emerging as major threats in urban, semi-urban and rural areas in many states/UTs.

Tuberculosis remains another public health problem, with India accounting for one-fifth of the world incidence. India, Bangladesh, Pakistan and the Philippines are among the countries in the Asia region with a high tuberculosis (TB) prevalence rate (more than 300 per 1,00,000 people). In addition, relatively high incidence of TB was observed among people of scheduled castes and tribes and religious minorities. Every year 1.8 million people in India develop tuberculosis, of which 0.8 million are infectious smear positive cases. The emergence of HIV-TB co-infection and multi-drug resistant tuberculosis has increased the severity and magnitude of the problem. India is experiencing a rapid epidemiological transition, with a large and rising burden of chronic diseases, which were estimated to account for 53 per cent of all deaths and 44 per cent of disability adjusted life years lost in 2005. Non-communicable diseases, especially diabetes, cancer, stroke, and chronic lung diseases have emerged as major public health problems due to an ageing population and environmentally-driven changes in behaviour. Cancer has become an important public health problem in India with an estimated 7 to 9 lakh cases occurring every year. At any point of time, it is estimated that there are nearly 25 lakh cases in the country. In India, tobacco-related cancers account for about half the total cancers among men and 20 per cent among women. One of the key factors in the spread of communicable diseases has been migration, which is also an important determinant of the achievement of health-related MDGs.

Constraints and Challenges of the Indian Health System

The important constraints of the health system of India are financial constraints, social constraints and health sector constraints. Health is largely financed by the private sector. Per capita public health expenditure is nearly $20 per annum. Shortage of funds has been primarily responsible for the non-availability of facilities per norms; provision of inputs such as drugs, equipment and facilities remain inadequate. Important social constraints are gender disparities and high in almost every segment of the health sector and in addition, there are spatial disparities such as between urban and rural areas, and across states. Because of the above all mentioned constraints, even poor people are forced to seek medical care from the private sector.

Important challenges of the Indian health care system are in critical areas like nutrition, child mortality, lifestyle and human resources. Malnutrition is a major problem in India, where 46 per cent of Indian children under-five are malnourished and 30 per cent of new born are significantly underweight. UNICEF report on "Childhood under Threat", speaking about India, states that millions of Indian children are equally deprived of the rights to survival, health, nutrition, education and safe drinking water. Thus, improving nutrition seems like the biggest task that may need inter-sectoral coordination and political commitment. In the case of child mortality, there is a considerable shortfall in the trend of reduced child mortality for achieving the MDG target; there is an urgent need for new approach and priorities in the overall strategy to achieve this MDG target. Intrapartum care, diarrhoeal diseases and acute respiratory infections need attention. Changing lifestyle may also be causing an increase in cases of coronary heart disease. Ageing of the population in any case is giving rise to a steep increase in the incidence of many chronic diseases, some of which are triggered by an adverse lifestyle. The number of doctors, nurses and other paramedical workers per 1,000 population is low particularly in rural areas and for deprived segments of the population. A large number of legal provisions exist in the health sector such as on smoking, drug abuse, waste disposal and protection of the environment but the level of enforcement is poor. There is a need to strengthen the implementation mechanism.

Some Policy Initiatives

A series of policies have been formulated since 2000, important among them are National Population Policy in 2000, the revised National Health Policy (2002), National Policy on Indian System of Medicine and Homeopathy (2002), and National Pharmaceutical Policy (2002), and introduction of Universal Health Insurance Schemes for the poor in 2003. The government recently launched a National Rural Health Mission to improve the availability of and access to quality health care by the people, especially those residing in rural areas, the poor, women and children. Under this scheme, each village will have a female Accredited Social Health Activist (ASHA) who will be the interface between the community and the public health system. The Ministry has constituted a task force under the chairmanship of the Director-General of Health Services to review and streamline the health information with feedback mechanism keeping in view the objectives of the National Rural Health Mission. NRHM seeks to improve access of rural people, to equitable, affordable, accountable and effective primary health care throughout the country. The Reproductive Health and Child Health Programme was launched in 2005 as a part of NRHM and is the principal vehicle for reducing infant mortality, maternal mortality and total fertility to meet the demands of the targeted population. In addition, the Integrated Child Development Services (ICDS) Programme, under the National Policy on Children, has attained some success over the past 30 years. However, it has not achieved significant reduction of child malnutrition in India because the programme has focused on food supplementation rather than on nutrition and health education and has lacked targeted interventions. Improvements in child and infant mortality are slowing and India is now off track for these MDG targets.

While rural poverty has fallen rapidly in some states, less progress has been achieved in the northern states. Pervasive gender inequalities, interacting with rural poverty and inequalities between states is undermining the potential for converting growth into human development. Recognizing the need for evidence-based information about various initiatives undertaken and their assessment as part of the health sector reform process, the Ministry of Family Welfare, in collaboration with the WHO Country Office, India, has undertaken a review and documentation of health sector reform initiatives. The important achievements of India's health care system are the literacy rate has shown a marked improvement and gender disparity has narrowed; there has been a decline in the under-five mortality rate but neonatal mortality continues to be high; leprosy has been virtually eliminated at the national level; the Public Health Foundation of India was recently launched to focus on management of health and try to fill up the gap in human resources appropriate for the health problems India is facing; and the government has notified the Cigarettes and Other Tobacco Products Act 2003 (No. 34 of 2003) that prohibits advertisement of tobacco products, and regulates their trade, commerce, production, supply and distribution.

The National Health Policy (2002) envisages the important recommendations are: to increase public expenditure on health from 0.9 per cent to 2.0 per cent of GDP by 2010; levy user charges for certain secondary and tertiary level public health services for those who can afford to pay; and promoting public health discipline and appreciating the role of the private sector in health. The Eleventh Five-Year Plan will provide an opportunity to restructure policies to achieve a new vision based on faster, broad-based, and inclusive growth. The plan will give special attention to the health of marginalized groups like adolescent girls, women of all ages, children below the age of three, older persons, disabled, and primitive tribal groups. Time-bound goals for the Eleventh Five-Year Plan are reducing maternal mortality ratio (MMR) to 1 per 1,000 live births; to reducing infant mortality rate (IMR) to 28 per 1,000 live births; to reducing total fertility rate (TFR) to 2.1; to providing clean drinking water for all by 2009; to reducing malnutrition among children of age group 0–3 to half its present level; to reducing anaemia among women and girls by 50 per cent; and to raising the sex ratio for age group 0–6 to 935 by 2011–12 and 950 by 2016–17.

Conclusion

In conclusion, Millennium Development Goals (MDGs) provide a focus and a way for global development agenda. Among all the goals health assumes centre of the development agenda. Improvements in health are important in their own right and a prerequisite for economic growth and social cohesion. Targets set in the National Health Policy, National Population Policy and the Eleventh Five-Year Plan are in tune with those under the MDGs. In fact, some of the Indian targets of health-related MDGs are more ambitious. Although some progress has been made towards achieving these targets, much more is still required. The recently launched NRHM is expected to provide the much needed stimulus and strengthen the capacity of the health infrastructure towards attaining the MDGs by 2015. Targeted programmes for vulnerable and marginalized groups are required with increased public investment, especially in the education and health sectors. Furthermore, domestic mobilization of resources and funding through pro-poor policies and public private partnerships are necessary to accelerate progress towards achieving MDGs.

References

Central Bureau of Health Intelligence (2005): "Health Information of India 2005", Central Bureau of Health Intelligence, Directorate General of Health Services, Ministry of Health and Family Welfare, Govt. of India.

Gangadharan, K. and K.P. Vipin Chandran (2008): "Nutritional Deprivation among Indian Children: Distributional Profile and Implications", *Journal of the Institute for Research in Social Sciences and Humanities*, 3 (1), pp. 85–97.

Government of India (2005): Report of the National Commission on Macroeconomics and Health, Ministry of Health and Family Welfare, Government of India, New Delhi.

—— (2007): "Millennium Development Goals: India Country Report", Ministry of Statistics and Programme Implementation, Central Statistical Organization, New Delhi. http://mospi.nic.in

—— (2008): "Planning Commission, Eleventh Five-Year Plan 2007–2012", Volume 11, Social Sector, Oxford University Press, New Delhi.

IIPS (2007): "National Family Health Survey (NFHS–III), 2005–06: India" Volume I, Mumbai.

Lule, Elizabeth, G.N.V. Ramana, Nandini Ooman, Joanne Epp, Dale Huntington and James E. Rosen (2005): "Achieving the Millennium

Development Goal of Improving Maternal Health: Determinants, Interventions and Challenges", HNP Discussion Paper, World Bank.

Menon, Purnima, et al. (2008): "The India State of Hunger Index: Comparisons of Hunger across States", International Food Policy Research Institute (IFPRI), pp. 1–18.

Ministry of Health and Family Welfare (2000): "National Population Policy 2000", Ministry of Health and Family Welfare, Government of India.

Planning Commission (2006): "Towards Faster and More Inclusive Growth: An Approach to the 11th Five-Year Plan", Planning Commission, Govt. of India: New Delhi.

UNICEF (2006): "The Millennium Development Goals: Progress and Challenges in South Asia", UNICEF, Nepal.

Vipin Chandran, K.P. (2009): "Hunger and Malnutrition among Indian Children and MDGs: Issues and Options", Paper presented in 6th International Conference on "Health, Equity and Human Rights", Organized by Indian Association of Social Sciences and Health (IASSH), held at Pondicherry, March 7–8, 2009.

Von, Grebmer, K., Fritschel, H., Nestorova, B. and Yahannes. Y., (2008), *Global Hunger Index: The Challenge of Hunger 2008*, International Food Policy Research Institute, Washington, D.C.

Wiesmann, D. (2007): "Global Hunger Index: Progress Towards the Millennium Development Goals", IFPRI, Washington D.C.

World Bank (2004), The World Health Report 2004, The World Health Organization, Geneva.

World Health Organization (2003): "En-gendering the Millennium Development Goals (MDGs) on Health", Department of Gender and Women's Health, World Health Organization.

9

Economic Valuation of Impact of Air Pollution in Manali Industrial Area of Chennai, Tamil Nadu

J. SACRATEES

Environmental pollution is a serious and growing issue in both industrialized and developing countries. The primary cause of air pollution in the study area of Manali is industrial operations. The health effects of certain air pollutants have been documented in numerous studies (Cropper et al., 1997a and Cropper et al., 1997b) and high concentrations of these substances in many developing countries are known to lead to increased incidence of illness (morbidity), especially among individuals suffering from respiratory problems which cause premature death (mortality). Air pollution causes various types of damages that are normally inflicted on society at large, rather than on those directly responsible. In the past these external impacts were mostly ignored but recently emphasis has been placed on the fact that such effects do involve an economic cost. In recent years, quantitative health risk assessment and comparative health risk assessment (CRA) procedures have been used to quantify human health risks associated with particular environmental exposures and rank them according to the magnitude and severity of health damages. The World Bank (Brandon and Homman, 1995) has initiated such efforts, whereby the economic costs of environmental degradation have been estimated for several cities in India.

Atmospheric pollution has been increasing at an alarming rate all over the globe. Most of the traditional pollutants directly affect the respiratory and cardiovascular systems and are more serious for certain sections of the population that may be at greater risk, for example, the young and the elderly, who are already suffering from respiratory and cardiopulmonary disease with hypertension (WHO/UNEP, 1992). Increased mortality, morbidity and impaired pulmonary functions are associated with elevated levels of particulate matter. Exposure to SO_2 causes impairment of respiratory function, aggravation of existing respiratory disease and decreased ability of lungs to clear foreign particles (Godish, 1991; USEPA, 2004). The studies from many countries confirm that long-term exposure to common air pollutants and living in urban as compared with rural areas, may be associated with increased prevalence of respiratory symptoms, lung function disturbances, cardiovascular irregularities and increased adult and infant mortality (Gilliland et al., 1999; Jedrychowski and Flak, 1995; Seaton and MacNee, 1995; Tango, 1994; Toulomi and Pocock, 1994; WHO, 1994).

Core Argument

The existing legal measures with regard to air pollution controls are unhelpful not because laws are particularly ineffective but because the law enforcement mechanism is spineless due to reckless monitoring mechanism, corrupt governance and institutional vacuum, which triggers up environmental issues. Under these vulnerable circumstances and when everything fails, what one needs to bring out is that the real scenario of the existing problems of air pollution in Manali Industrial Area is enormous and alarming. The basic motivation behind this research is threefold: one is to discuss what exactly is the real impact of air pollution on human health; second, is to assess the cost of health damage due to air pollution in Manali Industrial Area of Chennai; and third, is to introduce willingness to pay (WTP) to control air pollution.

Scope of the Study

The purpose of the study is to provide a new framework to strengthen the air quality control mechanism and mitigate the air pollution factor on disease burden. The principal core aim of the study is to assess human health risks associated with air pollution exposures using previously established dose-response information and cross sectional epidemiological information collected during the course of the study. The economic costs associated with these health risks are then evaluated using available economic information to enable us to rank particular environmental concerns on the basis of health and economic risks. The study is mainly focused on the area of Manali industrial corridors of Chennai based on national air quality monitoring programme since 1999 to 2001.

Methodology

The present study is descriptive based on both primary and secondary sources of data. Primary data are collected through questionnaire administration. Time-series data on the number of deaths that might be due to air pollution was collected from the Primary Health Centres of Manali industrial area of Chennai. The secondary data of air pollution induced mortality and morbidity data were collected from vital statistics department. This study focused on selected areas over a period of three years from 1999–2002. The other factors that are often thought to influence the health of the population, such as percentage of smokers, income level, occupational exposure to pollutants, access to medical care and age distribution, socio-economic status and location of the house where they are living were incorporated into the analysis. Stratified random samplings of different income categories respondents of 100 samples were used for analysing the data with minimum 500 metres of distance from the air quality monitoring point. Secondary sources of Ambient Air Quality Monitoring (AAQM) data were collected from Tamil Nadu Pollution Control Board (TNPCB) and National Environmental Engineering Research Institute (NEERI) Chennai. In addition to that other information relating to economic costs like cost of hospitalization, average wages, wage days lost, costs of medication and defensive expenditure to prevent illness, etc., were also collected through sophisticated survey questionnaire. The health costs of morbidity and mortality were estimated by taking into account all the above information for the research. A household survey was conducted continuously for a period of three months to ascertain the type and incidence of illness and average health costs. A few regression models were run to arrive at willingness to pay to reduce air pollution and to improve the health status of community.

Impact of Air Pollution on Human Health

An important reason for controlling air pollution is the damaging effects they have on human health, particularly the increasing particulate matter or sulphur dioxide. In recent years, the morbidity and mortality rates are increasing tremendously due to increase in pollution levels. One cornerstone of the Clean Air Act and its subsequent amendments is that improved air quality leads to better human health. These health benefits of improved environmental quality are usually obtained by combining epidemiological evidence, linking pollution levels to health outcomes with the value of avoiding such outcomes (Alberini and Krupnick, 1997; Cropper et al., 1997). Unfortunately, very few original epidemiological or willingness to pay studies have been conducted in developing countries, leading the analysts to offer recommendations based on extrapolating both concentration-response functions and the value of avoiding illness from US studies (Ostro et al., 1996).

Cost of Air Pollution in Manali Industrial Area of Chennai

The Manali industrial area of Chennai has witnessed high levels of air pollution in the past few decades. No effort has been made to curb the increasing level of air pollution in the industrial corridor of Manali since this area is not only covered by industries but also by the residentials. This study presents an economic valuation of benefits from reducing pollution in the industrial area as the main economic rationale for controlling emissions is the welfare gain from improvements in air quality. The current study focuses on the three most important economic impacts of air pollution namely health impacts and restrictions imposed on economic activities through environmental contingencies and people's willingness to pay to improve the health status of the people in the study area. The health hazards associated with SO_2, NO_X, RDP and PM_{10} are studied because these substances are the most important in terms of violating pollution standards. The concentration levels depend on the amount and location of emitted pollutants, geographical characteristics and industrial activities.

The pollution loads are still far above current air quality standards (see Table 1). We estimated the willingness to pay to avoid health damages due to air pollution of Manali industrial residents based on the classification done by Tamil Nadu Pollution Control Board (TNPCB). The respondents filled out daily questionnaire about minor respiratory symptoms and the actions taken to relieve these symptoms. Air pollution induced health effects were recorded from the respondents of industrial area of Manali.

Table 1

Annual Mean Concentration of various Air Pollutants during the Years 1999–2001

In 1999					*Descriptive Statistics*				
Various Pollutants	N	Range	Minimum	Maximum	Sum	Mean	Std. Error	S.D.	Variance
SO_2 μ/m^3	98	74.46	0.70	75.16	1501.91	15.33	1.38	13.64	185.92
NO_X μ/m^3	98	47.13	2.45	49.58	1285.49	13.12	0.75	7.43	55.24
SPM μ/m^3 (>10μ)	98	213	29	242	11666	119.04	4.50	44.55	1984.49

In 2000					*Descriptive Statistics*				
Various Pollutants	N	Range	Mini	Maxi	Sum	Mean	Std. Error	S.D.	Variance
SO_2 μ/m^3	97	75.7	2.2	77.9	1613.5	16.63	1.17	11.49	132.11
NO_X μ/m^3	97	34.8	2.8	37.6	1473.0	15.19	0.77	7.58	57.53
SPM μ/m^3 (>10u)	97	368	0	368	15175	156.44	6.97	68.69	4717.81
RSPM μ/m^3 (<10μ)	39	133	17	150	3241	83.10	5.10	31.82	1012.25

In 2001					*Descriptive Statistics*				
Various Pollutants	N	Range	Mini	Maxi	Sum	Mean	Std. Error	S.D	Variance
SO_2 μ/m^3	97	63.0	2.7	65.7	1846.3	19.03	1.21	11.95	142.92
NO_X μ/m^3	97	45.10	3.40	48.50	2029.91	20.93	.99	9.83	96.70
SPM μ/m^3 (>10u)	97	248	0	248	15190	156.60	4.19	41.26	1702.41
RSPM μ/m^3 (<10μ)	97	149	0	149	9418	97.09	2.68	26.36	694.56

Source: Computed data of AAQM, TNPCB.

The above table shows that annual mean concentration of various air pollutants during the period from 1999 to 2001. The mean level of pollution with respect to SO_2 has gone up from 15.33 in 1999 to 19.03 microgram/cubic metre in 2001 based on 98 days air quality monitoring per year. Similarly, the SPM has gone up from 119.04 microgram/cubic metre to 156.60 μ/m^3 (>10μ) in 2001 based on 97 days in a year. It is common knowledge that chronic exposure to higher levels of RSPM and SPM will lead to respiratory diseases at an alarming rate in Manali Industrial Area of Chennai.

The average level of pollution with respect to RSPM has gone up from 42 microgram/cubic metre in 2005 to 71 mg/m^3 at MMC in 2006. Similarly, the SPM has gone up from 121 microgram/cubic metre to 171 mg/m^3 in a year. It is common knowledge that chronic exposure to higher levels of RSPM and SPM will lead to respiratory diseases. It is basically because of industrial and heavy vehicles which have been carry goods and services from industries. However, the Tamil Nadu Pollution Control Board has showed air pollution like sulphur dioxide and nitrogen dioxide within permissible limits in Manali industrial area but whereas these pollutants has been measured only in the day time since the industrialists will release the gases in the midnight when the city is sleeping. This statement has been made by the residents of the Manali area if the TNPCB revitalize the monitoring into 24 hours, we could see the real picture of the air quality status of the Manali.

Table 2

National Ambient Air Quality Standards (NAAQS)

Pollutants	*Time weight average*	*Concentration in ambient air*			*Methods of measurement*
		Industrial Area	*Residential area*	*Sensitive area*	
Sulphur dioxide (SO_2)	Annual average*	80 μ/m^3	60 μ/m^3	15 μ/m^3	Improved West-Geake Method
	24 hours	120 μ/m^3	80 μ/m^3	30 μ/m^3	
Oxides of Nitrogen (NO_X)	Annual average*	80 μ/m^3	60 μ/m^3	15 μ/m^3	Jacob and Hochheiser Method
	24 hours	120 μ/m^3	80 μ/m^3	30 μ/m^3	
Suspended Particulate Matter	Annual average*	360 μ/m^3	140 μ/m^3	70 μ/m^3	Sampling (Average flow rate not less than 1.1 m^3/min.)
	24 hours	500 μ/m^3	200 μ/m^3	100 μ/m^3	
Respirable Dust Particles	Annual average*	120 μ/m^3	60 μ/m^3	50 μ/m^3	High volume sampling (Average flow rate not less than 1.1 m^3/min.)
	24 hours	150 μ/m^3	100 μ/m^3	75 μ/m^3	

Note: * Annual arithmetic means of minimum 104 measurements in a year or taken twice a week, 24 hourly at uniform interval.

Table 3

Manali Industrial Area Morbidity Data for the Year 1999

In 1999	*Adult*			*Children*		
1. Heart Diseases	*Male*	*Female*	*Total*	*Male*	*Female*	*Total*
(a) Congenital	—	—	—	3	6	9
(b) Rheumatic Heart Disease	—	3	3	—	4	4
(c) Heart Failure	3	1	4	1	1	2
(d) Ischaemic Heart Disease	4	1	5	—	—	—
(e) Hypertension	24	33	57	—	—	—
Total	31 (0.79)	38 (0.76)	69 (0.77)	4 (0.12)	11 (3.34)	15 (0.23)
2. Respiratory Diseases						
(a) Asthma	456	516	972	153	166	319
(b) Pneumonia	12	2	14	6	7	13
(c) Respiratory Tract Infection	1668	2580	4248	1980	1908	3888
(d) Puculota	—	—	—	—	—	—
Total	2136 (54.77)	3098 (61.60)	5234 (58.62)	2139 (62.65)	2081 (63.52)	4220 (63.08)
3. Skin Infection	349 (8.95)	702 (13.96)	1051 (11.77)	401 (11.75)	499 (15.23)	900 (13.45)
4. Cancer	0	4 (0.08)	4 (0.05)	—	—	—
5. Others	1384 (35.49)	1187 (23.60)	2571 (28.79)	870 (25.48)	685 (20.90)	1555 (23.24)
Grand Total	3900 (100.0)	5029 (100.0)	8929 (100.0)	3414 (100.0)	3276 (100.0)	6690 (100.0)

Note: Figures in the parenthesis are percentage to the total.

Source: Primary Health Centre, Manali.

The above table shows the morbidity data for the year 1999. The heart diseases have occurred in case of both males (0.79%) and females (0.76%). The highest ratio of respiratory diseases has been occurred among adults (58.62%) and children (63.08%) since children are the highly mitigate to the increasing air pollution in the study area.

Table 4
Manali Industrial Area Morbidity Data for the Year 2000
(Excluding of June and October)

In 2000	*Adult*			*Children*		
1. Heart Diseases	*Male*	*Female*	*Total*	*Male*	*Female*	*Total*
(a) Congenital	—	—	—	3	1	4
(b) Rheumatic Heart Disease	—	4	4	—	—	—
(c) Heart Failure	1	—	1	—	—	—
(d) Ischaemic Heart Disease	—	—	—	—	—	—
(e) Hypertension	16	31	47	—	—	—
Total	17(0.70)	35(0.86)	52(0.80)	3(0.13)	1(0.04)	4(0.08)
2. Respiratory Diseases						
(a) Asthma	296	422	718	126	178	304
(b) Pneumonia	4	—	4	15	18	33
(c) Respiratory Tract Infection	1183	1875	3058	1461	1623	3084
(d) Puculota	—	—	—	4	3	7
Total	1483 (60.93)	2297 (56.51)	3780 (58.16)	1606 (67.85)	1822 (71.39)	3428 (69.69)
3. Skin Infection	264 (10.85)	618 (15.20)	882 (13.57)	340 (14.36)	330 (12.93)	670 (13.62)
4. Cancer	1(0.04)	3(0.07)	4(0.06)	—	—	—
5. Others	669 (27.49)	1112 (27.36)	1781 (27.41)	418 (17.66)	399 (15.64)	817 (16.61)
Grand Total	2434 (100.0)	4065 (100.0)	6499 (100.0)	2367 (100.0)	2552 (100.0)	4919 (100.0)

Source: Primary Health Centre, Manali.

The above table shows that morbidity data for the year 2000, the total number of heart diseases has existed among both male 0.70 per cent and female 0.86 per cent. The highest ratio of respiratory diseases has been occurred about 58.16 per cent among the adults and 69.69 per cent among the children since children are the highly mitigate to the increasing air pollution in the study area. This statistics reveals that children and women are highly influenced by the air pollution. However, this figure is excluding of June and October due to non-availability of data.

Table 5

Manali Industrial Area Morbidity data for the year 2001 (Excluding of August)

In 2001	*Adult*			*Children*		
1. Heart Diseases	*Male*	*Female*	*Total*	*Male*	*Female*	*Total*
(a) Congenital	—	—	—	3	3	6
(b) Rheumatic Heart Disease	—	—	—	—	—	—
(c) Heart Failure	—	—	—	—	—	—
(d) Ischaemic Heart Disease	—	—	—	—	—	—
(e) Hypertension	184	200	384	10	10	20
Total	184 (6.87)	200 (4.00)	384 (5.01)	13 (0.44)	13 (0.44)	26 (0.44)
2. Respiratory Diseases						
(a) Asthma	304	347	651	135	151	286
(b) Pneumonia	—	—	—	—	—	—
(c) Respiratory Tract Infection	1115	2212	3327	1456	1340	2796
(d) Puculota	—	64	64	14	41	55
Total	1419 (52.97)	2623 (52.56)	4042 (52.70)	1605 (53.79)	1532 (51.93)	3137 (52.86)
3. Skin Infection	319 (11.91)	525 (10.52)	844 (11.00)	539 (18.06)	398 (13.93)	937 (15.79)
4. Cancer	—	—	—	—	—	—
5. Others	757 (28.26)	1643 (32.92)	2400 (31.29)	827 (27.71)	1007 (34.14)	1834 (30.91)
Grand Total	2679 (100.0)	4991 (100.0)	7670 (100.0)	2984 (100.0)	2950 (100.0)	5934 (100.0)

Source: Primary Health Centre, Manali.

The above table shows that morbidity data for the year 2001, the total number of heart diseases has been occurred among both male 6.87 per cent and female 4.00 per cent. The highest ratio of respiratory diseases has been occurred about 52.70 per cent among the adults and 52.86 per cent among the children since children are the highly mitigate to the increasing air pollution in the study area. This statistics reveals that children and women are highly influenced by the air pollution. However, this figure is excluding of August due to non-availability of data.

Table 6

Manali Industrial Area Morbidity Data for the Year 2002 (Excluding of Aug., Sep., Oct. Nov. and Dec.)

In 2002	*Adult*			*Children*		
1. Heart Diseases	*Male*	*Female*	*Total*	*Male*	*Female*	*Total*
(a) Congenital	—	—	—	—	—	—
(b) Rheumatic Heart Disease	—	—	—	—	—	—
(c) Heart Failure	—	—	—	—	—	—
(d) Ischaemic Heart Disease	—	—	—	—	—	—
(e) Hypertension	270	275	545	—	—	—
Total	270 (11.99)	275 (7.79)	545 (9.43)	—	—	—
2. Respiratory Diseases						
(a) Asthma	290	342	632	206	243	449
(b) Pneumonia	—	—	—	—	—	—
(c) Respiratory Tract Infection	606	1475	2081	572	732	1304
(d) Puculota	—	—	—	—	—	—
Total	896 (39.79)	1817 (51.50)	2713 (46.94)	778 (38.50)	975 (50.49)	1753 (44.36)
3. Skin Infection	331 (14.70)	372 (10.55)	703 (12.16)	309 (15.29)	272 (14.09)	581 (14.70)
4. Cancer	—	—	—	—	—	—
5. Others	755 (33.52)	1064 (30.16)	1819 (31.47)	934 (46.21)	684 (35.42)	1618 (40.94)
Grand Total	2252 (100.0)	3528 (100.0)	5780 (100.0)	2021 (100.0)	1931 (100.0)	3952 (100.0)

Source: Primary Health Centre, Manali.

The above table shows that morbidity data for the year 2002, the total number of heart diseases has been occurred among both male 11.99 per cent and female 7.79 per cent. The highest ratio of respiratory diseases has been occurred about 46.94 per cent among the adults and 44.36 per cent among the children since children are the highly mitigate to the increasing air pollution in the study area. This statistics reveals that children and women are highly influenced by the air pollution. However, this figure is excluding of August, September, October, November and December due to non-availability of data. Hence, the ratio of morbidity in Manali has been increasing manifolds during current years due to vast expansion of industrialization in urban Chennai.

Figure 1

Morbidity Data for Manali Industrial Area of Chennai since 1999 to 2002 (Adults)

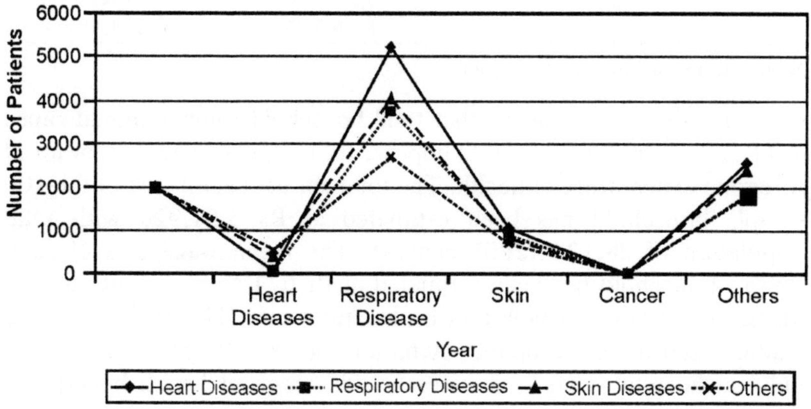

Figure 2

Morbidity Data for Manali Industrial Area of Chennai since 1999 to 2002 (Children)

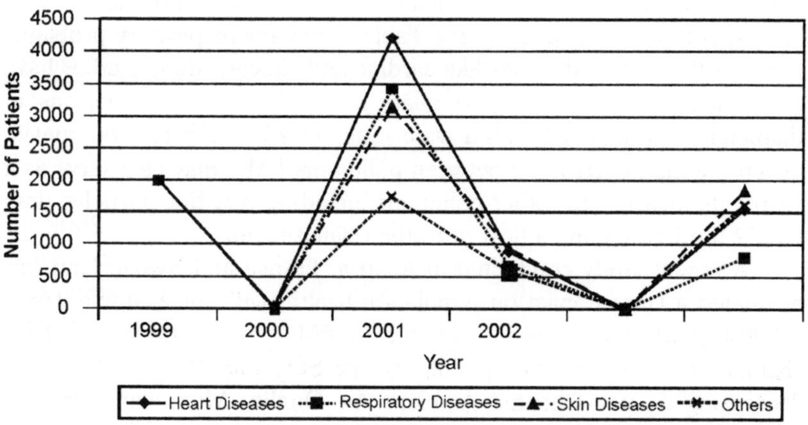

Table 7

Annual Mean Value of Rupee WTP, Health Cost, and Day's lost, Income, Per Capita Wage and Wage Loss Derived from the Statistical Analysis

Area	*Variables*	*Annual (Rs)*	*Sample Mean (Rs)*
Manali	Rupee WTP	1,36,800	1,368
	Health cost	3,91,920	3,919.2
	Days lost	1,685	16.85
	Annual income	22,73,132	22,731.32
	Wage	8,762.73	87.63
	Wage loss	67,445.23	674.45

Source: Computed from Primary Data.

The above table shows that total household sample annual rupee WTP is Rs.1,36,800 in order to improve the air quality and thereby avoid foregone expenditure of health. The total annual health cost of the 100 sample household has been estimated at Rs 3,91,920 with total population of 28,174 (2001 census). The mean wage loss of each sample household has been estimated at Rs 674.45 per month due to increasing level of air pollution in the study area. This paper – unlike studies such as of Hernandez-Avila and others (1995), who focused only on hospital costs – assesses a wide range of health benefits of reducing air pollution.

The survey questionnaire also facilitated us to determine actual exposure to outdoor pollution concentration, such as the actual time the respondent exercised or maximum hours spent outdoor each day. The data diaries were then matched with pollution level and other related information taken from monitoring point within 500 metres of respondent's residence. The total cost incurred by the sample respondents who have spent has been stated in the Table 7 only for respiratory problems not for other major diseases like cardiac and cancer. Many studies have demonstrated that PM_{10} (particulate matter less than 10 microns in diameter) is associated with a wide range of adverse health outcomes. Given the high correlation between pollutants PM_{10} may also serve as a surrogate measure for other pollutants including very fine particles (less than 2.5 microns) and a host of traffic related toxins.

A recent study conducted in Austria, France and Switzerland has estimated a large impact on population health, with for example, some 40,000 deaths per year attributable to PM_{10} in the three countries (Kunzli et al., 1999). The pollutants like SO_2 and PM load has been decreasing as per Chennai Ambient Air Quality Monitoring data of

Tamil Nadu Pollution Control Board (TNPCB), in reality these figures are quite high due to alarming rate of increasing vehicular population in the recent days. The researcher has covered entire diseases like respiratory illness, cardiac and cancer diseases while administering the questionnaire but he has not included here the cost incurred for cardiac and cancer diseases. If we add the cost incurred for cardiac and cancer would be more than the respiratory diseases. Hence, the annual per capita health expenditure for treatment of respiratory problems alone has been taken into consideration. Hence, the derived information about the cost of illness exclusively for air pollution alone has been placed in the table. The income level of the respondents of Manali is very low when compared to urban areas. This shows that majority of the respondents depended on primary health centre rather than private clinics. Hence, this study is not statistically significant based on health cost due to air quality but morbidity data is highly significant due to increasing level of air pollution.

Empirical Analysis of WTP for Air Quality Improvement

Here, we have used regression models in which the dependent or response variable itself can be dichotomous in nature. Basically, it is a 'Yes' or 'No' type answer received from the respondents with regard to improvement of the air quality. We used 1 or 0 value to measure this. In this question, some of the respondents are willing to pay and some are not. To estimate and infer problems, we have used Logit model. We have classified all categories according to their actual contribution in terms of rupees to avoid air pollution. We have found nearly 15 per cent respondents are not willing to pay to reduce air pollution. To measure the actual contribution for the respondent's air quality improvement we have used Tobit model.

The specification of the Logit equation is,

$$WTP = \alpha + \beta_{1Age} + \beta_{2Sex} + \beta_{3Income} + \beta_{4Distance} + \beta_{5Hcost} + \beta_{6Wage\ loss} + \beta_{7Primary} + \beta_{8High} + \beta_{9Degree} + \beta_{10Private} + \beta_{11Govt} + \beta_{12Business} + \beta_{13Fairly} + \beta_{14Greatly} + u_i$$

Where,

Dependent variable WTP = 1; if willing to pay for air quality improvement = yes

0 = otherwise

Dummy Independent variables (description)

β_1 = Age of the respondent (years)

β_2 = 1 if Sex=Male, 0=otherwise

β_7 = 1 if primary educated, 0=otherwise

β_8 = 1 if high school educated, 0=otherwise

β_9 = 1 if graduated, 0=otherwise

*Base Category – Illiterates (for education)

β_{10} = 1 if private employee, 0=otherwise

β_{11} = if government employee, 0=otherwise

β_{12} = 1 if business, 0=otherwise

**Base category – Unemployed

β_{13} = 1 if the person is fairly affected by air pollution, 0 = otherwise

β_{14} = 1 if the person is highly affected by air pollution, 0 = otherwise

***Base category – not at all affected by air pollution

Table 8

Logit Estimates of WTP for Environmental Improvement Dependent Variable: WTP (Willingness to Pay for Air Quality Improvement)

Independent variable	*Co-efficient*	*Marginal effects*
Constant	6.23617 (2.47)	0.0134
Age	–0.0505 (–1.53) **	0.1269
Sex	–2.0587 (–2.45) ***	0.0142
Income	.00025 (1.58) **	0.1149
Distance	–0.0046 (–2.14) ***	0.03198
Health cost	1.7624 (0.104) *	0.91638
Wage loss	–8.1117 (–0.48) *	0.6305
Primary	–1. 9483 (–1.37) ***	0.1707
High	2.1435 (2.07) **	0.03805
Degree	2.3783 (1.43) *	0.151951
Private	–1.2044 (–0.85) *	0.39675
Government	–1.4314 (–0.87) **	0.384699
Business	1.4187 (0.73) ***	0.468276
Fairly	–0.9635 (–0.59) **	0.548631
Greatly	–0.6408 (–0.39) *	0.690165
Log likelihood	–31.72202	
Restricted log likelihood	–43.96699	

Cont'd...

Cont'd...

Chi-square	24.48994
Pseudo R2	0.279
N	100

Source: Computed from Primary Data.

Note: Figures in parenthesis show the t-values.
*Statistically significant at the 1 per cent level;
** Statistically significant at the 5 per cent level;
*** Statistically significant at the 10 per cent level.

This study reports a survey of willingness to pay for the improvement of air quality in Manali industrial area of Chennai. (Table 8) Data from various income categories were pooled together to get a willingness to pay group. Out of 100 samples 85 samples, i.e., 85 per cent of the respondents have given positive answers towards willingness to pay and the rest of the respondents have given negative answer for willingness to pay for improving air quality. These results have several noteworthy features. First of all, the model is having a good fit. The chi-square value is 23.10, which is highly significant at 1 per cent level. Pseudo R^2 value is 24.48, which means that about 24 per cent of the variables in the WTP are explained by the included independent variables. Almost all the independent variables have positive influence on WTP. Hence all the variables are highly statistically significant. Age variable is positively related to WTP. As the age goes up the probability of WTP also increases. Variables sex, income, education and distance have higher probability of influencing willingness to pay for improving the environment. In the case of variable sex, male respondents have higher probability towards improving air quality compared to female and they have more awareness compared to female respondents. Their income level also is high compared to female respondents. When the respondent's income level has risen by 1 per cent, the probability of WTP for better air quality would also be raised by 0.1149 per cent. Age, sex, income have the positive sign and significance at 5 and 10 per cent level. The variable distance has the negative sign and it has the expected sign and significance showing that if the distance is closer to the monitoring stations (traffic point) the probability of WTP for air quality improvement goes up and if farther the probability of WTP drops down. The variable health cost also plays a vital role in determining WTP. If the health cost is more the probability of WTP for air quality improvement goes up at 1 per cent level of significance. The wage loss is the major deciding criteria for WTP among the respondents. It directly influences the WTP. It indicates a positive sign and significance at 1 per cent level. It is a good sign of awareness among respondents that their health deterioration is due to air pollution and something has to be done to improve the air quality in order to protect them from the air pollution induced illness and enjoy a healthy life. The variable education at primary and high school level has the negative sign and significance. Thus, education may also be interpreted as a proxy for the environmental awareness of the respondents and it clearly highlights the importance of education for environmental awareness. As the education level goes up the probability of WTP for air quality improvement rises up. This is very evident at degree level education. It has got positive sign and significance at 1 per cent level confirming the earlier results obtained through various studies (Alberini and Krupnick, 1997).

The variable occupation at private and business group is having negative impact on WTP. Private employees are working for less wage and they may not afford to pay for air quality improvement. The business group is affluent enough to use air cooler, A/C car, and good ventilated houses with exhaust fan, gas fuels, etc., to avoid the ill effects of air pollution. This is highly influencing WTP. As expected only private employees especially those who are working currently in various industries in Manali are more concerned and thus it has positive response for WTP. The personal health loss due to ambient air quality created lot of awareness among public. Irrespective of the degree of health loss due to environmental degradation, the results have positive significance at 5 per cent level. Thus, all the observations and results greatly influence each other and give positive result.

Table 9

Tobit Estimates of WTP for Air Quality Improvement Dependent Variable: Willingness to Pay (WTP)

Independent variables	*Co-efficient*	*Marginal effects*
Constant	1.3729 (5.01) ***	5.40
Age	–0.0069 (–1.93) **	0.50
Sex	–0.2494 (–2.65) ***	0.01
Income	1.1419 (1.28) *	0.20
Distance	–0.0005 (–1.89) **	0.05
Health cost	–5.2404 (–0.27) **	0.78
Wage loss	3.2491 (0.19) *	0.84
Primary	–0.2203 (–1.18) **	0.23
High school	0.2808 (1.99) *	0.04

Cont'd...

Cont'd...

Degree	0.2788 (1.45) *	0.14
Private	−0.2086 (−1.46) **	0.14
Government	−0.2239 (−1.38) **	0.16
Business	0.0175 (0.10) *	0.91
Fairly affected	−0.0279 (−0.32) **	0.74
Highly affected	0.0272 (0.31) *	0.75
Sigma	0.381665	—
Likelihood function	−58.5408	—
N	100	—

Source: Computed Primary Data.

Note: Figures in parentheses show the z-value.
*Statistically significant at the 1 per cent level;
**Statistically significant at the 5 per cent level;
***Statistically significant at the 10 per cent level.

Under this Tobit model, each variable has its own significance (Table 9) In this model, the actual value of WTP is directly linked with the respondent's willingness to improve air quality. If the coefficient sign is positive, one unit increases in age when other things remaining constant, would increase the WTP amount by about 0.50 per cent. Sigma value (0.3816) is highly significant. Because of this OLS is an unbiased estimate, which is highly significant, and it shows that leaving the sample lead to selection bias. Same is the case with that of the variable sex. It would increase the probability of WTP by about 0.01 percentages for 1 per cent increase in sex ratio. Income has a probability of increasing WTP by about 0.20 per cent. If the distance decreases, the probability of WTP increases by 0.09 per cent. Health cost and wage loss have got direct influence on WTP. It would increase the probability by 0.108 per cent and 0.011 per cent respectively. Education has much influence. As expected it had improved the WTP amount at each level of education namely primary, high school and degree level by about 0.23 per cent, 0.04 per cent and 0.14 per cent respectively. Occupation as private employee has negative influence on WTP amount. Private employees are less worried about the deterioration of air quality and less concerned to improve the air quality due to low wages. So, as predicted in theory so many reasons influence them to deviate. It has negative sign and insignificant too. But the variables, government employees and business group has positive effect on WTP. In contrast, business group variable one unit increase would influence the WTP by 0.91 per cent as against the government employee variable, which is just 0.16 per cent. The respondents have responded to the personal health loss due to air pollution as a subjective variable which influences an increase in WTP amount by 0.74 and 0.75 per cent respectively for fairly affected and highly affected variables. Thus, the Tobit model is a good model fit enough to explain the results.

Conclusion

The increasing threat posed to human health as a consequence of deteriorating air quality in Manali industrial area of Chennai has become a burning issue in recent years. This research paper has attempted to introduce environmental tax in order to improve air quality by the way of WTP. The results of the WTP indicate that health cost and preventive cost per household has increased drastically due to air pollution. The survey result shows that the respondents are well aware of present air quality and the necessity of their participation to restore the same. The study results also give a positive scope for introducing environmental tax. Most of the WTP studies carried out in developing countries in the past have been mainly limited to the estimation of user's mean WTP and sometimes been controversial. This research has attempted to extend the use of WTP survey results indicating that charging for improving the air quality for Manali may not have negative impact amongst the public. In this case of observed behaviour method, the assumptions made about the use of WTP for air quality improvement services may be far from true in the developing countries. Also, there could be difficulties in charging excessive amounts as WTP because of low levels of education and incomplete perception about environmental values due to lack of awareness. The paucity of adequate data on the degree of air pollution and its effects on people's health cannot screen the fact. Generally, the community and nature in general can only be speculated but the fast deteriorating trend of the air quality of the Manali Industrial Area can never be denied. It has been shown that nearly 85 per cent of the pollution comes from industrial activities as a result of which the cost of medication was estimated to be Rs 3,91,920 only for sample population. If the present quantum of air pollution continues to exist in future without taking preventive steps to control it, the society's cost of health expenditure may give huge burden among the people. The most important requirement is to do the design of environmental management plans. A tremendous air quality database needs to be revitalized for public domain for further research. Hence, the prevalence of diseases is more compared to developed countries. On top of that, air quality must be monitored round the clock and real data will be displayed for public domain for further research.

References

Alberini, Anna and Alan Krupnick (1997), "Air Pollution and Acute Respiratory Illness: Evidence from Taiwan and Loss Angeles", *American Journal of Agricultural Economics*, 79, No. 5, p.1620.

—— (2000), "Cost-of-Illness and WTP Estimates of the Benefits of Improved Air Quality: Evidence from Taiwan", *Land Economics*, 76, (1), February 2000.

Brandon, Carter and Kirsten Homman (1995), *The Cost of Inaction: Valuing the Economy-wide Cost of Environmental Degradation in India*, World Bank.

Carlsson, Fredrik and Peter Martinsson (2001), "Willingness to Pay for Reduction in Air Pollution: A Multilevel Analysis", *Environmental Economics and Policy Studies*, No. 4, p.17.

Chestnut, L.G., B.D. Ostro and N. Vichit-Vadakan (1997), "Transferability of Air Pollution Control Health Benefits Estimates from the United States to Developing Countries: Evidence from the Bangkok Study", *American Journal of Agricultural Economics*, No. 79, pp.1630–35.

Cropper, Maureen et al. (1997a), "The Health Benefits of Air Pollution Control in Delhi", *American Journal of Agricultural Economics*, No. 79, pp.1625–29.

Cropper, Maureen et al. (1997b), "Valuing Health Effects of Air Pollution in Developing Countries: The Case of Taiwan", *Journal of Environmental Economics and Management*, No. 34, pp.107–26.

Eskelund, Gunnar S. (1997), "Air Pollution Requires Multi-pollutant Analysis: The Case of Santiago, Chile", *American Journal of Agricultural Economics*, 79: pp.1636–41.

Gilliland, F.D. , Mc Conell, R., Peters, J. and Gong, H. Jr (1999), "A Theoretical Basis for Investigating Ambient Air Polution and Children's Respiratory Health", *Environ Health Prespectives*, Vol. 107, pp. 403–407.

Godish, T. (1991), *Air Quality*, Second Edition, Chelsea, Lewis Publishers, pp. 339-385.

Gupta Indrani (2000), "Willingness to Avoid Health Costs Results from a Delhi Study", Discussion paper funded by Ford Foundation and AETNA Insurance Company.

Jedrychowski,W. and E. Flak (1995), "Prospective Epidemiologic Study on Respiratory Diseases in Children in Cracow", *Przeglael-Epidemiologiczny*, Vol. 49, pp. 331–339.

Kunzli, N., M. Jerrett, W.J. Mack et al. (2005), "Ambient Air Pollution and Atherosclerosis in Los Angeles", *Environ Health Perspectives*, Vol. 113, pp. 201–06.

Larson, Bruce A. et al. (1999), "The Economics of Air Pollution Health Risks in Russia: A Case Study of Volgograd", *World Development*, 10, pp.1803–19.

Mexico Air Quality Management Team Policy Research Working Paper No. 2785, "Improving Air Quality in Metropolitan Mexico City: An Economic Valuation", The World Bank, Latin America and the Caribbean

Environmentally and Socially Sustainable Development Sector Unit, February, 2002, pp.1–62.

Ostro, B. et al. (1996), "Air Pollution and Mortality: Results from a Study of Santiago, Chile", *Journal of Exposure Analysis and Environmental Epidemiological*, No. 6, pp. 97–114.

Pearce, David (1996), "Economic Valuation and Health Damage from Air Pollution in the Developing World", *Energy Policy*, 24 (7): pp. 627–30.

Sacratees, J. (2009), "Economics of Air Pollution in Chennai City, India", *Journal of Social and Economic Development*, 11, No.1.

Seaton, A. and MacNee (1995), "Particulate Air Pollution and Acute Health Effects", *Lancet*, 345, 176-178.

Tango, T. (1994), "Effects of Air Pollution on Lung Cancer: A Poission Regression Model", *Environ Health Perspectives*, Vol. 102, pp. 41–45.

Toulomi, G. and J. Pocock (1994) "Short Term Effects of Air Pollution on Daily Mortality in Athens: A Time Series Analysis", *International Journal of Epidemiology*, Vol. 23, pp. 957–67.

USEPA (2004), "Region I: New England, Flotable Debris, The Problem", Washington, US Environmental Protection Agency.

WHO (1994), World Health Statistics Annual 1993, Geneva, World Health Organizaion.

WHO/UNEP (1992), *Urban Air Pollution in Megacitites of the World*, Blackwell, Oxford.

10

Availability of ICDS Facilities and Its Association with Child Nutrition in Rural India

ANAND PARIHAR AND USHA RAM

India is the second most populous country of the world and has changing socio-political-demographic and morbidity patterns that have been drawing global attention in recent years. Despite several growth-orientated policies adopted by the government, the widening economic, regional and gender disparities are posing challenges for the health sector. About 75 per cent of health infrastructure, medical man power and other health resources are concentrated in urban areas where 27 per cent of the populations live. Contagious, infectious and waterborne diseases such as diarrhoea, typhoid, infectious hepatitis, measles, malaria, tuberculosis, respiratory infections, and reproductive tract infections dominate the morbidity pattern, especially in rural areas.

Human resource is a key factor in development. The foundations of man's physical, mental and social development are laid in early childhood. Whatever one gets in formative years of life contributes much for the effective adjustment as adult during the later part of life. A child having understanding and encouraging parents, congenial family atmosphere, nutritious food and proper socialization will certainty score better when compared to others who are not having these facilities. But, because of poverty, ignorance and other reasons, our children are deprived (disadvantage, poor) of the basic facilities of good nutrition, health and education. Nutrition is an important determinant of health. The first six years of life are the most crucial period of the life and have a great and lasting influence on the quality of life of a human being.

This chapter is concerned with the basic rights of children under the age of six years, especially their right to nutrition, health and education. It focuses on the Integrated Child Development Services (ICDS) as a crucial means of protecting these rights. Of course, other interventions are also necessary to protect the rights of children under six. These include, for instance, crèche facilities and maternity entitlements, which are virtually non-existent today. Crèche facilities at the workplace are needed to ensure continued breastfeeding as well as emotional security for the young child. Maternity entitlements, for their part, are essential to enable the mother to recuperate (recover) after giving birth, and to give adequate time to the fragile infant. Health services, of course, are equally critical. The protection of children's rights also calls for far-reaching action in fields such as elementary education, gender relations and even property rights. The special role of ICDS, which is the main focus of this chapter, must be seen in this larger context.

There are a number of factors, which affect child nutrition, either directly or indirectly. The most common cited factors are food availability and dietary intake, breastfeeding, prevalence of infectious diseases, access to health care, immunization against major childhood diseases, vitamin A supplementation, maternal care during pregnancy, water supply and sanitation, socio-economic status, and health seeking behaviour. Demographic characteristics such as child's age and sex, birth intervals (both preceding and following) and mother's age at childbirth are also associated with child undernutrition (Sommerfelt and Stewart, 1994).

The recently released results of the Third National Family Health Survey (NFHS–III) show not only the poor state of children under six years of age but also slow progress of their development. Almost half (46%) of all children under age three are underweight. Only 23 per cent of babies are breastfed within one hour of birth, and just about 46 per cent are exclusively breastfed (for the first six months). The proportion of children who are severely undernourished is also notable 24 per cent according to height-for-age and 16 per cent according to weight-for-age and under nutrition is substantially higher in rural areas than in urban areas. Only 44 per cent of all children in the 12–23 months age group have received all recommended vaccines and only half the pregnant women had at least three antenatal check-ups (NFHS–III). In India breastfeeding initiated at least 24 hours after birth and often after 48 or 72 hours (Sandhya,1991). The breastfeeding practice varies by the different social cultural and demographical background characteristics such as mother's age at birth, education level, birth order, religion (Hinde and Mturi, 1996) and sex of child. United Nations World Food Programme (UNWFP) says that most of rural India is under the grip of malnourished. In addition, most rural Indians are victims of malnutrition, despite the introduction of several government schemes to end the problem (UNWFP Report Category: Indian Health News, Sunday, February 22, 2009).

The ICDS is such a scheme. It is a national level scheme of the Government of India providing a package of services to children below six years and to pregnant and nursing mothers, such as supplementary nutrition, immunization, and health check-ups, referral services and pre-primary education. The scheme now covers almost all districts in the country: however this does not mean that all children below six years from poorer sections of society are covered by the scheme. There are still large areas left uncovered, especially in less densely populated areas or where population is more scattered and in 'undeclared' slums also.

Need for the Study

The major causes of infant and child deaths are premature birth, acute respiratory infections, diarrhoeal disease, vaccine-preventable diseases where immunization coverage has not reached optimal levels, and inadequate maternal and newborn care. A national study conducted in 1992 by the National Institute of Public Cooperation and Child Development confirmed the positive impact of ICDS. Where the programme was operating, there were lower percentages of low-birth-weight babies, lower infant mortality rates, higher immunization coverage, higher utilization rates for health services, and better child nutrition. The percentage of severely malnourished children declined, the positive effects of pre-school were evident, and a larger percentage of mothers were getting their children medically examined.

Evaluation studies have found that, despite some unevenness in the quality of services, the ICDS programme has had a positive impact on the survival, growth, and development of young children. For example, a study conducted in rural areas of three southern states (Tamil Nadu, Andhra Pradesh and Karnataka) found that the programme had a significant impact on the psycho-social development of children, for both boys and girls. The study also showed that undernourished ICDS beneficiaries attained higher developmental scores than well-nourished children who were not enrolled in the programme.

Today malnutrition is the most debilitating health problem affecting millions of children. According to National Family Health Survey (NFHS) report, published in 2005–06, this shows infant mortality rate of 57 deaths per 1,000 live births in the country. The tragedy of malnutrition in children in India is that it not only leads to high mortality, but also cripples the growing generation and damages them permanently. Among the many crippling effects of malnutrition, the most dangerous is the impairment of vision in children. Malnutrition affects not only the health of children, but also their attendance and performance in the school. Improperly/inadequately fed children cannot concentrate on their studies. Child malnutrition has devastating consequences. A malnourished child gets ill easily. The brain and body do not develop properly. The right amount and kind of nutrients needed for growth do not get to the child during the period of rapid development. Child deaths are a tragedy not only for the child but for the whole family. Moreover, insecurity about child survival often leads families to have many babies in succession, which further affects the health of women and children.

National Institute of Nutrition (1990) found that mean body weight and height in ICDS area were higher, nutritional status of children were better than their non-ICDS counterparts. Similar conclusions were drawn by the previous studies of Yegammai and Nivargi (1995) and Jayalakshmi and Naik (1996). National Institute of Nutrition (1990) found that overall nutritional status of children was better in ICDS centres than those children who were not attending ICDS centres. One study has found to identify variables in the family and child sub-system which determine child health status in two selected rural areas of Karnataka, India. The multivariate approach stresses the importance of controlling for age as 0–12 and 13–36 months. The results show that some of the variables which explain the differences in weight- for-age are the direct influence of socio-economic status and operate indirectly through morbidity and per capita expenditure on food (Ramprasad and Kulkarni, 1985).

Objectives

- To examine the level of nutritional status of children in rural India.
- To compare and find out whether nutrition status of children in villages with ICDS facilities differ from those living in villages that do not have ICDS facilities.

Data and Methodology

The basic data used for this study have been taken from National Family Health Survey (NFHS–III) 2005–06. The unit of analysis is children aged 0–59 months in India for whom complete information is available with regards to health and ICDS characteristics. In NFHS, child nutrition has been measured using anthropometric measures: a child's height-for-age, weight-for-height and weight-for-age are expressed in standard deviations (Z-scores) from the median of the reference population, this being the commonly used US National Center for Health Statistics (NCHS) standard as recommended for use by the World Health Organization (WHO). The height-for-age Z-score measures the child's height according to age, this being an indicator that reflects the cumulative effects of growth deficiency and so is designed to measure long-term nutrition. The weight-for-height Z-score measures the child's weight according to height, where this indicator has been used to monitor the growth of children and is typically regarded as a measure of short-term rather than long-term health status. One of the preferred and commonly used anthropometrical indices for assessing nutritional status is the weight-for-age (underweight). This index reflects the body mass relative to chronological age. It influenced by both the height of the child and his/her weight. This index is often taken as a composite measure of two other anthropometrical measures, height-for-age (stunting) and weight-for-height (wasting). Stunting is an indicator of chronic deficiency whereas wasting is of acute under nutrition and underweight is a composite index of both. The classification of a child as undernourished is based on the comparison of its weight-for-age with the child of same sex and age from the NCHS/WHO international reference population. The comparison is done using Z scores or SD scores.

In the present study, the Z scores for weight-for-age are used to assess the status of malnourishment. Deviations of Z scores less than –2 SD from the international reference population are used to classify the children as moderately malnourished whereas deviation of Z scores less than –3 SD put the children in the severely malnourished category. However, these anthropometric measures are widely regarded by nutritionists as a reliable indicator of malnutrition.

To fulfil the proposed objectives, bivariate analysis has been carried out. In addition to that, multivariate regression analysis has also been carried out to understand the influencing factors on nutritional status of children. The dependent variables are nutritional status of children and other variable such as women's education, wealth index, residence, caste, etc., have been taken as independent variables.

Findings and Discussion

Table 1 shows the nutritional status of children by selected background characteristics. In rural India, about 26 per cent children are severely stunted whereas 7 per cent children are severely wasted and 18 per cent children are severely underweight. About 49, 79 and 54 per cent children are average among stunted, wasted and underweight. About 32 per cent of children living in rural India are severely stunted belonging to age group 25–36. Severe wasting is observed among children under 12 months of age, whereas severe underweight children range between 13 to 48 months of age.

Table 1

Percentage of Children Under Five Years Classified by Nutritional Status and Selected Background Characteristics for Rural India, 2005–06

Age in Month	*Height-for-Age*			*Weight-for-Height*			*Weight-for-Age*			*No. of Children*
	Normal	*Moderate*	*Severe*	*Normal*	*Moderate*	*Severe*	*Normal*	*Moderate*	*Severe*	
0–12	72.9	15.9	11.3	69.2	18.8	12.0	64.0	22.1	13.9	7,143
13–24	42.6	27.4	30.1	75.9	16.5	7.6	52.1	28.7	19.2	6,989
25–36	40.5	28.0	31.5	82.5	12.4	5.1	50.8	29.3	19.9	7,111
37–48	42.1	27.0	30.9	84.0	11.2	4.8	50.9	30.4	18.7	7,251
49–59	46.7	27.7	25.5	83.6	12.0	4.4	52.1	31.2	16.7	6,825
Sex										
Male	49.1	24.7	26.1	78.3	14.6	7.1	54.8	28.3	16.9	18,355
Female	48.8	25.6	25.5	79.9	13.7	6.4	53.2	28.3	18.5	16,963
Religion										
Hindu	49.2	25.3	25.6	78.5	14.5	7.0	53.2	28.8	17.9	28,326
Muslim	46.8	25.2	28.1	81.4	12.6	6.0	55.5	27.4	17.1	5,475
Others	54.2	23.3	22.5	81.6	12.9	5.5	63.2	21.6	15.2	1,518
Caste										
SC	44.0	26.3	29.7	78.0	15.1	6.9	49.0	30.8	20.2	7,434
ST	45.2	24.2	30.7	71.3	18.8	9.9	43.5	30.4	26.1	3,984
OBC	48.5	25.0	26.5	79.4	13.7	6.9	53.9	28.6	17.5	14,723
Other	55.9	24.5	19.6	82.6	12.1	5.3	63.0	24.5	12.4	8,173

Cont'd...

Cont'd...

Wealth Index										
Poorest	39.8	25.8	34.3	74.9	16.3	8.8	43.2	31.8	25.1	11,149
Poorer	45.8	26.3	27.9	77.5	15.6	6.9	50.4	30.0	19.6	9,492
Middle	51.4	25.5	23.1	81.0	12.9	6.1	58.7	27.0	14.3	7,531
Richer	60.6	24.3	15.1	84.1	11.4	4.6	66.8	24.7	8.6	5,099
Richest	75.7	17.1	7.2	88.6	7.6	3.9	80.9	15.2	4.0	2,049
Mother's Education										
No education	42.1	25.8	32.1	76.6	15.2	8.2	47.1	30.0	22.9	19,609
Primary	50.3	26.1	23.7	79.6	14.6	5.8	55.5	29.4	15.2	5,119
Secondary	60.3	24.0	15.7	83.2	12.1	4.7	65.4	25.4	9.2	9,226
Higher	66.6	19.9	13.5	83.7	11.6	4.7	71.4	19.1	9.5	1,364
Overall	49.0	25.2	25.8	79.0	14.2	6.8	54.0	28.3	17.7	35,320

Sex of the child does not bring out any clear picture. It has also been found that children belonging to Muslim religion show poor indicators whereas those belonging to others category show positive result. Higher proportion of average children is notably 64 per cent of those who are belonging to 37–48 age in months in weight-for-age as compare to other groups and overall percentage also. Higher percentage of male child (26.1) of severely malnourished are found to be in height-for-age from other category. Percentage of female child is higher from male child in weight-for-age category. Lower proportion of normal children are found in other category and higher proportion of severe children are also found in other category according to height-for-age and same study has been found in weight-for-age.

Children belonging to scheduled castes, scheduled tribes or other backwards classes have relatively high levels of undernutrition according to all three measures. Children from scheduled tribes have the poorest nutrition status on almost every measure.

Average children belonging to richest economic quintile, the percentage of undernourished children is low and higher proportions of severe malnourished children belonging to poorest economic quintile. This is true for all the three anthropometric measures. Indirect relation exits between level of educational attainment among mothers and severity of malnourishment. In short, it can be said that higher the educational level of mothers, better is the health of the child.

Table 2 reveals an inverted U-shaped pattern between age of children and underweight. Females are more prone to poor health than males. However, though the pattern is same for both villages, which are having ICDS facilities and which are no ICDS facilities, the magnitude varies. The villages with ICDS facilities show better result as compared to villages with no ICDS facilities. Another point to be noted is that availability of ICDS facilities nullifies the impact of religion whereas villages with no ICDS facilities shown that non-Hindu children are severely underweight (21%) compared to Muslim (17%) and others (15%). Lower proportion of underweight (weight-for-age) children are found to be severely as well as moderately malnourished in those villages having ICDS facilities as compared to villages with no ICDS facilities, irrespective of caste. In addition, children belonging to SC and ST have relatively high levels of undernutrition among all children.

Table 2

Percentage of Children Under Five Years Classified as Nutritional Status of Children Living in Villages having ICDS Facilities with those Living in Non-ICDS Facilities Villages in Rural India, 2005–06

Age in Month	*Weight-for-Age*							
	Children living in villages having ICDS facilities (ICDS)				*Children living in villages not having ICDS facilities (Non-ICDS)*			*No. of Children*
	Normal	*Moderate*	*Severe*	*Number*	*Normal*	*Moderate*	*Severe*	
0–12	64.0	22.1	13.9	6,526	63.8	22.6	13.6	616
13–24	52.3	28.9	18.9	6,457	50.6	25.8	23.7	532
25–36	51.1	29.1	19.8	6,545	47.3	32.3	20.3	567
37–48	51.4	30.4	18.2	6,619	45.7	30.5	23.7	633
49–59	52.5	30.9	16.6	6,240	47.6	34.4	18.0	585
Sex								
Male	55.1	28.1	16.8	16,827	50.7	30.5	18.9	1,528
Female	53.4	28.4	18.3	15,559	51.6	27.7	20.7	1,403
Religion								
Hindu	53.6	28.7	17.7	25,943	49.2	30.2	20.6	2,382
Muslim	55.3	27.5	17.2	5,089	58.3	25.1	16.6	386
Others	55.3	27.5	17.2	1,355	61.7	22.8	15.4	162
Caste								
SC	49.2	30.7	20.1	6,826	46.3	32.3	21.3	609
ST	43.4	30.6	26.1	3,396	44.2	29.4	26.5	587
OBC	54.2	28.5	17.3	13,614	50.6	30.0	19.4	1,108
Other	63.2	24.5	12.4	7,604	61.2	25.5	13.4	569

Cont'd...

Cont'd...

Wealth Index								
Poorest	43.5	31.7	24.8	10,076	40.0	32.8	27.1	1,073
Poorer	50.3	30.1	19.5	8,638	51.1	29.2	19.7	854
Middle	58.8	27.2	14.1	7,048	57.3	25.3	17.4	482
Richer	67.1	24.4	8.5	4,765	63.1	27.9	9.0	333
Richest	81.2	14.7	4.1	1,861	77.7	19.7	2.7	188
Mother's Education								
No education	47.2	29.9	22.9	17,767	46.2	30.9	22.9	1,842
Primary	56.1	29.3	14.7	4,688	49.1	30.5	20.5	430
Secondary	65.4	25.5	9.1	8,670	65.4	23.9	10.8	557
Higher	71.5	19.0	9.5	1,261	70.6	19.6	9.8	102
Over all	24.3	28.2	17.5	32,387	51.1	29.1	19.8	2,930

About 25 per cent children in poorest economic quintile are found to be severely malnourished and only 4 per cent children in richest economic quintile are found to be severely malnourished in villages having ICDS facilities. Moreover, about 27 per cent children in poorest economic quintile are found to be severely malnourished and only 3 per cent children to richest economic quintile are found to be severely malnourished in which villages with no ICDS facilities. All the measures decrease steadily with an increase in the wealth index of the household. Children from household with a low wealth index are twice as likely to be undernourished as children from households with a high wealth index.

Higher proportion of underweight (weight-for-age) children to the mothers with no education are found to be severe as well as moderate malnourished in both villages having ICDS facilities and which have no ICDS facilities and less proportion of underweight children to the mothers with higher education are found to be severe as well as moderate malnourished in both villages having ICDS facilities and which have no ICDS facilities. Undernutrition has a strong negative relationship with the mother's education.

Table 3 reveals that children who belong to age-group 37–48 months are significantly 12 times more likely to be severely malnourished as compared to children in 0–12 months in rural India. As compared to Hindu, severe and moderate malnourished are less likely to have underweight children in others category. Similarly, castewise distribution shows that compared to SC, severe and moderate malnourished are less likely to have underweight children in other category.

Table 3

Relative Risks Ratios from Multinomial Logistic Regression for Weight-for-age (underweight) by Selected Background Characteristics in Rural India, 2005–06.

Age in Month	*Severe*	*Moderate*
0–12 @		
13–24	9.57***	11.67***
25–36	11.56***	13.61***
37–48	12.1***	16.23***
49–59	8.09***	16.51***
Sex		
Male @		
Female	0.71**	–0.41
Religion		
Hindu @		
Muslim	3.67***	1.32
Others	–10.53***	–11.78***
Caste		
SC @		
ST	1.08	–2.06**
OBC	–3.33***	–2.81***
Other	–8.91***	–8.27***
Wealth Index		
Poorest @		
Poorer	–9.39***	–5.15***
Middle	–18.14***	–11.22***
Richer	–26.67***	–18.11***
Richest	–33.86***	–29.17***
Education		
Illiterate @		
Literate	–2.36**	–1.25
Rural India		
Non-ICDS villages @		
ICDS villages	–7.39***	–2.9***

Note: @-reference category
***At 1% level of significance, ** At 5% level of significance, *At 10% level of significance
*education variable has been recorded due to co linearity.

Higher proportion of children belonging to richest category is significantly 34 and 29 times less likely to be severe and moderate malnourished as compared to those in poorest category. Education data shows that, education is significantly 2 times less likely to moderate and less likely to severe malnourished in rural India. It can be said also that education of mothers is negatively related to underweight of children. Those children belonging to villages having ICDS facilities, are less likely to have severe and moderate malnourished children as compared to those who are living in villages no ICDS facilities in rural India.

Summary and Conclusion

About 32 per cent of children are severely stunted belonging to age-group 25–36 months. Severe wasting is observed among children under 12 months of age whereas severe underweight children range between 13 to 48 months of age. Sex of the child does not bring out any clear picture. It has also been found that children belonging to Muslim religion show poor indicators, whereas those belonging to others category show positive result. Females are more prone to poor health than males. However, though the pattern is same for both types of villages, those having ICDS facilities and those with no ICDS facilities. Lower proportion of underweight (weight-for-age) children are found to be severely as well as moderately malnourished in villages having ICDS facilities as compared to villages with no ICDS facilities, irrespective of caste.

All the measures decrease steadily with an increase in the wealth index of the household. Children from household with a low wealth index are twice as likely to be undernourished as children from households with a high wealth index. Higher proportion of children belonging to richest economic quintile are significantly less likely to be moderately malnourished and less likely to be severely malnourished as compared to those in poorest economic quintile in both villages, those having ICDS facilities and those with no ICDS facilities. Education of mothers is negatively related to underweight of children. Those villages having ICDS facilities of children are less likely to be severely and moderate malnourished as compared to those villages with no ICDS facilities.

References

Hinde, P.R. and A.J. Mturi (1996), "Social and Economic Factor Related to Breastfeeding Duration in Tanzania", *Journal of Biosocial Science,* Vol. 28, No. 3, July.

Jayalakshmi, H.K. and R.K. Naik (1996) "Impact of ICDS on Nutritional Status of Children in Dharwad Taluka, Karnataka", *Journal of Agriculture Science,* 9 (3): 493–98.

National Family Health Survey (2005–06), State Level Household Survey, Report, International Institute for Population Sciences, (Deemed University) Mumbai.

National Institute of Nutrition (1990), Annual Report on Nutrition, Hyderabad, Indian Council of Medical Research: 3–10.

Ramprasad, V. and P.M. Kulkarni (1985), "Determinants of Child Health Status: A Study in Rural Karnataka (India)", *Journal of Tropical Pediatrics*, October, 31 (5): 276–81.

Sandhya, S. (1991), "Socioeconomic and Culture Correlates of Infant Mortality: A Demographic Appraisal", New Delhi.

Sommerfelt, A.E. and M.K. Stewart (1994), "Children's Nutritional Status", *Demographic and Health Survey Comparative Studies,* 12, Calverton, Maryland: Macro International and Demographic and Surveys.

Yegammai, C. and R. Nivargi (1995), "Knowledge, Attitude, Practice of KAP and Nutritional Status of Beneficiaries of ICDS Program in Coimbatore and Hyderabad, India", *Journal of Nutrition and Dietetics*, 30 (6): 61–65.

Section III

Equity and Health

11

Rich-Poor Divide in Health Status in India

MANJU S. NAIR

Poverty and ill-health are interrelated. People get ill because they are poor; they also get poorer because they are ill. Bad health ensures that a person will not be able to break the shackles of poverty. Improving the health of the poor can be the first step towards fighting poverty. This has been widely recognized by government and international organizations. In the 1970s for instances the World Health Organization (WHO) led a global effort to achieve health for all by the year 2000. Representatives from more than 130 governments met in 1978 in Alma Ata and signed a declaration stating that "inequality in the health status of people, particularly between developed and developing countries as well as within countries, is politically, socially and economically unacceptable" (WHO, 1978). Nearly 40 years after the Alma Ata declaration, however, health for all remains an elusive goal. Large disparities in health persist both within and between countries, health problems including parasitic and infectious diseases, nutritional deficiencies, birth complication, etc. are concentrated among the poor (WHO, 2001). Even after conscious efforts to adopt policies to increase the health status of the poor, the situation is pathetic. For instance, even in healthy places such as the Netherlands, Finland and UK the poor die 5 to 10 years before the rich. (Gwatkin, 2003) The rich-poor divide is alarming in the case of all major indicators in the case of developing countries.[1]

The case within India is not different. One of the major objectives of India's plans has been to raise the standard of living and subsequently the health status of all its population. Even after five decades of our planning there exists alarming disparities in the health status between the rich and the poor in the country. This study attempts to shed light on how India's poorest people are faring, demonstrating the persistence and pervasiveness of inequalities in health. The remaining part of the study is organized into four sections. Section I analyses the rich-poor divide in health status in India. Section II provides the explanation for the divide and Section III focuses on the approaches for improving the health status of the poor. Section IV concludes the study.

I

Rich-Poor Divide in Health Status in India

The poor are heavily disadvantaged in health, relative to the better-offs within India. A number of dimensions of health status, including health risk, care seeking behaviour, incidence of disease, treatment and death are analysed to understand the quantum of inequality.

How a Poor is Identified?

The study uses NFHS–III[2] data to understand the difference in health status among the poor and rich in India. The poor is identified using the concept of wealth index[3] used in NFHS. Wealth index is an index of economic status of households. The wealth index has been developed and tested in a large number of countries in relation to inequalities in household income, use of health services, and health outcomes. It is an indicator of the level of wealth that is consistent with expenditure and income measures. The economic index was constructed using household asset data and housing characteristics. Each household asset is assigned a weight (factor score) generated through principal components analysis, and the resulting asset scores are standardized in relation to a normal distribution with a mean of zero and standard deviation of one. Each household is then assigned a score for each asset, and the scores were summed for each household; individuals are ranked according to the score of the household in which they reside. The sample is then divided into quintiles, i.e., five groups with an equal number of individuals in each. In NFHS–III, one wealth index has been developed for the whole sample and for the country as a whole. The lowest quintile represents the poorest and the highest quintile represents the richest.

The study uses several variables such as infant and child mortality, nutrition and anaemia, maternal and child health and fertility indices to examine how the poor are discriminated in health status against the rich. Each of these indicators is analysed below.

Infant and Child Mortality

Infant and child mortality rates are relevant to a demographic assessment of the population and are an important measure of a country's level of socio-economic development and quality of life. They can also be used for monitoring and evaluating population and health programmes. Differentials in neonatal, post-neonatal, infant, child and under-five mortality between the poorest and the richest is given in the table below.

Table 1

Rich-Poor Divide in Infant Mortality Indices in India

*Early childhood mortality rates**	*Poorest*	*Richest*
Neonatal mortality	48.4	22.0
Post-neonatal mortality	22.0	7.2
Infant mortality	70.4	29.2
Child mortality	32.3	4.8
Under-five mortality	100.5	88.8

*Neonatal mortality: The probability of dying in the first month of life.
Post-neonatal mortality: The probability of dying after the first month of life but before the first birthday.
Infant mortality: The probability of dying before the first birthday.
Child mortality: The probability of dying between the first and fifth birthdays.
Under-five mortality: The probability of dying before the fifth birthday

Source: National Family Health Survey, (NFHS–III), 2005–06, India, Volume I, International Institute for Population Sciences (IIPS) and Macro International, Mumbai, 2007.

The infant mortality rate is 70 among children in households in the lowest wealth quintile, 58 in middle wealth quintile households, and only 29 in the highest wealth quintile households. Households in the highest wealth quintile experience only one-third the under-five mortality rate of households in the lowest quintile. The ratio between the highest and lowest quintiles in child mortality is lowest in the neonatal phase (1: 2) and highest in the age interval 1–4 years (1: 7).

Maternal and Child Health

Maternal and child health has remained an integral part of the Family Welfare Programme of India since the time of the First and Second

Five-Year Plans (1951–56 and 1956–61) when the Government of India took steps to strengthen maternal and child health services. Several of the national socio-demographic goals for 2010 specified by the policy pertain to safe motherhood. For 2010, the goals are that 80 per cent of all deliveries should take place in institutions, 100 per cent of deliveries should be attended by trained personnel, and the maternal mortality ratio should be reduced to a level below 100 per 1,00,000 live births. To improve the availability of and access to quality health care, especially for those residing in rural areas, the poor, women, and children, the government recently launched the National Rural Health Mission for the 2005–12 period. Table 2 provides the differences in the coverage of delivery care and antenatal and postnatal care given to the poor and rich women of age group 20–49.

Table 2

Rich-Poor Divide in Maternal and Child Health Indices

Maternal and child health indices	*Poorest*	*Richest*
ANC by doctor	22.5	86.2
ANC by ANM/nurse, midwife	29.6	10.0
ANC by other health personnel	1.8	0.3
No one	41.3	2.6
Ultrasound testing during pregnancy	4.3	61.7
Doctor providing assistance during delivery	11.7	78.1
Delivery in a health facility institution	12.8	83.6
Delivery at home	87.2	16.4
No postnatal check-up	80.7	20.7
Child's size at birth		
Very small and smaller than average	23.5	13.4
Average or larger	74.6	83.0
All basic vaccination coverage	24.4	71.0

Source: same as Table 1.

Antenatal care (ANC) refers to pregnancy-related health care, which is usually provided by a doctor, an ANM, or another health professional. Ideally, antenatal care should monitor a pregnancy for signs of complications, detect and treat pre-existing and concurrent problems of pregnancy, and provide advice and counselling on preventive care, diet during pregnancy, delivery care, postnatal care, and related issues. In India, the Reproductive and Child Health Programme aims at providing at least three antenatal check-ups which should include a weight and blood pressure check, abdominal examination, immunization against tetanus, iron and folic acid prophylaxis, as well as anaemia management.

The likelihood of having received antenatal care at all, as well as antenatal care from a doctor, increases sharply with the household's wealth index. Among mothers in households with the lowest wealth quintile, 54 per cent received antenatal care and only 23 per cent received antenatal care from a doctor. By contrast, among mothers in households in the highest wealth quintile, 97 per cent received antenatal care and 86 per cent received antenatal care from doctors. Only 4.3 per cent of the pregnant women in the poorest quintile received ultrasound scanning as against 61.7 per cent in the richest quintile. It is equally important that deliveries take place in proper hygienic condition under the supervision of trained health professionals. The proportion of birth occurring in a health facility is too low for the poorest people (only 12.8%) as compared to 83.6 per cent in the richest quintile. Mother's wealth has a strong negative correlation in the deliveries at home. Obstetric care from a trained provider during delivery is recognized as critical for the conduction of maternal and neonatal mortality. Only 11.7 per cent of the poorest received the assistance of doctor as against 78.1 per cent in the richest quintile. The health of a mother and her newborn child depends not only on the health care she receives during her pregnancy and delivery, but also on the care she and her infant receive during the first few weeks after delivery. Eighty-one per cent of the poorest quintile did not receive any postnatal care as against 20.7 per cent in the richest quintile.

NFHS also gives information regarding various aspects of child health; there exists wide disparities between the richest and the poorest quintile in aspects of child health also. Birth weight is an important indicator of a child's vulnerability to the risk of childhood illness and chances of survival. Children whose birth weight is less than 2.5 kilograms, or children reported to be very small or smaller than average are considered to have a higher than average risk of early childhood death. Around 23.5 per cent of all time births of lowest quintile had low birth weight as against 13.4 for the highest quintile. Universal immunization of children against six vaccine-preventable diseases (TB, diphtheria, whooping cough, tetanus, polio and measles) is crucial to reducing infant and child mortality. Difference in vaccination coverage among the poorest quintile and richest quintile is alarming. Only 24.4 per cent of the poorest give immunization to their children as against 71 per cent for richer group.

Nutrition and Anaemia

Nutrition is critical to children and adults. Lack of adequate nutrition in children results in growth retardation, micronutrient deficiencies, and childhood illness. Malnutrition in women can result in reduced poverty, slow recovery from illness, and heightened risk of adverse pregnancy outcomes. Table 3 below gives details of nutritional status difference among the poor and rich in India.

Table 3

Rich-Poor Divide in Nutrition and Anaemia

Nutrition and Anaemia Levels	*Poorest*	*Richest*
Children		
Severely Stunted	59.9	25.3
Severely Wasted	25.0	12.7
Severely Underweight	56.6	19.7
Anaemia	76.4	56.2
Women		
Malnutritioned (BMI<18.5)	51.5	18.2
Height below 145 cm	15.9	6.5
Anaemia	64.3	46.1

Source: Same as Table 1.

Three standard indices of physical growth that describe the nutritional status of children are:

(a) Height-for-age (stunting)
(b) Weight-for-height (wasting)
(c) Weight-for-age (underweight)

All these measures decrease steadily with the increase in wealth index as shown in the Table. Anaemia is characterized by a low level of haemoglobin in the blood. Haemoglobin is necessary for transporting oxygen from the lungs to other tissues and organs of the body. Anaemia in young children is a serious concern because it can result in impaired cognitive performance, behavioural and motor development, coordination, language development, and scholastic achievement, as well as increased morbidity from infectious diseases. Presence of any anaemia (mild/moderate/severe) is as high as 76.4 in the poorest quintile as against 56.2 for the richest quintiles. Regarding the nutritional status of women, data shows that 51.5 per cent of the poorest quintile are under-nutritioned as against 18.2 per cent in the richest group. Anaemia level is also highly prevalent among the poor women. It is 64.3 per cent in the poorest quintile as against 46.1 per cent in the richest quintile.

Fertility Indices

Three fertility indices are selected to understand the fertility differences among the poor and rich in India. They are TFR, median age at first birth and teenage pregnancy (see Table 4). The TFR decreases steeply by the household's wealth index, from 3.9 children for women living in households in the lowest wealth quintile to 1.8 children for women living in households in the highest wealth quintile. The median age at first birth increases steadily with wealth index quintiles. The median is more than three years higher for women in households in the highest wealth quintile than for women in households in the lowest wealth quintile. The marriage of girls at young ages in India leads to teenage pregnancy and motherhood. Young women who become pregnant and have births experience a number of health, social, economic, and emotional problems. In addition to the relatively high level of pregnancy complications among young mothers because of physiological immaturity, inexperience associated with child care practices also influences maternal and infant health. Moreover, an early start to childbearing greatly reduces the educational and employment opportunities of women and is associated with higher levels of fertility.

Table 4
Rich-Poor Divide in Fertility Indices

Fertility indices	*Poorest*	*Richest*
Total fertility rates	3.89	1.78
Median age at first birth among women aged 20–49	5.17	2.98
Current age		
20–24	19	Nc
25–29	18.3	23
30–34	18.5	22.4
35–39	18.8	21.7
40–44	18.8	21.3
45–49	19.5	21.3
Teenage pregnancy	19.2	3.3

Source: same as Table 1.

Of the poorest quintile 19.2 per cent had teenage pregnancy as against only 3.3 in the richest quintile, i.e., the level of teenage pregnancy and motherhood is five times as high for women in households with the lowest wealth index than for women in households with the highest wealth index. Thus, the poor in India are disadvantaged in all major aspects of health. Researchers have developed a framework specially focused on explaining disparities, and strategies to solve the disparities can be adopted only when we explain the reasons for the disparities.

II

Explaining Disparities

Four broad mechanisms contribute to disparities, including social stratification, differential exposure, differential susceptibility and differential social consequences of ill-health.

Social stratification: Refers to the social differences and the size of those differences among population groups. Social position influences health status and those with higher social status tend to enjoy better health. Policies that reduce stratification or enhance social mobility may reduce health disparities.

Differential exposure: Refers to the higher likelihood that people of lower socio-economic status will be exposed to conditions that adversely affect their health. Less advantaged people tend to have greater exposure to multiple health risks. That is, exposures "cluster" less advantaged people and hence they may be malnourished and face limited access to clean water and educational services.

Differential susceptibility: Refers to the greater vulnerability of disadvantaged groups to illness due to the interactions among multiple health risks. These interactions may account for why the poor become more ill than the better off when experiencing similar levels of exposure to risk.

Differential consequences: The less advantaged also experience differential consequences of disease or injury. An illness producing limited consequences for the better off can be catastrophic for the disadvantaged, resulting in a low of land or livestock, school dropout and other outcomes. Ill-health, in turn, can exacerbate social divisions or social stratification because of its socio-economic consequences.

III

Approaches for Benefiting the Poor

More than thirty years after the 'Health for All' declaration was signed, evidence suggests that improving the health of the poorest groups in India remains an immense challenge. Researchers tend to agree that the most effective responses to health disparities are multisectoral, involving health, education, labour and other sectors (Evans, 2001). The approaches for improving the health status of the poor can be broadly classified as socio-economic approaches, health services approach and health financing approach.

Socio-economic Approaches

Factors outside the health sector including social, economic and environmental conditions are important determinants of health. Many of the determinants of ill-health, and thus the means for bringing about significant improvements in the health of the poor, will depend on developments beyond the health sector. Hence, poverty oriented health strategy should influence the determinants of health by shaping development policy in areas such as labour, trade, agriculture, micro-credit, education, rural developmental activities and pro-poor environmental policies.

Health Service Approaches

The health sector has an important role to play even though some important determinants of health inequalities may reside in the broader socio-economic environment. Equitable access to medical services could reduce rich-poor differences in the severity and lethality of disease. Greater access or exposure to public health measures, often preventive in focus could help reduce the occurrence of disease among the poor. Public health programmes may use 'targeting' strategies to direct of their benefits towards the poor. These strategies are often classified into two types, direct targeting and characteristic targeting. Direct targeting involves identifying particular individuals or households as poor so that they receive programme benefits. Targeting by characteristic involves directing programme benefits to population groups on the basis of factors such as residence, age, disease, employment, or nutritional status. In practice, many programmes employ multiple targeting methods to ensure that more benefits flow to the poor or to the targeted groups.

Health Financing Approaches

The costs associated with ill-health – including medical bills and indirect costs such as lost income – can be catastrophic for the poor. In India one study found that nearly 25 per cent of those hospitalized fell below the poverty line because of medical costs (World Bank, 2002). Analysts identify health problems as the single-most common trigger for the descent into poverty. Ill-health can deplete household savings and earnings and impair the capacity of adults and children to work and learn, fostering conditions that create and perpetuate poverty. Health care financing systems play an important role in determining whether the poor have access to health care services. Although insurance can provide protection from medical impoverishment, relatively few of the poor participate in these schemes. In India social or private insurance covers only a small proportion of the population working in the informal sector. The poor tend to work in the informal sector. Participation in community health care plans may be an option for poor rural people. The ultimate objective must be to attain larger, less fragmented insurance or prepayment plans because these ensure adequate sharing of risk, subsidization of the poor, larger financial reserves and more cost-effective administration.

IV

Conclusion

In examining the recent NFHS–III data in India, we find that the poorest people fare worse than the richest on a range of health outcomes including infant and childhood mortality, nutritional status and fertility indices. Widespread discrepancy exists in the use of health services like vaccination coverage, health care visits, maternity related services etc. In general, the poor in India are disadvantaged in all aspects of health. At the household level the poor are more vulnerable to disease because of lack of financial resources, limited knowledge of and education on health matters, limited use of health services and inadequate nutrition. Higher income and assets are especially important with regard to health. The better off tend to use health services more frequently, rely on trained health practitioners and have small better nourished families. Community factors also act as disadvantageous to poor in relation to health. The inhabitants of rural and remote areas tend to be poor and have less access to clean water, safe housing and efficient transportation. In poor communities, social norms are more likely to support behaviours associated with poor health including early age at marriage, large family size and discrimination against women. Also the poor receive fewer benefits from the health system than do the better off. The poor are more likely to find that the health services are unavailable, inaccessible, too expensive or of relatively low quality. Governmental spending also may not benefit the poor because many governments allocate the highest proportion of their health budgets to urban hospitals, leaving rural residents without adequate health facilities.

In the long term a comprehensive pro-poor approach needs to influence the multiple social and economic determinants of health disparities, improving access to vital services, opportunities and reducing discrimination and isolation. The health system can also institute more immediate changes that translate into better health quality of life for the people.

Notes

1. Under-five mortality rate for example is 155 for the poorest quintile and 64 for the highest quintile in Cambodia, malnutrition among women is 65 per cent for the poorest and 33 for the richest in Bangladesh and women receiving delivery assistance from a doctor or nurse is only 2 per cent for the poorest and 65 per cent for the richest in Haiti (Gwatkin, 2003).
2. The National Family Health Surveys (NFHS) programme, initiated in the early 1990s, has emerged as a nationally important source of data on population, health and nutrition for India and its states. The 2005–06 National Family Health Survey (NFHS–III), the third in the series of these national surveys, was preceded by NFHS–I in 1992–93 and NFHS–II in 1998–99. Like NFHS–I and NFHS–II, NFHS–III was designed to provide estimates of important indicators on family welfare, maternal and child health, and nutrition. In addition, NFHS–III provides information on several new and emerging issues, including family life education, safe injections, perinatal mortality, adolescent reproductive health, high-risk sexual behaviour, tuberculosis, and malaria. Further, unlike the earlier surveys in which only ever-married women age 15–49 were eligible for individual interviews, NFHS–III interviewed all women age 15–49 and all men age 15–54. Information on nutritional status, including the prevalence of anaemia, is provided in NFHS–III for women age 15–49, men age 15–54, and young children.
3. The NFHS–III wealth index is based on the following 33 assets and housing characteristics: household electrification; type of windows; drinking water source; type of toilet facility; type of flooring; material of exterior walls; type of roofing; cooking fuel; house ownership; number of household members per sleeping room; ownership of a bank or post-office account; and ownership of a mattress, a pressure cooker, a chair, a cot/bed, a table, an electric fan, a radio/transistor, a black and white television, a colour television, a sewing machine, a mobile telephone, any other telephone, a computer, a refrigerator, a watch or clock, a bicycle, a motorcycle or scooter, an animal-drawn cart, a car, a water pump, a thresher, and a tractor.

References

Evans, Timothy (2001) *Challenging Inequities in Health: from Ethics to Action*, Oxford University Press, New York.

Gwatkin, D. (2003) "Initial Country Level Information about Socio-Economic Differences in Health", *Nutrition and Population*, Volumes I and II.

IIPS (2007) "National Family Health Survey (NFHS–III), 2005–06: India, Volume I", Mumbai, 2007.

WHO (1978) "Alma Ata Declaration of International Conference on Primary Health Care", Alma Ata, USSR, accessed online at www who.int/hpr NPH/does.

WHO (2001) "Macro-Economics and Health: Investing in Health for Economic Development", Report of the Commission on Macro-economics and Health, Geneva.

World Bank (2002) "Raising the Sights: Better Health Systems for India's Poor", Washington D.C., World Bank.

12

Infant Mortality in India

Dimensions of Development

ANKUSH AGRAWAL

The United Nations Millennium Development Goals (MDGs), accepted through a UN declaration (UN Millennium Declaration, 2000), set forth targets to address world's major development challenges. These eight goals are to be achieved by 2015 through 18 quantifiable targets that are measured using 48 indicators. The goals encompass the different aspects of human development ranging from poverty, inequality, maternal and child health, education, environmental sustainability to developing global cooperation among the countries.

To track progress towards achieving the goal related to maternal, newborn and child survival, a movement named 'Countdown to 2015' was initiated by various stakeholders including governments, individuals and institutions. The countdown is aimed to stimulate country specific action by tracking coverage, health system performance measures, and policies and interventions needed to achieve these MDGs. It places India among a set of 68 countries having the highest burden of maternal and child mortality (UNICEF, 2008b). The *Lancet* published a series of articles highlighting the importance of reducing maternal and child mortality since 2003. In a recent article published in the *Lancet*, India's progress towards the fourth MDG has been termed 'insufficient' (Countdown Coverage Writing Group 2008). However, these global comparisons conceal the extent of disparity within a country or region.

The fourth MDG deals with health of children and one of its targets (Target–5) pertains to reducing by two-thirds, between 1990 and 2015, the level of mortality in children under-five (U5MR). The goal can be achieved through reduction in infant and child mortality, and increase in child immunization. In India, contribution of infant mortality rate (IMR) to overall mortality of children under-five is around 70 per cent. The percentage decline in U5MR in India during 1990–2006 was around 29 per cent, whereas the same for IMR was 25 per cent (UNICEF, 2008a). This means achieving the MDG would demand more than one-to-one decline in mortality rate of infants (0–1 years) compared to children of 1–5 years, for every one unit decline in CMR. Assuming one-to-one decline, this would mean reducing IMR to 27 per 1,000 live births by 2015 for the country as a whole. Sector-wise it should be 29 in rural and 17 in urban areas in 2015. But, this reduction in levels should not be achieved at the cost of increase in inequality. In a country with levels of IMR varying between 100 (Orissa) and 14 (Kerala), this is going to be a challenge; and needs careful exploration of underlying distribution and trends of IMR.

IMR, defined as number of infants dying per 1,000 live births in a given year, is a robust indicator of population health despite being limited to only a sub-group of population (those in the age group of 0–12 months). IMR reflects adequacy of nutrition available to infants and women of reproductive age-groups and utilization of protective health care services (Wermuth, 2003). The concave relationship between levels of living and life expectancy is well known in the form of Preston curve (Preston, 1975). IMR is a key indicator of inclusiveness of economic growth (Sen, 1998). Thus, IMR is an important indicator of level of human development and standards of levels of living and can be considered as an indicator of overall socio-economic development of a society. In this context, the inter-state differences in IMR reflects inter-state differences in socio-economic dimensions of development particularly health status and standards of living of the residents. To the extent health is state subject in India and state governments are responsible for provision of health infrastructure and services in a state, inequality in levels of IMR indicate commitment of the state governments towards health of its residents.

To study the progress towards reducing IMR in view of the commitments discussed above by examining the feasibility of achieving the MDGs using the past trend behaviour. We also study distribution of IMR across the Indian states to bring out inter-state inequalities in infant mortality. Specifically, this study seeks to examine:

(i) Trends in IMR at the national level given the targets mentioned above. We also examine trends in IMR at the state's level and compare performance of various states in reduction of IMR.

(ii) To analyse inter-sector inequality in IMR at the national and state's level. We also analyse inter-state distribution of IMR and explore the changes, if any, during past two decades.

(iii) Are the levels of IMR reducing faster in some of the states compared to others? Towards this end, we test for convergence. both unconditional on initial conditions prevailing in the states and conditional on initial level of per capita income in a state.

Inter-temporal comparison of IMR allows us to track effectiveness of government initiatives and programmes. Some of the programmes include Universal Immunization Programme (1985) and Reproductive and Child Health Programme (1997). It also serves as a guide towards programmes either yet to be implemented or implemented recently like National Rural Health Mission and National Urban Health Mission. Cross-sectional comparison allows us to examine the disparity prevailing in the country at one point of time. It also indicates extent of inequity in regional development of a country. Both comparisons help us to comment on the progress towards achieving the MDG and inclusiveness of the economic growth.

This study is organized as follows: next section briefs about methodology and database. Section III illustrates temporal dimensions of IMR, we also estimate rate of change of IMR for major states. Section IV explores inter-state distribution of IMR. We discuss the convergence in levels of IMR across the states in Section V. Last section concludes findings of the study.

II

Data and Methodology

We use vital statistics collected by the Registrar General of India through Sample Registration System (SRS) for data on IMR. The vital statistics provide information on demographic indicators including levels of IMR for major Indian states since 1970s. For some states however, data is available only from 1981 which restricts our analysis to 1981–2006 wherever mentioned.

In India, registration of births and deaths was voluntary till 1969 and there were problems of both underregistration and incomplete registration. Therefore, it was not possible to generate data on vital statistics.

Thus, SRS has become one of the most reliable sources to provide fertility and mortality estimates at the national and state level since its inception in 1969–70 (Office of the Registrar General, 2007a). SRS is a dual reporting system where field investigation involving continuous registration of births and deaths is done by an enumerator, and a separate independent survey covering similar demographic aspects is carried out every six months by a supervisor. Information obtained from the two sources is then matched and unmatched or partially matched records are verified again by an independent visit to the household under review. SRS is a representative sample of population. Sampling unit, viz., villages in rural areas and urban blocks in urban areas are periodically updated using census to preserve its representative nature. A study by Bhat shows that SRS is nearly complete in terms of coverage although death reporting between 1971–80 and 1981–90 has remained around 95 per cent for males and has fallen from 95 to 88 per cent for females (Bhat, 2002: 132). However, there are differences across the states. Given the variations in SRS annual estimates of birth and death rates, it is advisable to use three-year moving average for analysis (Office of the Registrar General, 1981). This means we will lose one observation at both the extremes leaving us with 34 observations when the analysis is for period 1971–2006. Owing to different characteristics, we analyse rural and urban sectors separately. This study is confined to the analysis of 15 major states defined on the basis of population by SRS.

We use per capita state domestic product (SDP) at constant (1993–94) prices as a proxy for level of economic development of a state, which we believe might affect the level of and progress towards reduction of IMR. Data on per capita state domestic product has been compiled from both "Handbook on Indian Economy" (Reserve Bank of India, 2006) and "Domestic Product of States of India" (EPWRF, 2003). These provide information on per capita income (PCI, hereafter) for Indian states at constant (1970–71, 1980–81 and 1993–94) prices. We then convert this series to a same base (1993–94 prices) by computing separate deflator for each state using some common observations for these three years. Instead of using PCI for single financial year we use two years average of PCI.

This is an exploratory study and we do not deal with determinants of either the inequality in or levels of infant mortality, though we use other studies and policy documents to explain the results at some places. We use statistical tools like correlation coefficients and box diagrams to summarize and study distribution of IMR. We estimate rate of change of IMR to compare relative performance of the states. The rate of change can be estimated by regressing IMR for each state on time trend. The dependent variable used is natural logarithm of IMR to account for non-linear decline in IMR. Thus for each state, we use the following log-linear (or semi-log) regression equation:

$$\ln(IMR_t) = \alpha + \beta t + \varepsilon_t \qquad \ldots(1)$$

where t ($t = 1, 2 \ldots 34$) denotes the time period 1972–2005. However for the states of Bihar and West Bengal, our analysis is restricted to period 1982–2005. β in above equation is average proportional or relative change in IMR between two adjacent periods and 100β is the corresponding per cent change in IMR (Gujarati, 2005). Thus, higher the coefficient of time trend t in magnitude, faster is change in IMR for a state.

We examine whether the levels of IMR across various states are converging or not. Two notions of convergence, more popular in the literature, are (Galor, 1996):

(i) *Absolute convergence:* It states that levels of IMR across the states tend to converge independently of their initial conditions.

(ii) *Conditional convergence:* It states that levels of IMR in states having identical structural characteristics and/or initial conditions converge.

There are two ways to examine the convergence. It can be studied either by examining the trend in the standard deviation or by regressing proportional growth rate in IMR on its initial value; the former is known as 'sigma-convergence' and the latter as 'beta-convergence'. If the dispersion in IMR across states (i.e., standard deviation) tends to decrease over time, IMRs across the states are converging in sigma-sense, whereas IMR converge in beta-sense if IMR declines at a faster rate in the states with high initial value of IMR than the states with low initial value. A necessary condition for existence of sigma-convergence is beta-convergence (Sala-i-Martin, 1996).

Conditional convergence can be examined either by using multiple regression equation which controls for structural characteristics/initial conditions of cross-sectional units or by segregating the data sets. We test for convergence of IMR across the major states conditional on their per capita income or per capita state domestic product. Following Islam (1995) and Durlauf et al., (2005), we use equation (2) to test for conditional convergence.

$$\ln IMR_{i,t} = (1+\beta)\ln IMR_{i,t-1} + \psi X_{i,t} + \alpha_i + \varepsilon_{i,t} \qquad \ldots(2)$$

where i denotes the state, X_{it} captures the structural characteristics for state i at time t (which is PCI for the present study), α_i is a state specific dummy and ε_{it} denotes zero mean random error term. Use of α_i allows for permanent difference in level of IMR between states that is not captured by X_{it}. For convergence, $(1+\beta)$ should be less than unity. Given the dynamic panel framework this equation uses, random effect estimation is unsuitable. We therefore use fixed effect estimator to estimate the above equation. Another way to examine convergence conditional on PCI is to classify the states in two or more groups based on their PCI and then examine the dispersion in IMR across these groups.

We use Stata/IC 10.0 and Microsoft Office Excel, 2003 for all the computations.

III

Infant Mortality: Temporal Dimensions

Figure 1 shows trends (1911–2005) in IMR for rural, urban and combined population of the country. IMR has declined by three-fourths during the past century. This decline though unstable in the initial half, seems to be sustained reduction in trend IMR. The IMR declined at an average of 1.5 per 1,000 live births per annum during 1911–2000. Since 1971, this average annual decline is about 2.1 in all-India, 2.2 in rural and 1.2 in urban sector respectively. The decline is faster in rural areas and as illustrated later, indicates reduction in rural-urban disparity in IMR. At this rate, IMR of the country in 2015 would be around 41 which would be well above the targets of the National Population Policy (NPP) and the MDG.

Figure 2 shows the trends in IMR (three-year moving average) for a relatively short period (1972–2005). We use three-year moving average

Figure 1

Long Term Trends in IMR: 1911–2005)

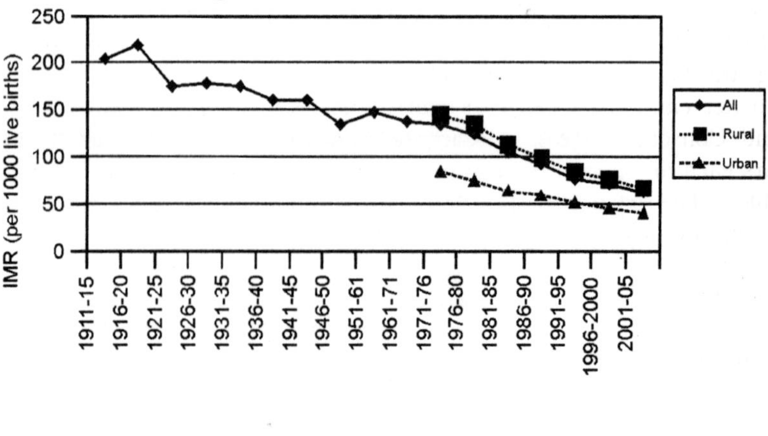

Figure 2

Trends in IMR: 1972–2005

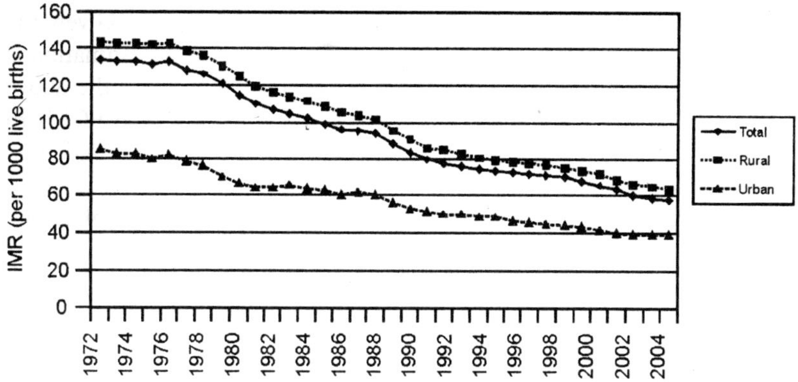

throughout this study (unless specified) to avoid the leverage that may arise due to presence of influential observations. Barring few initial years, there has been a sustained decline in IMR during the period of study. IMR seems to have declined faster in rural areas, hinting towards presence of convergence. An important thing to be noticed from this figure is discontinuity or non-smoothness of trend line even when the IMR is used as three-year average. This provides a basis for segregating the study period in small time periods. For instance, we see that even the three-year average trend line for IMR seems to deviate from its long-term trend during three years – 1977, 1989/90 and 1999/2000. We could not find much reason about 1977 except that the system was fully operational only in 1970 and IMR fluctuated a lot in initial years. Since 1989/90, some additional items recommended by a technical committee like mean age at marriage, interval between current and previous live births were also included in the survey questionnaire (Office of the Registrar General 1993). Since 1999, data on causes of birth is also being collected by introducing a VA (Verbal Autopsy) instrument with the same SRS questionnaire (Office of the Registrar General 2007b). The inclusion of more information may result in better canvassing of information from a household and change the trend. Consequently, we divide the period of study in three periods of nine years each and compute the annual average rate of decline as shown in Table 1. The rate of decline is the lowest during the phase 1990–98 at the national level though the picture is different across the sectors. The rate of reduction has been more volatile in urban areas than the rural. Further, stagnancy in IMR in urban areas during the last phase is a matter of concern. At this rate of reduction (1999–2005), IMR in 2015 would be 40, 46 and 33 in the combined, rural and urban population respectively missing the targets comprehensively. Using equation 1, average rate of IMR decline is 2.66 per cent per annum at the national level during 1972–2005. At this rate, IMR at the end of 2015 would be around 42.

Table 1

Annual Average Decline of IMR

Period	*Total*	*Rural*	*Urban*
1972–80	2.15	2.15	2.11
1981–89	2.37	2.63	0.81
1990–98	1.41	1.56	1.00
1999–2005	1.76	1.71	0.67
1972–2005	2.25	2.36	1.34

Source: Computed from various SRS bulletins.

IV

State-Level Trends

We now analyse the IMR at disaggregate (states') level. We use equation 1 to compute the rate of decline for each state and report the results in Table 2. Figure 3 shows distribution of IMRs at the states' level for both the sectors. We observe the following from the table and the figure:

- Levels of IMR are below the country average in most states except BIMARU states and Assam in 2003. Although, this is not true for the rate of decline. The high levels of IMR in some of the states indicate that there is enough scope to prevent the deaths of the infants in the country.
- IMR in each state shows a declining trend, but with wide variations in time path of decline. Kerala stands out as an outlier in both the sectors and is by far the best ¬ IMR declined at a rate of more than five per cent. In Gujarat, IMR declined at a rate of 3.34 per cent per annum. Initially in Gujarat, IMR was quite high which is below the national average now. On the other hand, Karnataka, Orissa and Rajasthan present a dismal picture with some of the lowest rates of decline.
- As observed earlier for the country as a whole, levels of IMR in most of the states seems to have declined very slowly during 1990s (Figure 3), this should be a worrying signal. For instance, IMR was stagnant for many years in urban areas of Andhra Pradesh, Assam, Karnataka and Madhya Pradesh, and in rural areas of Gujarat, Haryana, Kerala and Assam. Even the state of Kerala has achieved IMR of as low as 19 in early 1990s in rural sector which increased

to 15 in 2005 after being stagnant around 12 for some years. The slow pace of decline for MP is a concern given that the state already has high level of IMR.

Table 2

Rate of Decline (%) of IMR (1972–2005) by Sector

State	Obs.	Total	Rural	Urban	State	Obs.	Total	Rural	Urban
Andhra Pradesh	34	2.27	2.08	2.27	Maharashtra	34	2.96	2.76	3.15
Assam	34	2.18	2.18	3.25	Orissa	34	1.88	1.88	1.09
Bihar	24	2.76	2.76	1.29	Punjab	34	2.86	2.76	2.66
Gujarat	34	3.34	3.15	3.54	Rajasthan	33	1.88	2.27	1.29
Haryana	34	1.98	2.08	0.6	Tamil Nadu	34	3.25	3.34	2.57
Karnataka	34	1.69	1.49	2.57	Uttar Pradesh	34	3.15	3.15	2.66
Kerala	34	5.35	5.45	4.78	West Bengal	24	3.05	3.25	1.88
Madhya Pradesh	34	2.08	2.08	1.88	All-India	34	2.66	2.66	2.47

Notes: (1) 'Obs.' is number of years of observations used. For the states of West Bengal and Bihar, data is available from 1981 and for Rajasthan from 1972. (2) We have used three-year moving average of IMR in regression. Estimates presented here are compounded rate of growth. (3) All the coefficients are significant at five per cent level.

Figure 3

Distribution of IMR (1982–2005) by Major States and Sector

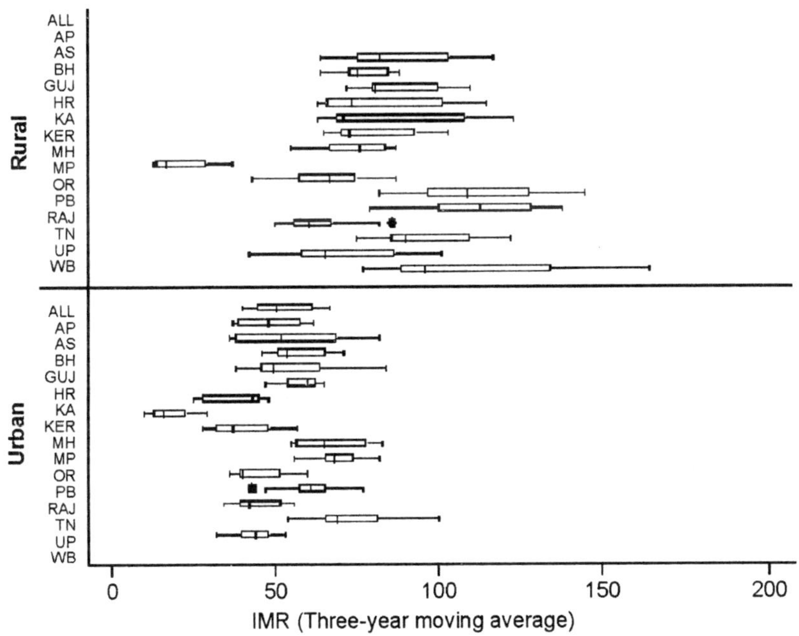

The decrease in the 1990s in the rate of decline of IMR needs careful investigation of the structural determinants of IMR. To the best of our knowledge, hardly any study has explored it carefully so far. However, some studies point out reduction in immunization coverage and other steps taken to improve child health (Visaria 2004; Claeson et al., 1999). Introduction of two programmes – Expanded Programme of Immunization in 1978, and Universal Immunization Programme in 1985–86 – was also partly responsible for higher decline in early 1990s. There were some changes in SRS sampling methodology and coverage that might change the estimates (Visaria, 2004). However, a recent report based on National Family Health Survey–III (NFHS–III) might rule out this possibility for, the estimates obtained from NFHS–III are quite close to that of SRS (IIPS and Macro International, 2007). It should also be noted that rate of decline of poverty too slowed down in India during the 1990s and income inequality (as captured by monthly per capita consumption expenditure) at the national as well as individual states' level has risen during 1993–94 to 1999–2000 (Deaton and Dreze, 2002).

Infant Mortality: Spatial Dimensions

We now examine the spatial distribution of IMR across the states. Figure 4 shows the sector-wise distribution of IMRs (three-year average) across the major states except Kerala for the years 1983, 1994 and 2005. It is noticed that:

- Dispersion in IMR has reduced over the years in both the sectors. The extent of reduction is higher in rural sector as revealed by the length of the box as well as the whiskers.
- While this reduction was higher in initial years, it slowed down with time. In urban areas, there does not seem to be any perceptible change in dispersion between 1994 and 2005 although the levels of IMR have declined.
- Inter-sector inequalities still exist in 2005, though their extent has declined in 2005 compared to 1982. The extent of inequality seems to be less in urban areas.

It may be noted that the reduction in dispersion of IMRs across the states is not so obvious despite the fact that levels of IMR have declined in most of the states. For instance, if IMR declines at a faster rate in the states with low levels of IMR compared to those with high levels of IMR, dispersion would increase despite reduction in levels of IMR. This would become clear when we examine convergence. In fact, this has not been the case with fertility. Although the fertility levels declined during 1972–98, inter-state differences widened (Visaria, 2004).

A state may be classified as a better state if IMR reduction took place at a higher pace despite the state having a lower level of IMR (Narayana, 2008). We rank the states based on their initial level of IMR and its rate of decline in Table 3. By construction, the states lying below the diagonal connecting B5–B5 are one of the worst performers. It is clear from the table that the states of Orissa and Madhya Pradesh need urgent attention. States of Haryana, Rajasthan and Bihar have not performed better either. These states not only have higher level of IMR, but their progress towards reducing IMR as measured by speed of decline is low as well. Except Haryana, all these states are relatively poor states. Karnataka despite being among the five states with lowest IMR has performed poorly in reduction of IMR. Position of states in various cells of the table is broadly similar for urban and combined (and thus rural) population. In few cases, a state belonging to a particular cell in one sector belongs to one of its adjacent cells in the other sector.

Table 3

Performance of States towards IMR Reduction

Rate of decline/ Level of IMR		*Rate of decline*					
		Combined			*Urban*		
		T5	*M5*	*B5*	*T5*	*M5*	*B5*
Level	T5	KER	MAH, PB, AP	KA	KER, MAH	KA, AP, WB	
	M5	TN, WB	AS	HR, RAJ	PB	TN	HR, RAJ, BIH
	B5	UP, GUJ	BIH	MP, OR	AS, GUJ, UP	MP	OR

Notes: (1) Row indicates the ranking of states by rate of decline as in Table 1 and column by the level of IMR (three-year average) in 1982. The year 1982 is used for initial IMR to ensure comparability across all the states. The state with lowest level of IMR is ranked first in terms of level. (2) T5, M5 and B5 indicate top, middle and bottom five states ranked as per the respective criteria (row/column). (3) Ranking for rural sector is omitted as positions of states are same as that for combined population. In other words, given its share in population, pattern of rural sector governs the pattern of combined population.

Rural-Urban Disparities

Rural areas have higher IMR than urban although the gap in absolute terms seems to be narrowing over time (Figure 1 and 2). The disparities can also be examined by computing the ratio of rural to urban IMR. Figure 5 shows the disparity between the sectors in absolute and relative

Figure 4

Distribution of IMR across Major States (excluding Kerala) by Sector

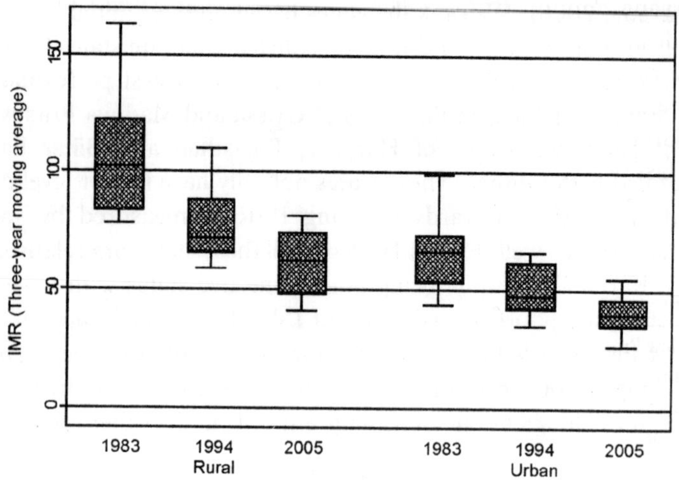

Figure 5

Rural-urban Disparities in IMR: All-India

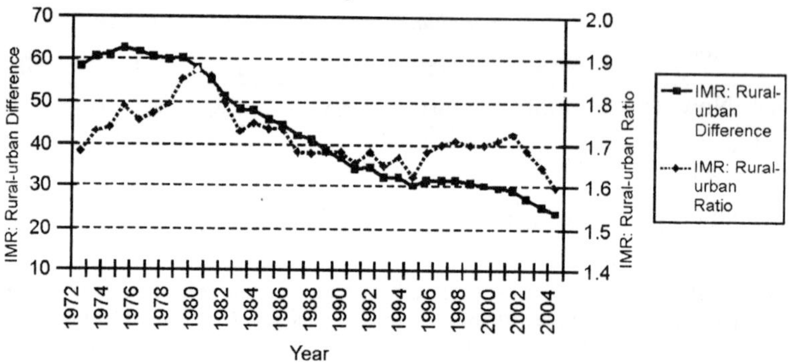

terms at the national level. This gap in absolute terms although halved during 1972–94, was stagnant during 1995–2002 before it started declining again in 2003. However, disparity as measured by rural-urban ratio increased till 1980, have shown declining trend till 1991, again increased during 1991–2003 before finally declining from 2003. Thus, during last three years the disparity indeed has declined. Table 4 shows rural-urban disparity ratio for IMR for 1972, 1983, 1994 and 2005 for major states. In 2005; IMR in rural areas was 160 per cent more than that in urban areas and rural-urban disparity was the highest in

Rajasthan and Assam and the lowest in Tamil Nadu. Disparity between 1994 and 2005 increased in the states Andhra Pradesh, Assam, Gujarat, Haryana and Rajasthan; decreased in the states Karnataka, Madhya Pradesh, Maharashtra, Orissa, Punjab, Tamil Nadu and West Bengal; and remained nearly constant in Bihar, Kerala and Uttar Pradesh. Compared to 1972, rural-urban gap in 2005 has widened in Assam, Gujarat, Maharashtra, Haryana and Kerala (increment is marginal for the last two states).

Table 4

Rural-urban Disparity Ratio for IMR

State	*1972*	*1983*	*1994*	*2005*	*State*	*1972*	*1983*	*1994*	*2005*
Andhra Pradesh	1.86	1.46	1.51	1.62	Maharashtra	1.39	1.50	1.89	1.56
Assam	1.68	1.36	1.23	1.75	Orissa	1.78	1.82	1.67	1.42
Bihar	—	1.54	1.36	1.35	Punjab	1.52	1.56	1.55	1.36
Gujarat	1.48	1.69	1.45	1.68	Rajasthan	1.71†	1.69	1.49	1.76
Haryana	1.35	1.62	1.13	1.39	Tamil Nadu	1.67	1.78	1.49	1.21
Karnataka	1.60	1.77	1.64	1.42	Uttar Pradesh	1.52	1.65	1.41	1.43
Kerala	1.33	1.23	1.33	1.36	West Bengal	—	1.75	1.47	1.32
Madhya Pradesh	1.60	1.78	1.73	1.50	All-India	1.69	1.73	1.69	1.58

Notes: (1) For Bihar, West Bengal data is available only from 1981 onwards. (2) † implies for Rajasthan, we use 1973 data (i.e., 1972–74 average).

Now, a relevant question to ask is whether IMR tend to be concentrated in some states? Or in other words, do the states with high/low IMR in rural areas have high/low IMR in urban areas as well and what has happened to this relationship over time? We estimate the rank correlation coefficient across the states for the two sectors. We find that the null hypothesis that IMR between the two sectors is independently distributed across the major states could be comfortably rejected for each of the years under study. The coefficient varies (over time) between 0.68–0.93 hinting that IMR tends to be concentrated in certain states/regions of states. Persistence of high value of coefficient means states performing poor/better continues to do so, and IMR seems to depend on state specific characteristics as well.

The annual average decline in IMR has been higher in rural areas than the urban (Table 1). The rate of decline too is higher in rural areas hinting towards presence of unconditional convergence, although this pattern is not uniform across states (Table 2). To understand progress towards eliminating these disparities prevailing across the two sectors, we form the grid as shown in Table 5 classifying the states according to the rate of reduction of IMR based on Table 2. We call the compounded annual rate of decline for a state as high, medium and low if that state's rank is among top-five, middle-five and bottom-five respectively. The disparity between the two sectors is minimal if a state belongs to one of three diagonal cells (High-High, Med-Med, and Low-Low). The grid highlights the following features:

- In general, south Indian states have recorded a high/medium rate of decline in urban sector. Barring Uttar Pradesh, BIMARU states have the medium/low rate of decline in both the sectors.
- Haryana and Orissa need serious attention for having slowest rates of decline in both the sectors. In these states, rural-urban disparities are one of the minimum (Table 4). This implies that merely elimination of disparities is not enough unless it is accompanied by sustained improvement in the level as well. In urban Haryana, IMR is almost stagnant since 1990s. The state started with lower than national average IMR in 1972 and ended up with IMR in 2003 that the country has achieved a decade earlier. Haryana is one of states with very uneven sex ratio. IMR in urban Haryana was 67 for girls against 30 for boys (Office of the Registrar General, 2007b). This probably indicates bias towards girl child.
- On the other extreme, Kerala, Gujarat and Uttar Pradesh have witnessed one of fastest decline in both the sectors and need to sustain it.

Two states of South-India, Andhra Pradesh and Karnataka have registered slower decline in rural areas. In rural sector, Karnataka has almost bridged the negative gap between its IMR and national average since 1972.

Table 5

Rural-urban Disparities in IMR Decline

Sector/Rate of decline		*Urban*		
		High	Med	Low
Rural	High	KER, GUJ, UP	TN, WB	
	Med	MAH, PB, AS		BIH, RAJ
	Low		AP, MP, KA	HR, OR

Notes: (1) High, medium and low in each sector refers to top, medium and bottom five states in terms of rate of decline of IMR.

V

Convergence in Infant Mortality

We examine both the absolute and conditional convergence across the states.

Absolute Convergence

Absolute convergence can be examined using time path of the standard deviation of IMR across the states as shown in Figure 6, separately for rural, urban and combined population. The figure indicates that the dispersion across states has reduced to almost half for rural as well as urban population during 1972–2005. In both the sectors the time path of dispersion has followed same pattern except the period 1986–93, during which the decline was 20 per cent in rural areas and merely four in urban. The figure also shows that dispersion in both sectors did not decline during 1995–2001 though it has declined in the following years.

Figure 6

Absolute Convergence across States: 1972–2005

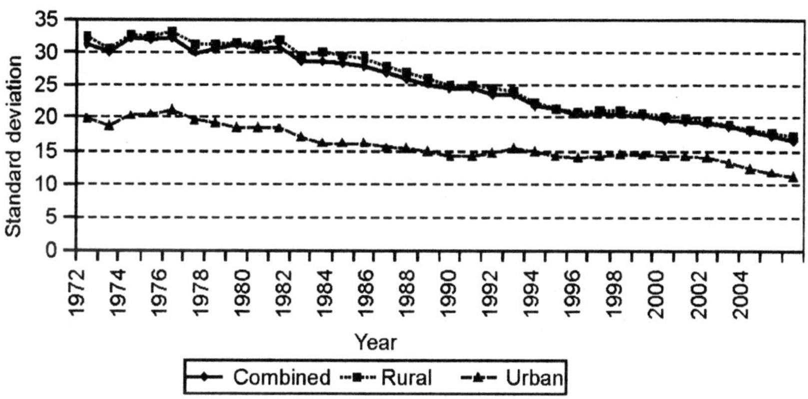

In sum, states show sign of sigma-convergence in IMR. This implies that levels of IMR across the states tend to converge independent of their structural characteristics/initial conditions. Given the fact that necessary condition for existence of sigma-convergence is beta-convergence; it implies that on average, IMR is declining faster in the states with lower level of IMR than the states with higher level of IMR. However, slow pace of IMR during the last decade is of concern.

Conditional Convergence

The conditional convergence controls for structural characteristics by taking into account some of these in the regression equation as discussed earlier (see equation 2). We use an unbalanced panel from 1972–2005 to test for conditional-convergence across the states. It is unbalanced for number of observations for each state and differs as pointed out earlier. Greene (2003) discusses some modifications needed while estimating parameters in such unbalanced panels. However, no correction for the coefficient is necessary in a LSDV model. Table 6 reports the fixed effect results for the period 1972–2005. The results provide evidence for existence of the conditional convergence. Here, PCI is included just as a control variable and because this is not a structural model for determinants of IMR; we do not bother to interpret it.

Table 6

Conditional Convergence: Fixed Effect Regression (1972–2005)

Variable	*Coefficient*	*Standard Error*
IMR (lag)	0.95	0.01
Ln (Per Capita Income)	–2.70	1.06
Const	26.12	10.28
R^2	0.99	
No of Observations	474	
No of Groups	15	

Notes: (1) dependent variable is three-year averaged IMR of the current period. (2) All the coefficients are statistically significant at five per cent level.

In another approach to test convergence, we classify the states based on their rank in PCI in two groups such that each group contains seven states. Similar states should be grouped in same group (Sala-i-Martin, 1996). We exclude Kerala from this analysis for it is an outlier as discussed earlier and its presence can affect our conclusions. Group A consists of poorest seven states – BIMARU states, Assam and West Bengal; remaining states excluding Kerala are clubbed in Group B (richer states). Figure 7 shows the dispersion in IMR for the two groups during 1982–2005. It highlights the following features:

1. The dispersion is higher in poor states than the rich. It implies that the IMR among the rich states vary less than that among the poor states. In other words, ability of per capita income in explaining the variation in IMR across the states might differ with the level of

Figure 7

Conditional Convergence across States: 1982–2005

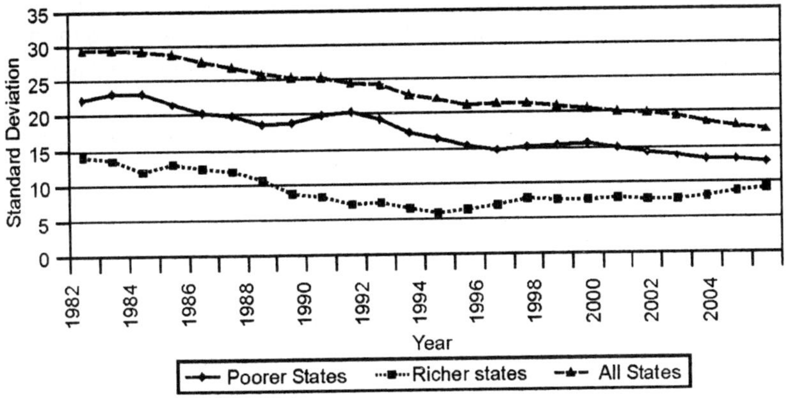

income. PCI may be more closely associated with IMR at higher level of income.

2. The dispersion across the poor states is declining steadily whereas for the richer states it increased in recent years after declining initially. This might be because of the fact that the level of IMR being higher in poor states continues to decline faster than the level of IMR in richer states.
3. Narrowing of the curves for the poorer and richer states indicates towards presence of convergence. But this convergence has not been uniform and during 1987–91, the gap between the two increased.

VI

Conclusions

We study disparities prevailing across the states and sectors in IMR and how does it correlate to the PCI. We do neither aim to determine structural or any other factors explaining variations in IMR nor aim to find out why certain states have phenomenally reduced the IMR. We, however study how the IMR changes over the years. Major conclusions from this study that need further exploration are the following:

1. With current rate of decline, the country is most likely to miss the target of IMR/child mortality as quantified in MDGs and other policy documents.

2. Reducing IMR is important to stabilize population. However, recent deceleration in IMR across states is likely to have implications for population policy for (i) contribution of IMR is about 20 per cent in explaining the high population growth, and (ii) decline in mortality usually precedes fertility decline (Planning Commission, 2006 and Ministry of Health and Family Welfare, 2002). If steps are not taken at appropriate time, it may hinder the goal of achieving a stable population by 2045.
3. States of Orissa and Madhya Pradesh need urgent attention. Not only the level of IMR is higher in these states, but the rate of reduction of IMR too is slow. Similar is the case with Haryana, Rajasthan and Bihar.
4. Rural areas have done well in reducing IMR both at the aggregate and at the states' level and thus there are signs of inter-sector convergence. However, during 1994–2003 the inter-sector disparity has increased.
5. Persistence of high IMR in some of the states is of concern. States having high IMR in 1970s continue to have the same in 2000 also and this is true for both the sectors.
6. We find evidence for inter-sector convergence both absolute and conditional. Presence of unconditional convergence means that dispersion of IMR across the states have declined over time and on an average, states with higher level of IMR show high rate of decline. Presence of convergence conditional on SDP per capita implies that the levels of IMR among initially poor and richer group of states tend to converge over time.

References

Agarwal, S.P. 2005. "Towards Achieving Millennium Development Goals in the Health Sector in India", *Journal, Indian Academy of Clinical Medicine* 6:4 (October-December), pp. 268–74.

Barro, Robert J. and Xavier Sala-i-Martin. 1995. *Economic Growth*, The MIT Press.

Bhat, P.N. Mari. 2002. "Completeness of India's Sample Registration System: An Assessment Using the General Growth Balance Method", *Population Studies*, 56:2, pp. 119–34.

Central Bureau of Health Intelligence. 2005. "Health Information of India 2005", Central Bureau of Health Intelligence, Directorate General of Health Services, Ministry of Health and Family Welfare, Govt. of India.

Claeson, Mariam, Eduard Bos and Indra Pathmanathan. 1999. "Reducing Child Mortality in India: Keeping Up the Pace", Health, Nutrition and Population (HNP) Discussion Paper, World Bank, Washington, DC.

Countdown Coverage Writing Group. 2008. "Countdown to 2015 for Maternal, Newborn, and Child Survival: The 2008 Report on Tracking Coverage of Interventions", *The Lancet*, 371, pp. 1247–58.

Deaton, Angus and Jean Dreze. 2002. "Poverty and Inequality in India: A Re-Examination", *Economic and Political Weekly,* September 7.

Durlauf, S.N., P.A. Johnson and Temple J.R.W. 2005. "Growth Econometrics", in P. Aghion and S.N. Durlauf (eds.), *Handbook of Economic Growth,* North Holland.

EPWRF. 2003. "Domestic Products of States of India: 1960–61 to 2000–01", *Economic and Political Weekly,* Research Foundation, Mumbai.

Galor, Oded. 1996. "Convergence? Inferences from Theoretical Models", *The Economic Journal*, 106:437, July, pp. 1056–69.

Greene, William. 2003. *Econometric Analysis* (Fifth Edition), Pearson Education, Inc.

Gujarati, Damodar N. 2005. *Basic Econometrics* (Fourth Edition). New Delhi: Tata McGraw-Hill.

International Institute for Population Sciences (IIPS) and Macro International. 2007. National Family Health Survey (NFHS–III), 2005–06: India, Volume I. Mumbai: IIPS.

Islam, Nazrul. 1995. "Growth Empirics: A Panel Data Approach", *Quarterly Journal of Economics,* CX, pp. 1127–70.

Ministry of Health and Family Welfare. 2000. "National Population Policy 2000", Ministry of Health and Family Welfare, Government of India. Accessed at www.mohfw.nic.in on March 1, 2008.

Narayana, D. 2008. "Intensifying Infant Mortality Inequality in India and a Reversal by Policy Intervention", *Journal of Human Development*, 9: 2, pp. 265–81.

Office of the Registrar General, India. 1981. "Sampling Variability of SRS Vital Rates: 1975–77", Ministry of Home Affairs, Government of India: New Delhi.

Office of the Registrar General, India. 1993. "Sample Registration System: Fertility and Mortality Indicators 1991", Ministry of Home Affairs, Government of India: New Delhi.

Office of the Registrar General, India. 2007a. "Baseline Survey Report 2004", Ministry of Home Affairs, Government of India: New Delhi.

Office of the Registrar General, India. 2007b. "Sample Registration System: Statistical Report 2006", Ministry of Home Affairs, Government of India: New Delhi.

Planning Commission. "Report of the Working Group on Population Stabilization for the Eleventh Five-Year Plan (2007–12)", Planning Commission, Govt. of India: New Delhi.

Planning Commission. 2006. "Towards Faster and More Inclusive Growth: An Approach to the 11th Five-Year Plan", Planning Commission, Government of India: New Delhi.

Preston, Samuel H. 1975. "The Changing Relation between Mortality and Level of Economic Development", *Population Studies*, 29: 2, pp. 231–48.

Reserve Bank of India. 2006. "Handbook of Statistics on Indian Economy", Reserve Bank of India: Mumbai.

Sala-i-Martin, Xavier X. 1996. "The Classical Approach to Convergence Analysis", *The Economic Journal*, 106:437, July, pp. 1019–36.

Sen, Amartya. 1998. "Mortality as an Indicator of Economic Success and Failure", *The Economic Journal*, 108:446, Jan. pp. 1–25.

UNDP. 2007. "Human Development Report 2007/2008", United Nations Development Programme (UNDP), published by Palgrave Macmillan, New York.

UNICEF. 2008a. "The State of the World's Children 2008", United Nations Children's Fund (UNICEF), New York.

UNICEF. 2008b. "Tracking Progress in Maternal, Newborn and Child Survival: The 2008 Report, V2", Countdown to 2015: Maternal, Newborn and Child Survival. United Nations Children's Fund (UNICEF), New York.

Visaria, Leela. 2004. "Mortality Trends and the Health Transition", in *Twenty-first Century India: Population, Economy, Human Development and the Environment,* Tim Dyson, Robert Cassen and Leela Visaria (eds.), Oxford University Press.

Wermuth, Laurie. 2003. *Global Inequality and Human Needs: Health and Illness in an Increasingly Unequal World,* Pearson Education, Inc.

Wooldridge, Jeffrey M. 2002. *Econometric Analysis of Cross Section and Panel Data,*. Cambridge, Massachusetts: The MIT Press.

World Bank. 2004. "Attaining the Millennium Development Goals in India: Role of Public Policy and Service Delivery", World Bank: Washington DC.

13

Gender Discrimination in Health Care

SAUMYA CHAND

In India, excess female mortality and a preference for sons has existed for centuries. In the past 100 years, population sex ratios from censuses have shown more or less a continuous decline from 972 females per 1,000 males in 1901 to 933 females per 1,000 males in 2001. Indian censuses since 1872 have noted masculine sex ratios. "In many parts of the world, women receive less attention and health care than men do, and particularly girls often receive very much less support than boys. As a result of this gender bias, the mortality rates of females often exceed those of males in these countries" (Sen, 2001).

This is an important issue because gender discrimination that contributes to poorer health status for girls than for boys is likely to be the main pathway for excess female child mortality. Such discrimination occurs in India was recognized at least as early as the 1901 census, which noted that "there is no doubt that, as a rule, she (a girl) receives less attention than would be bestowed upon a son. She is less warmly clad; she is probably not so well fed as a boy would be, and when ill, her parents are not likely to make the same strenuous efforts to ensure her recovery" (1901 census). There has been a growing international concern on the issue of higher female mortality, declining sex ratio and missing females in India (Sen, 1990; Das Gupta and Baht, 1997; Sudha and Rajan, 1998; Mayer, 1999; Bose, 2001; Guiliot, 1998; Patel, 2004; Arokiasamy, 2004)

The subordinate status of women in India is largely a result of patriarchy and its influences on the social, cultural and religious aspects of life. A patriarchal structure is based on the foundation that the family line runs through a male – that is, all descent and inheritance are traced through the male. This has resulted in an exalted status for the male and reduced the woman to a secondary position, dependent on and controlled by different men in the family – father, brother, husband, son – at the various stages of her life.

One of the main reasons why daughters are considered a liability is the dowry required to get them married. The perception that daughters belong to their marital home, families take this as double burden along with dowry. An investment in daughters is therefore considered one without returns. In a market-driven society and with the commercialization of the institution of marriage, the cost of marriage itself has gone up. In most cases, this cost is borne by the girls' family. Thus dowry – sometimes repeated demands for it, cost of marriage and an investment in bringing up a daughter who cannot carry forward the family name and offer old-age support, are factors that contribute to more and more families seeing sense in eliminating daughters. The most common logic being, it is better to invest Rs 5,000 now than Rs 50 lakh later. What is the cause of female foeticide? The answer is simple: girls are liabilities, boys are assets. Girls mean dowry and with growing greed (Bose, 2001).The exceedingly greater care and vigilance in raising daughters and in protecting their sexuality, in arranging for grooms, dowry, and life-long presentations and gifts, are conducive in making girls an avoidable proposition (Patel, 2004).

A preference for certain sex may affect the treatment of sons and daughters and even their chances of survival. Gender discrimination is believed to be the principal cause of excess female mortality that is often manifested during childhood.

Sex differentials in child mortality are much higher in the northern than the southern states of India. The main reason for the relatively high sex ratio in the northern part of the country is higher female mortality due to the discrimination against females in access to food and medical care (Dyson and Moore, 1983).

Objectives

The main objectives of this paper are:

- To emphasize the practice of gender discrimination in health care facilities such as antenatal care, maternal care, and impact of gender discrimination in health care facilities, especially on female mortality and sex ratio.
- To analyse regional variations in health care facilities, female mortality and sex ratio.
- To make suggestions for improvization of better health facilities for women in India to reduce excess female mortality.

Sources of Data

- Data for the present study has been taken from Census of India, National Family Health Surveys and Bulletin of Sample Registration System. To study the regional variation in sex ratio, mortality and health care facilities states/UTs are grouped into four regions:
- North/North-West India
- South India
- East/North-East India
- Central and Western India

There has been a pronounced difference between male and female childhood mortality rate. Infant and child mortality in India is higher for girls. Thus, while there has been improvement in overall female mortality over time, the discrimination against the girl child has continued in Indian society. There is no clear pattern in the difference between the female and male mortality rate hence part of the decline in sex ratio seems to be result of this discrimination.

Gender discrimination and son preference are closely associated with the declining sex ratio and infant and child mortality. Socio-cultural and biological factors together influence the overall demographic composition of a population and its sex ratio (SR). As a key demographic indicator, sex ratio generally depicts the number of males per 100 females in a given population. In international demographic terms, a "high sex-ratio" society is defined as one that has disproportionately more males, and a "low sex-ratio" society that has disproportionately less females.

However, in India, the sex ratio is expressed as the number of females per 1,000 males in a given population. Thus here a declining sex ratio indicates that the number of females is getting disproportionately less. In India, as per the last census, there are 933 females per 1,000 males. In India, the last century was marked by an almost continual decline in the country's SR. The beginning of the 21st century has shown a marginal increase of 6 points (from 927 in 1991 to 933 in 2001).

Regional variations in the sex ratio reflect the diverse levels of social obstacles that girls and women face in different parts of the country. These factors have affected the natural balance of the male and female population. The greater the obstacles the lower the sex ratio. The situation is worse in the north-western states of India, in this region the most affected states/UTs are Punjab, Haryana, Himachal Pradesh and Chandigarh, in central and western India there was sharp decline in the overall sex ratio with respect to Dadra and Nagar Haveli and Daman and Diu.

Sex Ratio in India

Table 1 shows the sex ratio pattern in India over the census 1991–2001.

Table 1

Overall Sex Ratio in India for 1991 and 2001

Regions	*States/UTs*	*Sex ratio*		*Changes*
		1991	*2001*	
India		927	933	6
North/North-West India	Chandigarh	790	777	–13
	Delhi	827	821	–6
	Haryana	865	861	–4
	Himachal Pradesh	976	968	–8
	Jammu & Kashmir	923	892	–31
	Punjab	882	876	–6
	Rajasthan	910	921	11
	Uttarakhand	NA	962	—
	Uttar Pradesh	879	898	19
South India	Andaman & Nicobar Islands	818	846	28
	Andhra Pradesh	972	978	6
	Karnataka	960	965	5
	Kerala	1036	1058	22
	Lakshadweep	943	948	5
	Pondicherry	979	1001	22
	Tamil Nadu	974	987	13
East/North-East India	Arunachal Pradesh	859	893	34
	Assam	923	935	12
	Bihar	911	919	8
	Jharkhand	NA	941	—
	Manipur	958	978	20

Cont'd...

Cont'd...

	Meghalaya	955	972	17
	Mizoram	921	935	14
	Nagaland	886	900	14
	Sikkim	878	875	–3
	Tripura	945	948	3
	West Bengal	917	934	17
Central and Western India	Chhattisgarh	NA	989	—
	Dadra & Nagar Haveli	952	812	–140
	Daman & Diu	969	710	–259
	Goa	967	961	–6
	Gujarat	934	999	65
	Madhya Pradesh	931	919	–12
	Maharashtra	934	922	–12
	Orissa	971	972	1

Source: Census of India, 2001.

Table 1 shows that situation is worse in the north-western states of India, in this region the most affected states/UTs are Punjab, Haryana, Himachal Pradesh and Chandigarh. In central and western India there was sharp decline in the overall sex ratio with respect to Dadra and Nagar Haveli and Daman and Diu which shows the decline of 140 and 259 points respectively.

In India, sex preference is mainly manifested in the form of excessive mortality of female child. The excessive mortality of female relatively to males is found to be due to the discrimination against females in the allocation of food and health care within the household.

Differentials in Early Childhood Mortality Rates by Sex

Table 2 shows differentials in mortality rates for the males and females. Considering the data it is seen that the infant mortality rate is marginally

Table 2

Neonatal, Postnatal, Child and Under-Five Mortality Rates in India for the NFHS–I, NFHS–II and NFHS–III

	NFHS–I		*NFHS–II*		*NFHS–III*	
	Male	*Female*	*Male*	*Female*	*Male*	*Female*
Neonatal mortality	57.0	48.1	50.7	44.6	40.9	36.8
Postnatal mortality	31.7	35.8	24.2	26.6	15.4	20.9
Child mortality	29.4	42.0	14.6	19.7	14.2	22.9
Under five mortality	115.4	122.4	97.9	105.2	69.7	79.2

Source: National Family Health Survey I, II and III. Department of Family Welfare, Government of India.

higher for females than males. However, in the neonatal period, mortality is lower for females than for males. As children get older, females are exposed to higher mortality than males due to discrimination against girls and greater parental care and favoured treatment with regard to food and medical attention for male children.

Infant mortality rate is marginally higher for females and there is great and significant variation in infant mortality rate across states. Table 3 shows infant mortality of males and females for 2006 by states. F-M gap shows the gap between male and female infant mortality rate. It has been firmly established that the main reason for the relatively low sex ratio in India is higher female mortality which is influenced by practice of discrimination against females in access to food and medical care facilities.

Table 3

Infant Mortality Rate by Sex in India and States for 2006

Regions	*States/UTs*	*Total*	*Male*	*Female*	*F-M (Gap)*
India		57	56	59	3
North/North-West India	Chandigarh	23	20	27	7
	Delhi	37	36	39	3
	Haryana	57	57	58	1
	Himachal Pradesh	50	45	55	10
	Jammu & Kashmir	52	51	53	2
	Punjab	44	39	50	11
	Rajasthan	67	65	69	4
	Uttarakhand	43	42	44	2
	Uttar Pradesh	71	70	73	3
South India	Andaman & Nicobar Islands	31	27	36	9
	Andhra Pradesh	56	55	58	3
	Karnataka	48	46	50	4
	Kerala	15	14	16	2
	Lakshadweep	25	29	21	–8
	Pondicherry	28	20	36	16
	Tamil Nadu	37	36	37	1
East/North-East India	Arunachal Pradesh	40	38	43	5
	Assam	67	67	68	1
	Bihar	60	58	63	5
	Jharkhand	49	46	52	6
	Manipur	11	10	13	3

Cont'd...

Cont'd...

	Meghalaya	53	53	52	–1
	Mizoram	25	24	25	1
	Nagaland	20	17	23	6
	Sikkim	33	26	40	14
	Tripura	36	31	41	10
	West Bengal	38	37	40	3
Central and Western India	Chhattisgarh	61	59	62	3
	Dadra & Nagar Haveli	35	28	27	1
	Daman & Diu	28	28	28	0
	Goa	15	16	14	–2
	Gujarat	53	52	54	2
	Madhya Pradesh	74	72	77	5
	Maharashtra	35	35	36	1
	Orissa	73	73	74	1

Source: SRS Bulletin (2007), Sample Registration System, Registrar General of India, Vol. 42.

Considering the data for India as a whole, it is seen that the infant mortality rate is marginally higher for females (59) than males (56). Difference is higher in northern and north-west Indian states like Punjab, Himachal Pradesh. Himachal Pradesh shows high F-M gap of 10, Punjab shows 11. In east and north-east regions Sikkim and Tripura shows high F-M gap which are 14 and 10 correspondingly. Table 3 shows that infant mortality for the 2006 is higher for females than for males and F-M gap shows the gap between male and female infant mortality rate.

The long-term moderately excess female mortality in the country over a period of time has been mainly due to the gender discrimination. It can be seen in the form of:

- A pronounced preference for a male child
- Bias in the intra-household distribution of food and nutritive elements
- Poor medical care facilities for women

A Pronounced Preference for a Male Child

Son preference is the desire to have a high proportion of sons as compared to daughters, which affects the child mortality, sex ratio and fertility. There are many factors related to the gender preference. Theses factors can be classified into micro and macro factors. Micro-level factor includes the individual characteristics of parents, socio-economic status of parents. Macro-level factor includes fertility rate, population policies, cultural setting and socio-economic factors. Rapid decline in fertility and two-child family norms has increased the concern of son preference among couples. In some cases, parents are prepared to accept the daughter if she happens to be the first child but thereafter they want only sons. A strong preference for sons has been found to be pervasive in Indian society, affecting both attitudes and behaviour with respect to children and the choice regarding number and sex composition of children. In NFHS–III, women aged 15–49 and men aged 15–54 who gave a numerical response to the question on the ideal number of children were asked how many of these children they would like to be boys, how many they would like to be girls, and for how many the sex would not matter. Table 4 shows the percentage who desire more sons than daughters, the percentage who desire more daughters than sons, in India and states over the period of 1998–99 and 2005–06. The tables shows a consistent preference for sons over daughters, although table, son preference has declined from NFHS–II to NFHS–III.

Indicators of Sex Preference by States

Table 4

Percentage of Women Who Want More Sons than Daughters and Percentage Who Want more Daughters than Son for Ever Married Women in India and States, NFHS–II (1998–99) and NFHS–III (2005–06)

Regions	*States/UTs*	*Percentage who want more sons than daughters*		*Percentage who want more daughters than sons*	
		NFHS–II	*NFHS–III*	*NFHS–II*	*NFHS–III*
India		33.2	22.4	2.2	2.6
North/North-West India	Delhi	23.1	11.7	2.6	2.1
	Haryana	37.5	22.0	0.5	1.2
	Himachal Pradesh	25.9	11.8	0.6	2.0
	Jammu & Kashmir	38	23.4	2.7	3.1
	Punjab	29.1	17.7	0.4	1.6
	Rajasthan	47.5	34.3	1.3	1.54
	Uttarakhand	N.A.	20.7	N.A.	2.1
	Uttar Pradesh	53.3	33.5	1.4	1.7
South India	Andhra Pradesh	19.8	9.3	2.7	2.6
	Karnataka	13.0	11.6	1.9	4.6
	Kerala	14.6	11.0	5.2	5.7
	Lakshadweep	N.A.	N.A.	N.A.	N.A.
	Pondicherry	N.A.	N.A.	N.A	N.A.
	Tamil Nadu	9.6	5.7	1.9	3.1

Cont'd...

Cont'd...

East/North-East India	Arunachal Pradesh	41.9	28.3	2.5	5.0
	Assam	38.2	24.1	2.9	2.1
	Bihar	47.9	39.2	2.1	1.2
	Jharkhand	N.A.	28.1	N.A.	2.3
	Manipur	36.5	28.5	4.8	4.2
	Meghalaya	20.9	11.9	16.9	17.0
	Mizoram	26.0	29.0	19.0	22.7
	Nagaland	32.7	21.4	6.3	9.8
	Sikkim	22.4	15.5	3.1	5.9
	Tripura	N.A.	17.7	N.A.	3.4
	West Bengal	20.7	16.5	3.4	3.5
Central and Western India	Chhattisgarh	N.A.	32.8	N.A.	3.6
	Dadra & Nagar Haveli	N.A.	N.A.	N.A.	N.A.
	Daman & Diu	N.A.	N.A.	N.A.	N.A.
	Goa	17.0	8.7	5.1	4.1
	Gujarat	33.2	22.7	1.8	2.3
	Madhya Pradesh	42.5	30.8	2.9	1.8
	Maharashtra	27.1	14.1	1.9	2.9
	Orissa	20.7	24.2	3.4	2.4

Sources: National Family Health Survey–III (2005–06).

Table 4 presents strong preference for sons among women age 15–49 by state. According to NFHS–II, 32 per cent of women want more sons than daughters and only 2 per cent of women want more daughters than sons. According to NFHS–III, 22 per cent of women want more sons than daughters, but only 3 per cent want more daughters than sons.

Twenty per cent of men want more sons than daughters, but only 2 per cent want more daughters than sons. According to this table, son preference has declined from NFHS–II to NFHS–III. The data shows son preference attitudes among women age 15–49 by states. The strength of son preference varies substantially across the states. Son preference tends to be stronger in the northern part of the country, especially in Bihar, Uttar Pradesh, and Rajasthan. Other states with a particularly high son preference include Arunachal Pradesh, Madhya Pradesh, Chhattisgarh, Manipur, Jharkhand, and Jammu & Kashmir. The weakest son preference is found in the South and West Regions and parts of the Northeast Region. States with particularly low, but still discernible, son preference include Tamil Nadu, Goa, Kerala, Karnataka, Himachal Pradesh and Delhi.

Poor Medical Care Facilities for Women

According to NFHS–III almost one out of every five women in India did not receive any antenatal care for their last birth in the five years preceding the survey. There is wide variation in the use of antenatal care services among the states. Utilization of antenatal care is almost universal in Kerala, Tamil Nadu and Goa. In addition, more than 90 per cent of women received ANC in Andhra Pradesh, Maharashtra, West Bengal, Karnataka, Delhi and Punjab. The percentage of women receiving antenatal care was lowest in Bihar.

Table 5

Indicators of Health Care Facilities for Women in India and States (2005–06)

Regions	*States/UTs*	*Antenatal care*		*Maternity care*	
		Mothers who had at least 3 antenatal care visits for their last birth (%)	*Mothers who consumed IFA for 90 days or more when they were pregnant with their last child (%)*	*Birth assisted by a doctor/ nurse/other health personnel (%)*	*Institutional births (%)*
India		52.0	23.1	48.2	40.7
North/North-West India	Chandigarh	N.A.	N.A.	N.A.	N.A.
	Delhi	75.1	39.5	65.1	60.7
	Haryana	59.2	26.7	54.2	39.4
	Himachal Pradesh	62.6	37.9	50.2	45.3
	Jammu & Kashmir	73.5	27	60.5	54.3
	Punjab	74.8	27.9	68.6	52.5
	Rajasthan	41.2	13.1	43.2	32.2
	Uttarakhand	44.9	26.4	29.2	22.0
	Uttar Pradesh	26.6	8.8	41.5	36.0

Cont'd...

Cont'd...

South India	Andaman & Nicobar Islands	N.A.	N.A.	N.A.	N.A.
	Andhra Pradesh	85.4	41.2	74.2	68.6
	Karnataka	79.5	39.3	71.3	66.9
	Kerala	93.6	75.1	99.7	99.5
	Lakshadweep	N.A.	N.A.	N.A.	N.A.
	Pondicherry	N.A.	N.A.	N.A.	N.A.
	Tamil Nadu	95.9	41.6	93.2	90.4
East/North-East India	Arunachal Pradesh	35.5	11.2	74.2	68.6
	Assam	39.3	16.2	31.2	22.7
	Bihar	17.0	9.7	30.9	22.0
	Jharkhand	35.9	14.2	28.7	19.2
	Manipur	69.6	13.1	61.7	49.3
	Meghalaya	54.0	16.7	31.7	29.7
	Mizoram	59.3	24.7	69.4	64.6
	Nagaland	32.7	3.5	725.9	12.2
	Sikkim	70.1	38.7	55.8	49.0
	Tripura	60.0	18.0	50.0	48.9
	West Bengal	62	25.7	45.7	43.1
Central and Western India	Chhattisgarh	54.2	20.7	44.3	15.7
	Dadra & Nagar Haveli	N.A.	N.A.	N.A.	N.A.
	Daman & Diu	N.A.	N.A.	N.A.	N.A.
	Goa	94.9	69.6	94.3	92.6
	Gujarat	67.5	37.9	64.7	54.6
	Madhya Pradesh	40.7	12.4	37.1	29.7
	Maharashtra	75.1	31.4	70.7	66.1
	Orissa	61.8	33.8	46.4	38.7

Source: National Family Health Survey–III (2005–06).

Table 5 shows antenatal and maternity care indicators by states. Columns 3 and 4 present percentage of live births during the five years preceding the survey whose mothers received different types of antenatal care for their most recent birth. The utilization of antenatal care services differs greatly by states. Goa, Kerala and Tamil Nadu rank in the top five states in the country in the terms of their performance on almost all of the indicators. In these three states, mothers 94–96 per cent had three or more visits, 42–75 per cent took IFA tablets for at least 90 days. Bihar ranks the lowest of the antenatal care indicators. Uttar Pradesh, Jharkhand and Rajasthan also perform poorly on health care indicators. Fifth and sixth column presents maternal care indicators which shows that in India only 48 per cent births are delivered by doctors, nurse or other health personnel and 40 per cent births are delivered in medical institutions.

Nutritional Status of Women and Men in India

For women, weight and height measurement can be used to access health risks. A widely used indicator of nutritional status is the body mass index (BMI), which is defined as the weight in kilograms divided by height in metres squared (kg/m^2). This indicator is used to assess both thinness and obesity. It is helpful in detecting the risk of health or nutritional disorders. A BMI of less than 18.5 indicates chronic energy deficiency (CED). At the other end of the spectrum, women with a BMI of 25.0–29.9 are considered to be overweight and those with a BMI of 30.0 or above are identified as obese. Table 6 shows the percentage of women and men age 15–49 in India who have chronic energy deficiency and the percentage who are over weight. Around 36 per cent women have chronic energy deficiency and 13 per cent women are overweight.

Table 6

Indicators of Nutritional Status of Women in India and States

	States/UTs	*Women whose body mass index is below normal %*	*Women who are overweight or obesity %*
India		35.6	12.6
North/North-West India	Chandigarh	N.A.	N.A.
	Delhi	14.8	26.4
	Haryana	31.3	17.4
	Himachal Pradesh	29.9	13.5
	Jammu & Kashmir	24.6	16.7
	Punjab	18.9	29.9
	Rajasthan	36.7	8.9
	Uttarakhand	30.0	12.8
	Uttar Pradesh	36.0	9.2
South India	Andaman & Nicobar Islands	N.A.	N.A.
	Andhra Pradesh	33.5	12.6

Cont'd...

Cont'd...

	Karnataka	33.5	15.3
	Kerala	19.0	29.1
	Lakshadweep	N.A.	N.A.
	Pondicherry	N.A.	N.A.
	Tamil Nadu	28.4	20.9
East/North-East India	Arunachal Pradesh	16.4	8.8
	Assam	36.5	7.8
	Bihar	45.1	4.5
	Jharkhand	43.0	5.4
	Manipur	14.8	13.3
	Meghalaya	14.6	5.3
	Mizoram	14.0	10.6
	Nagaland	17.4	6.4
	Sikkim	11.2	15.4
	Tripura	36.9	7.1
	West Bengal	39.1	11.4
Central and Western India	Chhattisgarh	43.4	5.6
	Dadra & Nagar Haveli	N.A.	N.A.
	Daman & Diu	N.A.	N.A.
	Goa	27.9	20.2
	Gujarat	36.3	16.7
	Madhya Pradesh	41.7	7.6
	Maharashtra	36.2	14.5
	Orissa	41.4	6.6

Source: National Family Health Survey–III (2005–06).

Table 6 shows that 36 per cent women in India have chronic energy deficiency and 13 per cent women are overweight. Level of CED is high in the states of Chhattisgarh, Orissa, Madhya Pradesh, Bihar, and Jharkhand and Uttar Pradesh. CED is particularly pronounced for rural women, illiterate women, and women living in households with a low standard of living and among those women who do not consume proper nutritious food.

Bias in the Intra-household Distribution of Food and Nutritive Elements

In India, sex preference is mainly manifested in the form of excessive mortality of female child. The excessive mortality of female relatively to males is found to be due to the discrimination against females in the allocation of food and health care within household. Table 7 presents the difference in male and female food consumption. It is clear that men consume more nutritious food than women.

Table 7

Percentage Distribution of Women and Men aged 15–49 Consuming Specific Foods at Least Once a Week in India, 2005–06

Type of food	*Men*	*Women*
Milk or curd	67.2	55.4
Pulses or beans	90.7	89.5
Dark green leafy vegetables	93.6	92.9
Fruits	47.4	39.8
Eggs	41.	32.3
Fish	31.3	28.2
Chicken or meat	28.3	22.7
Fish or chicken/meat	40.9	35.4

Sources: National Family Health Survey–III (2005–06), Department of Family Welfare, Government of India

Table 7 shows that women consume less nutritious food than man.

Differentials in Vaccination of Children by Sex in India and States

Table 8

Percentage of Children aged 12–33 Months Who Receive Specific Vaccine

		Male	*Female*
BCG		80.2	75.8
DPT	1	78.4	73.2
	2	69.2	63.8
	3	57.4	53.0
Polio	0	50.4	46.2
	1	94.1	91.9
	2	89.5	88.0
	3	79.3	77.1
Measles		61.4	55.8
All Basic Vaccination		45.3	41.5
No Vaccination		4.3	6.0

Sources: National Family Health Survey–III (2005–06).

There is difference in percentage of men and women who received vaccines, women received less number of vaccination than men over the period of 2005–06.

What should be done?

The high number of "missing girls" is indicative of the poor status of the girl child and of women. The overpowering desire to have a male child stems from perceived economic and social benefits that are not rooted in current reality: a son does not have to be married off with a dowry; he will grow up to be the breadwinner and support his parents (the fact that this is not always true is another matter!), he will carry the family name forward. A daughter is seen as a burden from day one. While the pregnant women herself may sometimes be a willing participant in this exercise, most often she is forced to opt for prenatal sex determination and made to get rid of the female foetus under tremendous social and family pressure to deliver a male child. She does so at considerable risk to her own life, as such abortions are usually performed in the fourth or fifth month of pregnancy. The woman's own status and survival within the household is dependent on whether or not she gives the family its heir. Consequences of not doing so are often desertion, abandonment and unending mental and sometimes physical trauma.

Such elimination of the girl child points to a rot in the social and cultural fabric of societies. It is imperative that all sectors join in to change the mindset and attitude that allows and encourages this crime and discrimination. And both doctors and the general public have an equal responsibility in helping bring about this change.

The falling sex ratio is definitely a matter of concern. The situation is definitely a matter of concern. In Indian context there is a strong preference for sons. This preference is influenced by various social cultural and economic factors, such as the son being responsible for carrying forward the family name and occupation especially in agricultural sector.

The practice of dowry and daughter being viewed as "Paraya Dhan" is yet another reason why sons are preferred to daughters. If this phenomenon continues, than a stage will reach when it would difficult to make up for the missing girls. Society needs to recognize this discrimination. Girls have a right to live just as boys do.

From the foregoing discussion it has been firmly established that the main reason for the relatively low sex ratio and higher female mortality in India is influenced by practice of discrimination against females in access to food and medical care facilities.

Also, it seems that the increasing new medical technologies and facilities may provide more availability for induced abortions in future which may cause a decline in the family size norms in rear future. Unfortunately, several medical practitioners have become witting or unwitting facilitators of foeticide, colluding with parents and other relatives of the unborn child to do sex determination tests. Easy, quick money was a motivation for some of them; and a few others simply saw it as another medical service or even a way of helping parents and stopping female infanticide. As a consequence, sex determination centres have mushroomed all over the country, even in small and remote towns. In many cases, these centres are not manned by qualified doctors but by technicians. What started as a trickle soon became a flood. Alarm bells started ringing when the census and other statistics revealed a drastic fall in the sex ratio, especially in urban areas and among educated population segments. In 1994, after intensive public debate all over India, Parliament enacted the Pre-Natal Diagnostic Techniques (Regulation and Prevention of Misuse) Act on September 20, 1994. The Act, which came into operation from January 1, 1996, provided for:

- The regulation of the use of prenatal diagnostic techniques for the purpose of detecting genetic or metabolic disorders or chromosomal abnormalities or certain congenital mal-formations or sex linked disorders; and
- The prevention of the misuse of such techniques for the purpose of prenatal sex determination leading to female foeticide.

The Act has been amended with effect from February 14, 2003 with a view to make it more comprehensive and renamed as Pre-Conception and Pre-Natal Diagnostic Techniques (Prohibition of Sex Selection) Act, 1994 (PNDT Act). It brought within its ambit the techniques of pre-conception sex selection to pre-empt the misuse of such technologies. It has explicit provisions for the use, regulation and monitoring of ultrasound machines to curb their misuse for detection of the sex of the foetus.

Some of the steps that the government has been taking, in partnership with international bodies, NGOs and other groups, to stop the elimination of the girl child and give her an equal status is really progressive and praiseworthy.

The decisive battle against gender discrimination has to be fought in the minds of people since son preference has its roots in prejudices and an anti-women mindset. The answer lies in creating awareness about the true worth of women, the irrelevance and also the illegality of sex selection, and the need to question old and outdated rituals and social behaviour. The Ministry of Health and Family Welfare works with a variety of partners including civil society groups, the National

Commission for Women (NCW), Centre for Social Research (CSR), CEHAT, Population Foundation of India (PFI), NGOs as well as development partners such as UNFPA, to raise the level of public discourse and build alliances to highlight the issue of sex selection.

Recent activities included the following:

Valuing the girl child: The solution of the problem of gender discrimination, female infanticide and foeticide is inextricably linked to enhancing the status of women and, more specifically, the girl child. The efforts of the government and its partners in this girl-saving exercise, therefore, focus on making families value the girl child and convincing them of the need to treat daughters at par with sons, give girls equal opportunity for education and equal right in the property.

One of the government's efforts in this direction is the 'Save the Girl Child Campaign', highlighting the achievements of girls. In 2003–04 and 2004–05, tennis star Sania Mirza and CBSC topper Aruna Kesavan were brand ambassadors for the Campaign. Joshna Chinnappa, Jr., Senior National Asian Squash Champion, is the brand ambassador for 2005–2006. In line with the same approach, the theme of the tableau of the Department of Family Welfare at the 2004 Republic Day parade was 'Save the Girl Child'. The idea of such initiatives is to make people aware that today girls can achieve as much, if not more than boys; that girls can make a family/a village/a nation proud; that girls matter ... that a girl is not a liability but an asset.

Working with the media and entertainment industry: Apart from organizing workshops and seminars through voluntary organizations at the state/regional/district/block levels to create awareness against the practice of prenatal sex selection, the government is using the outreach of the broadcast, electronic and print media to do the same.

Reaching the masses through religious/spiritual leaders: Keeping in mind the vast multitudes that India's religious and spiritual leaders reach out to, UNFPA made an effort to get them involved in spreading awareness on the issue of sex selection.

Connecting with young persons: It is the youth that will shape tomorrow, it is essential to see that their attitudes to gender issues are not coloured by old prejudices and social behaviour. UNFPA's efforts to reach out to young people included collaborations with HT Pace (a division of the Hindustan Times Group of Newspapers), Delhi Public Schools (DPS) Society and the National Institute of Information Technology (NIIT).

Conclusion

A number of all these efforts at spreading awareness and sensitivity on the issue, coupled with the firm determination to implement the provisions of the PNDT Act in spirit and tone, are bound to have an impact on the situation and will, hopefully, be reflected in the sex ratio in the next census. If we can improve the socio-economic and demographic status, then over the period of time, it is likely that wider societal acceptance of education, health, etc., will occur owing to the demonstration effect of the benefits of these services to families and the community at large. This would contribute to the elimination of sex discrimination and enable couples to resolve the conflict between the achievement of small family and sex preference with the balance in sex ratio.

The constitution, law agencies and enforcement authorities are trying hard to remove such social and ethical sin but these laws are meant to empower men not to women. Further, the acceptance of women as their equal partner is a much bigger problem. If males themselves become ready to accept and acknowledge the significance of their counterparts, this discrimination against so-called a different species "Women" can be minimized, if not completely eradicated.

References

Annual Report of Implementation of Pre-Conception and PreNatal Diagnostic Techniques, (2005), PNDT Division, Ministry of Health and Family Welfare, Government of India, New Delhi.

Arokiasamy, Perianayagam (2004), "Regional Patterns of Sex Bias and Excess Female Child Mortality", *Population-E*, 59 (6).

Bose, Asish (2001), "Fighting Female Foeticide", *Economic and Political Weekly*.

Census of India (2001), Office of the Registrar General and Census Commissioner, India.

Das Gupta, Monica and P.N. Mari Bhat (1997), "Fertility Decline and Increased Manifestation of Sex Bias in India", *Population Studies*, 51.

Dyson, Tim and Mick Moore (1983), "On Kingship Structure, Female Autonomy and Demographic Behaviour in India", *Population and Development Review*, 9.

Guilot, Michel (2002), "The Dynamics of the Population Sex Ratio in India, 1971–96", *Population Studies*, 56.

Mayer, Peter (1999), "India's Falling Sex Ratio", *Population and Development Review*, 25 (2).

National Family Health Survey (NFHS–I), India, 1992–1993, NFHS–II (1998–99) and NFHS–III (2005–06), Department of Family Welfare, Government of India, International Institute for Population Sciences.

Patel, Tulsi (2004), "Missing Girls in India", *Economic and Political Weekly*.

Sen, Amartya (1990), "More Than 100 Million Women are Missing", *New Review of Books*, 37.

—— (2001), "Many Faces of Gender Inequality", *The Hindu*, 18 (22).

SRS Bulletin (2007), Sample Registration System, Registrar General of India, Vol. 42.

Sudha, S. and Irudaya Rajan, S. (1998), "Intensifying Masculinity of Sex Ratio in India: New Evidence 1981–1991", Centre for Development Studies, Thiruvananthapuram.

14

Health of the Workers in Plantation Economy

A Study of Cardamom Plantations in Kerala

ANNS ISSAC

Plantation industry is significant in Kerala in terms of both the number of people dependent on it for livelihood and in terms of its contribution to GDP. Last few decades saw a shift in the large-scale plantation to small grower plantations and increased employment of temporary and seasonal labour. Given the heterogeneity of crops and changing structure of plantations, it is hypothesized that it accentuates the vulnerability of workers in plantations. But it has never been part of any large scale discussion in the plantation sector, in the backdrop of globalization. The forces operating in the production process like nature of employer-employee relationship, the type of industry, i.e., small, medium or large in respect to capital investment, the demand for the product and the type of market along with the bargaining power of the people attached to the industry, all have an influence on the welfare of the workers. Very few scholars have pointed out the interrelatedness of working and living conditions on the health of the people. For instance, Qadeer and Roy have pointed out the influence of the nature of the industrializing process, social stratification, welfare services, legal processes and trade union movements on the health of the population (Qadeer and Roy, 1989).

This paper aims at a comprehensive and critical reflection of the present status of workers in the cardamom plantations in Idukki with a view to highlight its implications on their health. The study presented here is based on a fieldwork done among the cardamom plantation workers in Idukki district during October 2006–January 2007. A total of seven plantations are selected for the present study after a preliminary visit to the various plantations in Udumbanchola. All the available workers in the plantations during the period of study are taken as sample population and it consists of 95 workers. The data is collected through interviews and in-depth discussions with workers, planters, trade union leaders, political activists, forest department staff, spices board officials, plantation officers, health service personnel and local environmental activists. The secondary data is collected from journals and newspapers, books and theses, plantation enquiry committee reports and records from panchayat office, primary health centre and spices board.

Idukki is the major cardamom grower with about 79 per cent of the total area under cardamom in the state and contributes to about 92 per cent of the total production of cardamom (Government of India, 2006). Udumbanchola is one of the major cardamom cultivating regions in the district. About 70 per cent of the population in Udumbanchola panchayat consists of labourers in the cardamom plantations (GoK, 2005). Majority of cardamom plantations belong to the category of small and medium scale holdings. It is estimated that besides the large number (about 20,000) of smallholders, about 17,000 workers are also employed in cardamom cultivation. No proper data regarding the number of workers in cardamom plantations are available since the available figures have not counted the temporary and seasonal workers.

Socio-Economic Profile of the Plantation Labourers

The study covers three small and medium plantations each and one large plantation of cardamom in Udumbanchola. Details regarding the size of the holdings and the distribution of labourers of the survey are given below:

Table 1

Distribution of Labourers according to the Size of Holdings

Size of the holding (hectares)	*Number of holdings*	*Number of labourers*
5–10	3	12
11–20	3	29
Above 50	1	54

Source: Primary Survey.

The sample population include 12 labourers from three small holding plantations, 29 from three medium scale holdings and 54 from one large scale holding. The sample population consists of a total of 95 labourers including 28 males and 67 females. There is a concentration of female labourers irrespective of the size of plantations. The producers give preference for females because, as explained by one of the owners, "they are regular, sincere, hard working, obedient and less unionized". The age and sexwise categorization of the labour force under study is given in Table 2 below:

Table 2

Age and Sexwise Distribution of Sample Population

Age group	*Male*	*Female*	*Total Persons*	*Total Percentage*
18–28	3	16	19	20
29–39	14	32	46	49
40–50	9	13	22	23
51–61	2	4	6	6
Above 61	—	2	2	2
Total	28	67	95	100

Source: Primary Survey.

It is evident from the table that majority of the labourers belong to 29–39 age group which consists of 49 per cent of the total labourers in the plantations. Around 20 per cent fall into 18–28 age group even though a few of them who reported their age as 18–19 seem to be less than that age. The 40–50 age group include 23 per cent of the labourers while 6 per cent are in 51–61 range. There are two female labourers who are above the age of 61.

In the younger age group, comparatively fewer males are opting for work in plantations than females. This may be due to the less attractive remuneration and non-sustainability of job in the plantations and availability of other works like construction work, shop assistant job, etc., in the nearby towns. Among the labourers interviewed, it is clearly brought out that the system of employing whole family is prevalent in cardamom industry. It is noted by many studies that family labourer's are major work force in plantation sector (for instance, Bhowmik, 1992; Sajhau and Muralt, 1987). In some case, whole family is employed in cardamom industry over the generations. Among the 95 labourers interviewed, they belong to 74 households. Of the total 95 labourers, six are unmarried, including one male and five female. All others are married and two are widows. The average size of the family is four among workers in the study region. But families with 3–4 children are not rare. Around 7 per cent of the household having a family size of six. The religion-wise distribution of sample population shows 67 Hindus, 26 Christians and 2 Muslims. The caste-wise break-up of study population is given in Table 3 below.

Table 3
Caste-wise Distribution of Sample Population

Category	*Number of workers*	*Percentage*
Scheduled Caste	32	34
Other Backward Caste	55	58
Forward Caste	8	8
Total	95	100

Source: Primary Survey.

The majority of the workers in the study population are from Other Backward Castes (OBCs) which includes Ezhava, Thevar, Muslim, CSI and Latin Catholics. The Scheduled Caste (SC) population, consists of Parayan, Chaklian, Pulayan and Pandi, ranks second. Forward caste includes Nair and Roman Catholics; constitute only 8 per cent of the study population.

An enquiry into the educational status of workers revealed that about 89 per cent has received formal education. Although not educated formally, another 8 per cent could read and write in Tamil, their mother tongue. Around 30 per cent labourers have got schooling till upper primary level, while 46 per cent labourers stopped their studies after lower primary level and 3 per cent of the workers have passed 10th standard.

The labourers are very keen to educate their children as much as possible and most of the respondents' children are attending schools. Some of the Tamil households send their children to their relative's houses in their native place for schooling as there are no Tamil medium schools in the locality. However, there is one Tamil medium school in the nearby village, which is only up to 7th standard. Children have to travel to far away place from Udumbanchola to attend the only higher secondary school, located at Anakkara. Further, the capacity of the school is inadequate to accommodate all the students. For higher education, they have to depend on other districts, as Idukki has only two government colleges. Some private unaided institutions and parallel colleges are working in Nedumkandam which serves very few students.

The Spices Board is giving educational scholarships to the children of labourers, but it can be availed only by the children of permanent plantation labourers. This prevents majority of children in availing those benefits. Discussion with the respondents also revealed that children of many labourers work in the cardamom plantations during the harvest time and vacations.

Employment Characteristics

Working time in the plantation is 8 am to 5 pm usually and in the case of pesticide application or in harvesting season, it may extend beyond these timings. There is a clear division of labour and the wages given to female workers and male workers are not equal. The kind of work that female labourers has to do include weeding, trashing, plucking the pods, mulching, manuring, spraying pesticide, etc., and they get an average of Rs 90 per day. Tree felling for shade regulation, digging pits, irrigation, spraying pesticides, collecting and chipping of fire woods, etc., are the duty of men. They get Rs 100 per day. In the harvesting season, males also engage in plucking the pods.

The wage settlements are on a weekly basis. Permanent workers are entitled to maternity benefit, casual leave, Employees' State Insurance (ESI) and Provident Fund (PF) facilities, but in practice these benefits are not reaching to the workers. Two types of woollen sheets are to be provided by the plantation owners to the labourers in a year. One sheet is a thick and rough one, meant to be used in the field. The other one is comparatively better one for use inside the house. In the big plantations, permanent labourers are said to be getting two woollen sheets while it is not provided in the other plantations.

The distribution of labourers according to their status of work is shown in Table 4. There are 72 temporary and 23 permanent labourers in the plantations under study.

Table 4

Distribution of Labourers according to the Status of Labour

Status of Labourers	*Number of Labourers*	*Per cent*
Temporary	72	76
Permanent	23	24
Migrant	68	72
Non-Migrant	27	28

Source: Primary Survey.

About 72 per cent of labour force consists of migrants from Tamil Nadu, and 43 per cent among them are first generation migrants who came to the plantations in Idukki through some relatives and neighbours from their own villages in Tamil Nadu. Children of many of the labourers followed their parent's path and 25 per cent among the present labour force are second generation migrants. Around 28 per cent are local labourers, mostly from other districts of Kerala neighbouring Idukki, like Pathanamthitta and Kottayam.

Material Conditions of Workers

The Plantation Labour Act 1951 (PLA, 1951) has laid down rules regarding housing, drinking water, sanitation, drainage and sewage arrangements. Of the 95 labourers interviewed, who belong to 74 households, only 31 per cent families are living in the houses provided by the management in the plantation premises. They are permanent labourers. The labour lines are rows of quarters constructed to provide shelter to the labourers and their families. Rest of the labourers are living in the rented houses (45%) and the remaining in own houses (24%). The Table 5 explains basic facilities of workers.

Table 5

Distribution of Labour Households according to Residential Facilities

Facilities	*Description*	*Total Number of houses*	*Percentage*
Roof	Tile	46	62
	Asbestos	26	35
	Concrete	2	3
Wall	Brick + Sheet	2	3
	Brick	72	97
Floor	Plastered with Cow dung	2	3
	Cement	72	97
Number of rooms including kitchen	No separate rooms	2	3
	2	9	12
	3	61	82
	4	2	3
Latrine	Pit latrine	2	3
	Septic tank	72	97
Bathroom	Common bathroom	21	28
	Attached to the house	53	72
Drinking water source	Well	17	23
	Tap water	57	77

Source: Primary Survey.

All the labour lines except five are with asbestoses sheet for the roof and concrete walls. The floors are also cemented. There are two rooms plus one kitchen in each line house. Toilets and bathrooms are common for each line. Many of the workers reported that since the size of the room is very small, they find it very difficult to live as there are many family members. Many houses have made their own bathrooms in the backyard, attached to the houses with sheets. Waste from the houses is dumped in a pit dug in the centre yard. Very little free space is available to each line. The source of drinking water is tap water provided by the management. Labourers reported water scarcity. All the lines are electrified and the electricity charge is to be paid by the labourer himself.

While three houses provided by the employer are with tile roofs, cemented floors and brick walls, the rooms are not separated. These houses are actually small sheds constructed for some other purpose and later converted into labourer houses. They lack proper toilet and they are forced to use the toilet-cum-bathroom much away from the house. The water source is the employer's well. The condition of the rest of the two houses is very bad, with sheet roofs and sheet walls. The floor is polished with cow dung. Cooking, eating and sleeping are in the same room. Only the husband and wife are living here and they have sent their children to their ancestral home for study. They are using pit latrine in the plantation premises and for water, depend on the owner's well. The house is not electrified.

About 24 per cent of the labourers are living in their own houses. Many of such houses are half way in construction. But all are tiled, with brick walls and cemented floor. Bathrooms and toilets are attached to the house. The land attached to the house is very small in most of the cases, but with the available land, they tried to manage a home garden. Water source is tap water for many but some of them use well water from the neighbour. Latrines are septic tank type and houses are with proper drainage facilities. These houses are with a small drawing-cum-dining hall, one or two bed rooms and a kitchen, in general. Rented houses are, in most of the cases, very congested and many of them are extensions from the already existing houses. They do not have proper drainage facilities, and little space for sleeping and cooking.

Labourers reported that the quality of the rice supplied through PDS is not good and hence for cooking purpose, most of the labourers have to buy rice from the open market. Use of intoxicants like toddy, beedi, pan, ganja, etc., is frequent among the labourers and illegal preparation of arrack is common in the area. Many of the jobless people in the area are turning to arrack making, as it is profitable.

Source of Income

The main source of income for majority of the households is the wage obtained from the plantations. For 69 per cent of the households under study, plantation labour is the only source of income. In 12 per cent of households, the spouses of plantation labourers are working as construction workers in Nedumkandam and Adimaly areas. About 19 per cent households are getting income from agricultural works other than the work in plantations. Additional sources of income for the labourers include earnings from animal husbandry, poultry, agriculture etc. Two of the sample households have cows while 12 of them have poultry. Around 32 per cent households in the sample have got some land attached to their house, and five of them got land above 10 cent. One person has got 1 acre land of his own. In some rented houses also, a few cents of land are attached to the house where the labourers are allowed to cultivate vegetables. All the labourers who are having their own land above 10 cents are cultivating cardamom along with some vegetables. Nearly 68 per cent of the labour households do not possess any land.

Savings and Indebtedness

Getting credit from registered banks is practically impossible, especially for the landless, migrant labourer who does not have anything to deposit as security. So their options of financial support are limited to employers and private moneylenders. The purpose of taking credit varies from marriage, health problems, construction and maintenance of houses, buying household goods, children's education, to buying land and repaying debt. Most of the labourers interviewed have taken money in credit either from the employer or private moneylenders. There are plenty of private moneylenders in high range area, most of them are from Theni in Tamil Nadu and a few Malayalees from the plains.

Table 6

Indebtedness of Labourers

Amount	*No. of people*	*Percentage*
Less than 1,000	30	32
1,001–10,000	22	23
10,001 –20,000	9	9
Above 20,001	2	2
Reported no debt	20	21
No answer	12	13
Total	95	100

Source: Primary Survey.

All the labourers except 21 per cent reported having taken money for different purposes. The amount varies from a few hundreds to more than Rs 20,000. Interest rates vary from Rs 125 to Rs 150 per thousand rupees per month. Suicide cases are reported among labourers and marginal farmers because of indebtedness and due to the threat of the private financiers. For repaying the debt, in many cases labourers have to sell their minimum assets like furniture in the house. In spite of the financial crisis, some of the labourers try to save money. It seems 12 permanent labourers in the large scale holding have PF deposits while rest of the labourers neither have taken any insurance scheme nor have any bank deposits.

Role of Trade Union in Cardamom Plantations

The trade unions entered into cardamom industry at the end of 1960s and there is little documentation on it. The extent of union participation among the labourers is very low. There are four unions working among the Cardamom Plantation labourers in the study area viz., CITU (Centre of Indian Trade Union), INTUC (Indian National Trade Union Congress), AITUC (All-India Trade Union Congress) and BMS (Bharathiya Mazdur Sangh). Among them, CITU has the maximum number of labourers and INTUC comes second. AITUC comes next and BMS has very few members. Among the seven landholdings under the study, these trade unions are having members only in the larger plantation and come around to total 15 members. Many workers are even reluctant to reveal that they are trade union members. The management always try to resist the trade union movement and it has succeeded to a certain extent.

In none of the trade unions, female members are in any important positions. One of the reasons as to why women are preferred by many managements is that "they are not union oriented and hence less troublesome". Though 70 per cent of the study population are females, the female participation in the trade union is only 9 per cent of the sample population. Even if they participate, it is restricted to mere membership and/or attending some protest marches, if any. They reported that union participation did not bring any visible changes in their life. Women's non-participation in trade union activities is also closely related to their under-representation in the political institution.

Health Care Services and Reported Health Issues

The small and medium scale cardamom plantation workers obtained no proper medical services as there is no legal compulsion for providing it to them. In the larger plantation, it is reported that there is a visit by a doctor once in three months. Apart from that, no medical services are provided to the labourers. So, workers have to rely on available health services in the locality.

As noted, the region is one of the backward districts in Kerala regarding the health services development. Posts of two doctors, one junior public health nurse and one lady health inspector are vacant in the PHC in Udumbanchola. The timings are not favourable for the workers to utilize the services. Apart from the routine vaccinations, no other activities are carried out in the PHC. There is no pharmacist in the PHC. The staff quarters are not in a condition to inhabit. The local people said that the PHC is not functioning regularly and most of the time staff is absent. There is a demand from the people to improve the services. The Taluk hospital is situated in Nedumkandam which is 16 km away from Udumbanchola panchayat area. There are five doctors, but only two are permanent and others are on deputation. One is a junior doctor on compulsory service for 6 months. Vacancies have not been filled for the post of a nurse and head nurse each. And there is no radiologist in the hospital. One ambulance and two mini buses are in the hospital, but there is only one driver.

The common diseases reported by the staff are diarrhoea, fever, asthma, skin diseases, common cold, cough etc. In the year 2005–06, there were 653 diarrhoea cases, mostly among the Tamil labourer households, two Hepatitis-A cases including one death, 10 chickenpox cases, four malaria cases, one leprosy and five tuberculosis cases were reported in the PHC. Though they do not have any statistics of cancer cases and patients suffering from heart diseases, the staff said that both are increasing in the population. Many cases are not reported here as the migrant labourers go to Madurai for treatment. There are reports that cancer of uterus and oral cancer are increasing. In association with the panchayat, PHC had conducted awareness classes among the people to stop using 'pan' products and on the safe handling of pesticides. There are four cases of delivery at home and all are among Tamil population. Three cases of still births were also reported last year among the labourers.

A number of private allopathic clinics and hospitals are there in the nearby town in Nedumkandam. The labourers mainly go to the private allopathic hospitals in Nedumkandam, as the timing is convenient for them and the services are far better than the government hospital. They added that even if they go to the government hospital, they have to buy medicine from outside.

The workers receive no guidelines or training in how to handle the pesticides. They do not have information about the quantity of the pesticide to be used per hectare. In different plantations, they follow differently according to the availability of the pesticide. They even mix different pesticides and sprays. The mixing of different pesticides alters its characteristics to an unpredictable extent. The impact of the pesticides on human being depends up on the toxicity of the pesticide, the length of the exposure, and the health status of the individual. The long-term effects of these pesticides are to be explored further.

The workers reported symptoms like over sweating, dizziness, nausea, skin irritation, headache, burning sensation in eyes, blurred vision, breathing difficulties, fatigue, loss of appetite, etc., while applying pesticides. But such cases do not generate wider discussion as the above symptoms persist only for a short time. So in most cases no medical help is sought. All the workers interviewed said that they have a vague idea regarding the hazards of the pesticides which they are handling, but most of them are not taking any precautionary measures such as using masks or gloves, or even do not wash their hands with soap after spraying. This is not due to the unwillingness of the workers but the non-availability of such protective devices and facilities. The workers reported that they do not have any other option as the situation is not different in other plantations also.

Asthma, cancer and infertility among the plantation workers are increasing as reported by activists. In Kanchiyar panchayat, 300 cancer cases are identified in a survey conducted by Indian Council of Medical Research (ICMR) and JRCS. It is reported that the same company which produces pesticides, carried out their drug trial in the cancer patients in high ranges through a prominent cancer research institute in the state capital. The particular drug costs Rs 1.20 lakh rupees and which is given at free of cost to these patients. The patients are forced to accept this 'treatment' because of their poor economic condition. Though it was reported in the local media it never captured attention of the government.

Discussion

The nature of the labour force is an important factor in understanding how the issues of workers are unaddressed in the ongoing debates on development in Kerala. The workforce in the plantations is primarily composed of migrant labour, predominantly females and most of them are on temporary basis. Their lower social and educational status interfered with their capacity to negotiate for their rights.

The existence of sexual division of labour is favoured by the producers since female workers are to be paid less than male workers. Though the Equal Remuneration Act (1976) ensures the provision of equal wage for equal work, none of the plantations found in survey follow it. The wage varies from Rs 80–90 for women and Rs 100–115 for men from different localities of cardamom plantations in Idukki. Women workers have to do continuous 'back bending' jobs while plucking the pods from the panicles of plants. Health-related problems of the workers, especially the problem of backache in female workers, attributed to the nature of the work they are performing in the plantation. There is no toilet facility in the plantations except in the labour lines. Females are forced to do hazardous jobs like spraying of pesticides which majority of the male labourers are reluctant to do. In all the reported cases of pesticide poisoning, the victims are either child labourers or women. Children are employed in the cardamom plantations, especially during harvesting seasons and they are mainly employed for spraying pesticides. They are paid only Rs 40–50 per day. In recent years it is noted that there is a trend to use temporary workers in plantation sector and there is no transform of this temporary status to a permanent one. Since most of the schemes and law including Plantation Labour Act (1951) are aimed at permanent workers, producers are not liable for any welfare measures to these temporary workers.

The wage obtained from their labour is not adequate to meet their basic requirements of the worker's family. There is no job security for migrant workers and they hardly find work in lean seasons. Increasing cost of living forces many workers to work on holidays in neighbouring plantations. Workers are demanding hike in their wage to Rs 135 from the present wage of Rs 92. Most of them complain that major share of their wage goes to local moneylenders as they are indebted to them for their basic expenses. Any health problem creates a burden on the family not only because of the cost for direct treatment but also loss of wage for those days. Since the area is entirely cash crop producing area, the food items has to come out from outside the area and the workers have to depend on the market.

Dominant political groups raised the issues of reduction in profits of producers in the plantation sector and their entire discussion focused on the welfare of producers. There are many other sources of income that exist for planters in the medium and large holdings. Many of them are also running a business, holding other land and buildings in the mainland. The earnings from the plantation form only a part of their income. Producers have formed several associations and are pressurizing the government to scrap the provisions for services and minimum wages to be given to the workers. The media also project the problems of the producers due to the price crash while they give very little attention to worker's issues.

The activities of trade unions in cardamom plantations are very limited. One can see a maximum of three or four protest marches, conducted jointly with all trade unions in tea, coffee and rubber plantations, against cutting down of dearness allowances of workers etc. Issues of pesticide deaths, child labour, unequal wage system for male and female labourers, ensuring minimum wages, sanitation and medical facilities, etc., have never been raised by the trade unions. Temporary and seasonal labourers are not at all represented in the trade unions who are the majority in cardamom plantations. Apart from the lack of political consciousness, another important factor hindering the unionization of workers is cultural heterogeneity. In the study area, the population is divided into migrant Tamil labourers and native Malayali labourers. Though they all are victims to more or less same kind of exploitation by the owners and the apathy of the state, these factors prevented them from forming a strong union. The difference in the operations is also another factor. Apart from a few big plantations, all other holdings in cardamom are small and marginal and scattered in a sparsely populated area.

During the interviews with different cross-sections of people including owners, trade union leaders, people's representatives, labour welfare officers, etc., they are always making a comparison with the situation in tea plantations in the district, many of which are facing severe crisis. They are repeatedly saying that the working and living conditions of labourers in cardamom plantation are much better than those of tea plantations. The producers are trying to justify the existing lack/denial of facilities to workers in the cardamom plantations on the backdrop of price crash of the crop. As members of organized sector labour force, the workers are entitled to enjoy these facilities and cannot be considered as a favour from the plantation owner.

Conclusion

The plantation region continues to be highly underdeveloped compared to other regions in the state. Plantation sector corner attention in development debates only when the industry is in crisis. Though the crisis had an impact on the overall industry, it affected mostly the workers who are devoid of any supportive services to cope with the crisis. Even at the times of prosperity in the industry, the benefits were not at all translated into the worker's life; in fact, the methods adopted for increasing productivity by using pesticides and fertilizers created major health problems for the workers. The trade unions have failed to represent the workers' interests. The interest of the government is solely focused on the commerce of the crop and it is favoured towards the planters. The discourse of public health in the state is more centred on attempts to reduce diseases, questions over increase in public expenditure on particular disease or supply of medicines rather than addressing the livelihood issues of people or conceiving development as freedom. The study emphasizes that formulation of health policies on the concept of health as 'absence of disease', is no more able to deal with the real problem in the state.

Acknowledgement

The researcher acknowledges her sincere thanks to Prof. K R Nayar for his valuable comments on this paper.

References

Bhowmik, Sharit K. (1992), "Plantation Labour Act and Child Labour", *Economic and Political Weekly*, 27 (42): 2287–89.

Government of India (1951), Plantation Labour Act 1951.

—— (2006), Spices Board Schemes, Ministry of Commerce and Industry, Cochin.

Government of Kerala (GoK) (2005), Panchayat Report, Udumbanchola Panchayat, Idukki.

Rajiv, K.T. (2004), "Trail on Patients Too: The Inaction of the Government", *Deshabhimani*, July 5.

Mathew, Binu (2005), "Idukki the Next Victim of International Pesticides Companies", Free Press, March.

"Plantation Sector for Price Related Wages", *Business Line*, September 27, 2004, Cochin Edition.

Prakash, P.K. (2004), "Cancer Drug Trial on Victims of Pesticide Poisoning", *Madhyamam*, July 1.

—— (2004), "Excessive Use of Pesticides: Agricultural Department and Cardamom Research Institute are Responsible", *Madhyamam*, June 30.

Qadeer, Imrana and Dunu Roy (1989), "Work, Wealth and Health: Sociology of Worker's Health in India", *Social Scientist*, 17: 45–92.

Sajhau, Jean Paul and Jurgen Von Muralt (1987), Plantations and Plantation Workers, International Labour Office, Geneva.

15

Poverty and Human Development in India

An Inter-State Analysis

K.V. VINESH KUMAR

Several significant changes have taken place in India since independence. Some of these changes are distinctly visible – especially in the economic sphere with adoption of new technologies, diversified production, and sophisticated management. Changes have also taken place in the social sphere – with affirmative action for disadvantaged communities, with the weakening of untouchability and caste discrimination, and with women enjoying by and large more freedom than ever before. On the political front, India has remained a vibrant democracy with increased participation by women and men in political decision-making. However, in terms of achievements, India's performance during the past 60 years has been decidedly mixed. From a human development perspective, the glass can be considered half-full or half-empty; much depends upon the eye of the beholder. The country has recorded impressive gains in many areas, significant reductions in the intensity of poverty, but there is still much ground to cover in terms of ending human deprivations.

The economic growth contributes to most of the poverty reduction, when it expands the employment productivity and wages of poor and public resourses are channelled to promote human development. As a result of increasing employment a virtuous cycle of economic growth and human development arises which culminates in the generation of human skill and improvement in health. Thus, within a decade, we have moved dramatically from earlier caloric intake measure of poverty and the UNDP introduced the concept of HDI, which went beyond the concept of income poverty to understand the extent and nature of poverty. Instead of examining the average state of human capabilities as in the human development index, capability poverty measure, the subsequent measure of poverty, conceived by UNDP, reflected the percentage of people who lack of basic minimal human capabilities, which are both ends in themselves and are needed to lift the poor income poverty to sustainable human development.

Data and Methodology

This present study analyses the estimate of human development indicators with special focus on multidimensional and deprivation indicators of poverty and this paper also deals with the deprivational perspective analysis of poverty among the Indian states. The study is based on the secondary data. The principal sources of data are the decennial censuses, the various rounds of National Sample Survey, NFHS, and Economic Survey. Indicators have been complied at national and state levels (Human Development Report by UNDP, UNFPA and various state government agencies), various articles and publications are used for this study.

Concept and Definition of Human Development Index

The concept of human development is complex and multidimensional. Human development index (HDI) is extensively used to measure the standard of living of a country. The measure has been enlarged with many related indices of human development like Gender Development Index (GDI), Gender Empowerment Index and Human Poverty Index (HPI). HDI is calculated based on three indices; life expectancy to measure longevity, educational attainment to represent knowledge and real gross domestic product (GDP) to represent income. The HDI constructed by the UNDP as a summary measure of well-being or human development, which combines countries achievements in health education and income. The UNDP uses life expectancy as a proxy for health, a combination of adult literacy and school enrolments as the education variable. GDP per capita in purchasing parity dollars as the income variable:

$$\text{Dimension index} = \frac{\text{Actual value} - \text{Minimum value}}{\text{Minimum value} - \text{Maximum value}}$$

The maximum and minimum values of life expectancy of birth is considered as 85 and 25 respectively. Knowledge as measured as the weighted average of adult literacy rate and the combined primary, secondary and tertiary gross enrolment ratio with two-thirds and one third weight respectively. The maximum and minimum value for the adult literacy rate and gross enrolment ratio are 100 per cent and 0 per cent respectively. The decent standard of living measured by Gross Domestic Product per capita calculated on purchasing power parity basis in US$ for the sake of international comparison. Maximum and minimum values of GDP per capita (purchasing power parity in dollar terms) are taken as 4,000 and 100 respectively. Then Gender Development Index adjusts average achievement to reflect the inequalities between men and women calculated in HDI dimensions. The human poverty index measures the average deprivation in three basic dimensions of HDI. The long and healthy life as the vulnerability to death at a relatively early age as measured by probability at birth not surviving to 40. Knowledge measured as the exclusion from the world of reading and communication on measured by adult literacy rate. The decent standard of living is the lack of access of overall provisioning.

Trends in Human Development Index in India

Human development is conceptualized at the national or the state level. Various indicators developed for its measurement are useful for cross-national comparisons but rarely give an idea of variations within a country. However, since in India desegregation to the state level has been possible at least for the major states for which relevant data are available, regional variations have been observed (EPW Research Foundation, 1994; Shariff, 1999). But there are variations within states as well. In addition to spatial variations (rural-urban, inter-district, inter-agro-climatic zones), differentials have been observed across social groups, notably, religion and caste groups. The inter-state variations in human development index are plausibly caused by differences in natural resources, cultural and historical factors and state specific policies and programmes. From the policy angle, it is necessary to assess to what extent the inter-state variations in both the levels and differentials in human development. India made progress on the HDI value that has gone up from 0.595 in 2002 to 0.619 in 2005 World Human

Development Report (HDR) 2007. On HDI ranking, India is again ranked at 128 of 177 countries. India's rank on the Human Poverty Index (HPI) is 58 in a universe of 103 developing countries. On the Gender Development Index (GDI), India's rank is 113 in a universe of 140 countries (Global Human Development Report, 2007). The variations in HDI could be socio-economic status (SES), demographic, health, and diet and nutrition indicators. Therefore, composite indexes of all these indicators can better represent the real human development and poverty status for Indian states.

The HDR Report 2005 warns that some of the most highly visible globalization 'success stories' including China and India are failing to convert wealth creation and rising incomes into more rapid progress on the social indicators. If India could close the gender gap in < 5 year age old mortality between girls and boys that would save an estimated 1,30,000 lives. Reducing gender inequality would have a catalytic effect on reducing gaps in primary education between girls and boys. Eliminating gender inequality could reduce the underweight rate among children less than three years old by 13 percentage points in South Asia, equal to 13.4 million fewer malnourished children. The Report warns that if the current trends continue, the promise to get every child into school and to close gender gaps in education will not be met. National Human Development Report 2001 for India reveals the vast difference in the human development and poverty between the states of India since 1981. The report notes wide disparities at the state level. The reports also notes that disparities amongst the states with respect to human poverty are quite striking. It is more alarming that over the decade there has been no reduction of such disparities.

While there has been improvements in the human development index and human poverty index since 1980s, the inter-state disparities have persisted through this decade.

At the national level, HDI, which takes a value between 0 and 1, has improved from 0.381 in 1991 to 0.472 in 2001. At the state level, Kerala, Punjab, Maharashtra and Haryana were among the states with better HDI at both points of time. States like Bihar, Uttar Pradesh, Madhya Pradesh, Rajasthan and Orissa were at the other end. Based on the latest available data the HDI has been estimated for 2001 for selected major states only. At the national level it has increased to 0.472. The gap between Kerala and next best state, i.e., Punjab remains quite significant, though it has declined. By and large the states maintained their relative position between 1991 and 2001.

Table 1
Statewise Human Development Index in India

States	*1991*		*2001*	
	Value	*Rank*	*Value*	*Rank*
Andhra Pradesh	0.377	9	0.416	10
Assam	0.348	10	0.386	14
Bihar	0.308	15	0.367	15
Gujarat	0.431	6	0.479	6
Haryana	0.443	5	0.509	5
Karnataka	0.412	7	0.478	7
Kerala	0.513	1	0.638	1
Madhya Pradesh	0.328	13	0.394	12
Maharashtra	0.452	4	0.523	4
Orissa	0.345	12	0.404	11
Punjab	0.475	2	0.537	2
Rajasthan	0.347	11	0.424	9
Tamil Nadu	0.466	3	0.531	3
Uttar Pradesh	0.314	14	0.388	13
West Bengal	0.404	8	0.472	8
India	0.381		0.472	

Source: National Human Development Report 2001, Planning Commission of India.

The economically better-off states, as well as for the poor states, attainments on HDI and income levels show a direct correspondence. In other words, the poor states are also the states with relatively poor performance on HDI. Similarly, the economically better-off states are also the ones with relatively better performance on the HDI. However, the relation between the HDI and the level of development does not show any correspondence among the middle-income states in the country. In this category of states, some states like Kerala have high attainments on HDI, at the same time; there are states like Andhra-Pradesh or even West Bengal where HDI values are not as high. Thirdly, though at the national level, the economic growth in the nineties was nearly one percentage point higher than the earlier decade, it has, perhaps, resulted in less human development in the nineties. This is primarily on account of performance of the outlier states and slower improvement in human development indicators for states already with higher HDI values. Finally, it turns out that inequality across states on the HDIs is less than the income inequality as captured in the per capita State Domestic Product.

Inter-state Comparison of Human Deprivation in India

The main aim of this study is to measure the state-wise human deprivation. Deprivational status of human development calculates in three dimensions: decent standard of living, education and health. The deprivational score of each indicator is measured on the basis of various components: the decent standard of living measured by poverty line, education deprivation measured by illiteracy and health deprivation measured by infant mortality rate. In general, poverty can be defined as a situation when people are unable to satisfy the basic needs of life. The definition and methods of measuring poverty differs from country to country. According to the definition by Planning Commission of India, poverty line is drawn with an intake of 2,400 calories in rural areas and 2,100 calories in urban areas. If a person is unable to get that much minimum level of calories, then he/she is considered as being below poverty. These poverty lines are then applied on the NSSO's household consumer expenditure distributions to estimate the proportion and number of poor at state level.

Literacy is a reasonably good indicator of development in a society. Spread and diffusion of literacy is generally associated with essential trait of today's civilization such as modernization, urbanization, industrialization, communication and commerce. It is the important measurement of HDI. Illiteracy is calculated as 100 minus literacy rate. Infant Mortality Rate (IMR) is regarded as an important and sensitive indicator of the health of a community. It also reflects the general standard of living of the people. It is commonly used as an indicator of welfare in poor countries. This vulnerable age is exposed to several exogenous and endogenous factors, which influence the health growth and development. Infant mortality rate is the number of infants who die before reaching the one-year of age expressed per 1,000 live births in a year.

On the basis of these three indicators human deprivation index were constructed. These three indicators had been given equal weightage to measure the human deprivational index of Indian states.

Human Deprivation Index = 1/3 (PL) +1/3 (IR) +1/3 (IMR)
where

PL = Poverty line
IR = Illiteracy rate
IMR = Infant mortality rate

Based on the above equation, the human deprivation index of different states in India given in the Table 2 has been constructed on the basis of the aforesaid equation

Table 2
Human Deprivation Index

States	*Poverty*		*Illiteracy rate*		*IMR*		*Deprivation Index*		*Rank*	
	1987–88	1999–00	1991	2001	1991	2001	1991	2001	1991	2001
Andhra Pradesh	25.86	15.77	55.9	38.89	55	66	45.58	40.21	10	6
Assam	36.21	33.47	47.1	45.26	92	44	58.43	40.89	5	5
Bihar	52.13	42.60	61.5	52.47	75	67	62.87	54.02	4	3
Gujarat	31.54	14.07	38.7	33.57	78	64	49.41	37.21	9	7
Haryana	16.54	8.74	44.2	31.41	52	69	37.58	36.38	13	10
Karnataka	37.53	20.04	44	32.96	74	58	51.84	36.99	6	8
Kerala	31.79	12.72	10.2	9.08	42	16	27.99	12.59	14	14
Madhya Pradesh	43.07	37.43	55.8	36.92	133	97	77.29	56.77	1	2
Maharashtra	40.41	25.02	35.1	28.73	74	49	49.83	34.24	7	11
Orissa	55.58	47.15	50.9	36.39	125	98	77.16	60.50	2	1
Punjab	13.20	6.16	41.5	30.05	74	54	42.9	30.06	12	12
Rajasthan	35.15	15.28	61.5	38.97	87	83	61.21	45.74	5	5
Tamil Nadu	43.39	21.12	37.3	26.58	54	53	44.89	23.54	11	13
Uttar Pradesh	41.45	31.15	58.4	42.64	99	85	66.28	52.92	3	4
West Bengal	44.72	27.02	42.3	30.78	62	53	49.67	36.92	8	9
India	38.86	26.10	47.8	34.80	77	71	54.55	43.96		

Source: National Human Development Report 2001.

The above analysis shows that Orissa is the first in human deprivation with 60.5 in the human deprivation index followed by Madhya Pradesh, Bihar, Uttar Pradesh and Assam. These five states are the most deprived states with their score higher than the national average in the last two decades. Kerala is the least deprived state in these two decades (27.99, 12.59). This means that it is tackling human development and reduction of poverty very well. Tamil Nadu has the best achievement in this period. In 1991 deprivation score was 44.89 which decreased to 23.54 in 2001. This shows the better position of Tamil Nadu in hunan development. It is also significant to note that compared to other states Andhra Pradesh has shown least deprivation during 2001.

The most deprived states need to take necessary steps to improve the human development. To achieve human development, deprivation should be eliminated. For this, overall economic growth is necessary, which can alleviate poverty and its evil consequences. With economic upliftment, good health and education can make an enormous difference in the lives of poor people and these are the main goals of development. The Development Radars, as well as the composite indices are, no doubt, useful tools in policy formulation and mapping progress in human development over time and across states. However, by their very construct, they have a limitation in capturing human development in all its facets.

Incidence of Poverty among Indian States

Poverty is a state of deprivation. In absolute terms it reflects the inability of an individual to satisfy certain basic minimum needs for a sustained, healthy and a reasonably productive living. Conceptually, any attempt at quantifying the incidence of poverty in any population requires taking into account the level and pattern of an individual's personal consumption expenditure, as well as their access to social transfers and public provisioning. However, it is not easy to measure the consumption shares of an individual in the publicly provided goods and services or the benefit he or she derives from the overall social contexts, for often it is not possible to price them or they are provided free of charge, even though it all adds up to the well-being of the concerned individual. In general, therefore, for identifying the poor one looks at the level of personal expenditure (or income) that enables the individual to satisfy a certain minimum consumption level. The proportion of population not able to attain the specified level of expenditure is then segregated as poor. Using such an approach the Planning Commission, Government of India has been estimating the Head Count Ratio of the poor at state level, separately for rural and urban areas for over three decades.

Table 3
Poverty Ratios among Indian States

States	*1993–94*	*1999–2000*
Andhra Pradesh	22.19	15.77
Assam	40.86	36.09
Bihar	54.96	42.60
Gujarat	24.21	14.07
Haryana	25.05	8.74
Karnataka	33.16	20.04
Kerala	25.43	12.72
Madhya Pradesh	42.52	37.43
Maharashtra	36.86	25.02
Orissa	48.56	47.15
Punjab	11.77	6.16
Rajasthan	27.41	15.28
Tamil Nadu	35.05	21.12
Uttar Pradesh	40.85	31.15
West Bengal	35.66	27.02
India	35.97	26.10

Source: National Human Development Report 2001, Planning Commission, India, National Sample Survey Organization, Ministry of Economics and Statistics, Government of India.

At the national level, the incidence of poverty on the Head Count Ratio declined from 35.97 per cent in 1993–94 to 26.10 per cent in 1999–2000. It was a decline of nearly 10 percentage points in the period between 1993–94 and 1999–2000. In absolute terms, the number of poor declined from about 320 million in 1993–94 to 260 million in 1999–2000. The decline has not been uniform either across states or across rural and urban areas. At state level, among the major states, Orissa, Bihar, Madhya Pradesh, had more than 40 per cent of their population below the poverty line in 1993–94. However, by 1999–2000, Bihar and Madhya Pradesh had a large level reduction of poverty ratios. The poverty is closely connected with human development index. In a high human development state, the poverty level is lower. The literacy, infant mortality, life expectancy and per capita state domestic product of these states is very low compared to the high HDI states. The lack of these factors causes poverty level in Indian states.

There is an inter-state comparison of socio-economic indicators in India. The performance of states is across various sub-sectors be it, poverty, health, education related. This disparity in performance between states may be accounted for by exogenous factors but largely can be attributed to government service. In the past, the efficacy of the trickle-down process for eradication of poverty has been questioned, and there is increasing awareness that governments have to implement active pro-poor policies. There is less public debate on the need for public intervention in the social sectors, although perhaps even that is changing. Perhaps the reluctance to follow more interventionist policies in the social sectors is due to the supposed high correlation between income growth and progress in the social sectors in cross-country regressions. Of course, a high correlation does not necessarily imply causation.

Conclusion

The main purpose of this paper is to analyse inter-state comparison of human deprivation. The main feature of Indian states is heterogeneous in character. The states cannot be classified as success or failure because some states are well in education but have a high rate of mortality but are poor achievers in education. There is no evidence of the richer states, that is those with higher per capita state domestic product, necessarily have higher levels of achievement in the social sectors. This is particularly true of achievements in the health sector. All states with low incidence of poverty have better levels of achievement in the social sectors. Mahatma Gandhi once remarked: India's salvation consists in unlearning what she has learned during the past fifty years. Similar changes are now required to living ad in cultivating a genuine public sprit. India need to get it priority to right. If human poverty has to be eradicated attention must shift from income poverty to the poverty and inequality of opportunities: economic, social and political. India needs a sustained public action to be guided by strong human development priorities.

Select References

Chandrasekhar, C.P. and Abhijit, Sen, (1996), "Statistical Truths: Economic Reform and Poverty" *Frontline*, Madras: February 23.

Datt, G. and M. Ravallion, (1993), "Regional Disparities, Targeting and Poverty in India", in Michael Lipton and J. van Der Gaag (eds.) *Including the Poor*, World Bank, Washington D.C.

EPW Research Foundation, (1994), "Social Indicators of Development for India-II, Inter-state Disparities", *Economic and Political Weekly,* 29 (21): pp. 1300–08.

Government of India, (2003), "Selected Socio-economic Statistics for India: 2003", Central Statistical Organization, Department of Statistics, Ministry of Planning and Programme Implementation, New Delhi.

Human Development Report, (2003), www.undp.org/hdr

"India", in Michael Lipton and J. van Der Gaag (eds.), *Including the Poor.* World Bank, Washington D.C.

Mehta, A.K. and A. Shah, (2003), "Chronic Poverty in India: Incidence, Causes and Policies", *World Development,* 31 (3), pp. 491–511.

Mehta, Jaya and Shata Venkataraman, (2000), "Poverty Statistics Bermicidis Fast", *EPW,* July 1, www.epw.org.in.

National Council for Applied Economic Research, (1996), "Human Development Profile of India", New Delhi.

Noorbakhsh, F., (1999), "Standards of Living, Human Development Indices and Structural Adjustments in Developing Countries: An Empirical Investigation", *Journal of International Development,* Vol.11, pp. 151–75.

PCGI (Planning Commission, Government of India), (2002), National Human Development Report, 2001, Planning Commission of India, New Delhi.

Ravallion, M. and G. Datt, (2002), "Why has Economic Growth been More Pro-poor in Some States in India than Others?", *Journal of Development Economics,* 68, pp. 381–400.

Rudra, A., (1974), "Minimum Level of Living: A Statistical Examination in Poverty and Income Distribution in India", *Sankhya, Indian Journal of Statistics,* 36 Series C, June-December, pp. 281–90.

Sen, Amartya, (1999), "Health in Development", *Bulletin of the World Health Organization* 2997, 77 (8) WHO, p. 623.

Shariff, Abusaleh (1999), *India: Human Development Report,* New Delhi: Oxford University Press.

Usha Devi, M.D., (2001), "Poverty Database in Education Strategies for Monitoring Poverty Reduction", *EPW,* July 21.

16

Refugee Health Care

Policy Options and Strategic Directions

G. SATHIS KUMAR AND S. RAMASWAMY

Of the many global issues, the world refugee problem is perhaps the most complex. Unlike the others, it has no dominant trait. Basically, it is a problem of individuals, but it also manifests itself in various forms on the societal, governmental and international levels. It is a humanitarian and moral issue, a security issue, a development issue and to a growing extent also an environmental and natural resources issue (Hakovirta, 1993). Most refugees are ordinary people living extraordinary lives: driven from their homes by fear, conflict and persecution, they have had to give up jobs, possessions, dreams, even families in their struggle to survive. They remain as the most vulnerable people in our societies (UNHCR, 2006). With the problem of refugees prevailing in the developing countries than the developed countries, every year, millions of people around the world flee their homes escape persecution, conflict, violence, and circumstances including an environmental component – from rising sea level to drought encroaching deserts. Such complex emergencies principally pose a great risk to the health of populations who are suddenly exposed to new risks and lose access to basic health services. Refugees are placed under great pressures, which can influence their status of well-being, especially living environment – where all health activities are also considered as positive state of social well-being in which harmonious development of mental and physical capacities of individuals' level to the enjoyment of the full life. Recent studies on refugee health and health-related issues (Strand and Jones, 1983;

Young et al., 1987; Hakovirta, 1993; Dolan et al., 1997; Pross, 1998; Ito, 1999; Burns et al., 2000; Hynes, 2002; and Palinkas et al., 2004) have generally eschewed the theoretical explanations of the relationship of culture and disease; and the significance of policy options and strategic directions. This paper does not deal with the former issues, but deals with the latter. Besides, it focuses on the emerging issues in refugee health care and policy options which necessitate the need for designing the refugee health strategy, and analyses the existing strategic and policy directions in refugee health care.

Some Insights on Refugee Health Care

The International Conferences on Health and Human Rights (1994) and Population and Development (1994) have offered a more comprehensive vision on health and highlighted the impact of health policies, programmes, and practices on human rights; and the impacts of human rights abuses on health; and the deeper and fundamental connections between realization of human rights and health promotion and protection (Dolan et al., 1997). Since then, local, regional, national and international, humanitarian and health communities have joined together to provide comprehensive health services to refugees and the displaced. Caring for and protecting the refugees in unstable and insecure environments is not an easy task, nor is meeting their health needs. Nevertheless, these are the major tasks that the governmental and non-governmental, CBOs are committed to undertake. While the health needs and demands of different populations vary, the questions for many are whether and how the health needs of refugees and internally displaced differ from those of populations living in non-refugee situations (Burns et al., 2000).

Knowing the similarities and differences between the populations living in refugee and non-refugee situations could help and guide the policy makers and programme planners, to consider the refugee health care, listen to the voice and demands of the refugees, and thus make following strategic decisions: (i) within humanitarian assistance, knowledge about health and the competence skills to provide health services have to be augmented; (ii) health services mostly be based on the needs and demands of the refugees; and (iii) refugee community must be involved in all aspects of programmes of health planning and implementation, so as to ensure that their needs are met and secure their investment in a programme's success; and the international refugee communities must continue to advocate for more funds for health development and for a greater commitment on the part of policy makers and governments (Burns et al., 2000). But, international refugee studies in general, refugee health studies in particular alarmed that the refugees receive only third class health care and while comparing to the other vulnerable sections, the refugees are facing number of difficulties to access the health care services. In addition, the recent studies on refugees' health care (Strand and Jones, 1983; Young et al., 1987; Hakovirta, 1993; Dolan et al., 1997; Pross, 1998; Ito, 1999; Burns et al., 2000; Hynes, 2002; and Palinkas et al., 2004) found that though refugees' right to health are rooted in international law, refugees' health care may sometimes vary by country and by organizational structure. Against this, the emerging issues of refugees is to be viewed from the multi-dimensions because the problem of refugees itself caused by multi-factors.

Emerging Issues in Refugee Health Care

The overwhelming majority of the world's refugees originate from countries where even the most basic resources required for health, such as safe drinking water, shelter, an adequate food supply and education, are scare (Foundation House, 2007). Upon arriving in a country, refugees are sent to camps which are usually disserted barracks and public buildings. The camps are often located in isolated areas, hard to reach by public transport, and surrounded by barbed wire with guards posted at the entrance. The services including health are provided to the refugees by physicians who offer only minimum care (Pross, 1998). Physicians who wish to give adequate care to refugees feel handcuffed. The conditions of the services provided to the refugees may vary from state to state. The current legal and institutional framework for addressing refugees' situations was, however, shaped in the crucible of twentieth century events. Throughout the century, coping with refugee problems has become increasingly formalized. This formalization was inevitable in a world where nation states jealously guard their authority. When people cross the borders on an emergency basis, outside the provisions of normal immigration controls, governments must be concerned. If people such under emergency circumstances, it is because governments have either violated their obligations to their residents or have not been able (whether it is due to war, natural disaster, famine, civil war and unrest, etc.) to protect or assist them at some minimum level (Gallagher, 1989) and in most cases, refugees are forced to sit idly in camps with no hope of attaining self-sufficiency in circumstances a long way from the aspirations of human dignity (Mann, 1985).

One common goal of international refugee laws and regimes is to find out the ways and means to solve the problem of refugees and illustrate and improve the status of refugees in terms of both physical and mental. Research communities of the world have already made several attempts to focus the issues of refugees and found quiet number of new issues for refugee research, viz., education, human rights, geography, history, war, ethnic problems, regional disparities, development etc. Studies on refugee health and health-related issues (Strand and Jones, 1983; Young et al., 1987; Hakovirta, 1993; Dolan et al., 1997; Pross, 1998; Ito, 1999; Burns et al., 2000; Hynes, 2002; and Palinkas et al., 2004) have generally eschewed theoretical explanations of the relationship of culture and disease and emphasized specific illness conditions, immunization levels, or the potential for disease outbreaks (Young et al., 1987). Further, it found that refugees generally experience a threefold challenge to their health and well-being, viz.,: (i) psychiatric disorders precipitated by the refugee experience; (ii) infectious and parasitic diseases endemic to countries of origin; and (iii) chronic diseases endemic to host countries (Palinkas et al., 2004); and research studies on refugees' health show that the stable population in long-term camp situations often enjoy better health and access to health care than people in either the country of origin or the host communities. The US Centers for Disease Control and Prevention conducted a research in 52 post-emergency phase camps in seven countries. The study concluded that refugees and internally displaced in most of these settings had better health outcomes than their respective host or country of origin populations (Hynes, 2002). These results suggest that investing in health programmes can make a measurable impact on the health of refugees and internally displaced. Present-day, international humanitarian agency like United Nations High Commission for Refugees (UNHCR), is working for the welfare of the refugees' community. UNHCR and other international organizations and institutions' research studies on refugees' health are alarmed that irrespective of nation, region, political belief, etc., refugees have very poor health status and they have always been experiencing difficulties in accessing and making use of the health services in the host countries. Providing health services and protecting the well-being of refugees are in the interests of both refugees and the local community at large. Good physical and mental health is vital for refugees to deal effectively with the challenges of settling in the host country and to participate fully in the economic, social and cultural life of their asylum countries. It is recognized that the physical and mental health and well-being of refugees depends on their access not only to health services, but also the delivery of effective health services to refugees may demand attention to social and economic issues in their lives. The

World Health Organization (WHO) has identified social and economic factors, such as employment, which are very influential in the quality of health, defined by WHO as "a state of complete physical, mental and social well-being and not merely the absence of disease or infirmity",

In general, addressing key social determinants of health such as employment and experience of discrimination is outside the traditional ambit of the health services system. However, national and international health service agencies can have significant roles to play in promoting refugee health and well-being generally by: linking refugees with services that can assist with concerns such as employment, education and housing; supporting the capacity building of refugee communities so that they are better able to assist settled and newly arrived members; and providing sites and spaces for social connection, an important social determinant of health, for example through their roles in offering recreational activities and support groups (Foundation House, 2004).

A seminar report by International Organization of Migration (IOM) says that in our new world order, an increasing number of refugees are likely to be caught in post-conflict or tenuous economic or political situations, and may have limited access to health care; they are therefore at great risk from infectious diseases and reproductive, mental, and other health problems. Further, the report exhibits that there is a need for a dynamic relationship and interdependence that exists between refugees and health, and the need for involvement of the various populations including the population of host countries. On one hand, the host countries' needs include: (i) Protection of native populations from disease threats which may be introduced, imported, or propagated by migrating populations; and (ii) Reduction of burden on publicly funded health and social services programmes that might be required by refugees before and after resettlement. On the other hand, refugee populations have certain priorities that include: (i) Need for timely and safe movement to resettlement; (ii) Access to appropriate medical treatments and health interventions, both to improve health during displacement and forced migration and to facilitate successful integration into resettlement communities; and (iii). Protection of civil society liberties. Clearly, one of the most important challenges we face today is producing development policies that integrate refugees and health needs of receiving and host countries and refugee populations (IOM, 2004). As against this, countries like Australia, New Zealand, and United State have developed a highly effective refugee health strategy and they have designed several policies to improve the health status of the refugees by removing the difficulties that prevailed in accessing the health services. Accordingly, the community of refugees' research stressed that in addition to the regular health services and strategies, it is need of the hour to adopt exclusive health strategies for refugees especially in the countries where the refuges flight is higher.

Refugee Health Strategy and Policy Options

While formulating any programmes and policies related to the welfare of the vulnerable group including refugees, it is suggested that the opinion and involvement of the respective vulnerable group is essential. On the subject of refugees, New Zealand Diversity Action Programme – a research project involving/consulting refugees in the policy decisions, promoted the following principles on health strategy/policy for the refugees and endorsed by the refugee communities: *Principle 1: Nothing about us is without us.* Refugee communities should be involved meaningfully and respectfully at all stages in health policy development and in health service delivery; *Principle 2: Focus on strengths not weaknesses.* Refugees must be integrated into this country knowledge, experience and many skills. This is the place where we live peacefully and we want to contribute for the development. We have confidence in capacity building to show our strength to the host communities; *Principle 3: Human rights are the basis for policy development and implementation.* A human rights approach should be the basis for policy development and service delivery; and *Principle 4: A shared voice is a strong voice.* There is much in common voices among the refugee communities that coming together and working together are common issues (New Zealand Diversity Action Programme, 2006).

Figure 1

Necessity of including Refugees as Beneficiary of Health System of Host Country

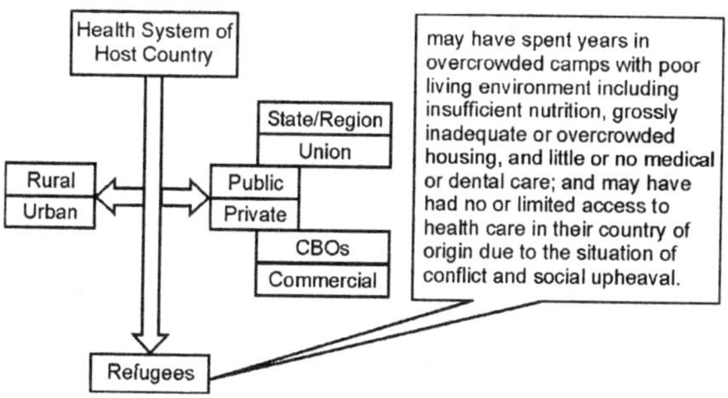

To build a sustainable model of refugee health strategy, it has been suggested that Community Based Organizations (CBOs) are better suited to act as the cultural intermediaries and interpreters of the medical message than the native clinic and clinical professionals. Effective arrangement for health funding would be a partnership between the health departments and the CBOs to develop health-related guidelines and materials for promoting health outreach activities. The health department of host country has the resources and specialized professionals to develop health materials, and the CBOs posses skills to translate and present materials for effective understanding of the refugee population. (Ito, 1999) Of course, the needs of refugees are diverse. Some refugees arrive with physical injuries, a diverse range of diseases and may be survivors of torture and trauma. On arrival they have no knowledge of the health delivery system of the host country, and they do not know what services and where the services are located. Accordingly, the effective model of refugee health strategy should enable the refugee communities to make choices which must be conducive to their health; improve access for refugees to a range of health services; enhance the health services directed to the refugees health, in partnership with community based organizations, and governmental agencies; and promote research into refugee health (NSW Health, 1999). Thus, there is a need for effective model for refugee health, because, refugees are one of the most vulnerable groups in our society; linking refugees into health services early on arrival is a mandatory to any nation since they are the signatory to a number of important international treaties on humanitarian and above all, there is a need to develop a clear framework to guide existing service provisions and to promote collaboration in the health service needs of refugees, for which sustainable health delivery model for refugees are recommended for taking care of the refugees.

Conclusion

It is an universally accepted fact that the right to environmental health and the right to safe living environment are necessary and essential conditions for secure and sustainable living of humans. These are equally applicable to both native and refugee population. Health in general and environmental health in particular is seldom found in the research areas of leading national and international institutions which should emphasize on refugee health, including quality of life – determined by physical, social and psycho-social factors of refugees. Besides, these institutions could assess, correct and prevent those factors which potentially affect the refugee health. Moreover, the research institutions which deal with refugee welfare are mostly located in the developed countries (UNHCR, Refugees Study Centre (London); Centre for Refugee

Studies) where the problems of refugee are less and scanty. None of the institutions in developing countries worried about the welfare of refugee and displaced population whose welfare and voices are unnoticed, uncared, and ignored by governments of host countries. Under these circumstances, the institutions in developing countries could come forward to establish the action-oriented research centres in collaboration with international research institutions so as to project the issues and problems of refugees which are caused by many critical factors such as racial and religious conflicts, ethnic and cultural conflicts, credo and ideological conflicts, political and demographic conflicts, social and economic conflicts, and ecological and developmental conflicts. These conflicts could be scientifically analysed, based on the information available both at the local to global levels. Globally acceptable development policies are to be designed by involving the various conflict victims, decision makers, policy makers and experts from CBOs who have to work together for the advancement of welfare (including environmental health services and health systems) of conflict victims in general and refugees in particular. In addition, providing appropriate health care facilities with acceptable training and development to refugee population could improve the quality of human capital. This could enhance the livelihood opportunities of refugees in the host countries where they are both directly or indirectly involved in the economic development of host countries. These initiatives on policy options and strategic directions could improve the welfare of refugees and their dependents.

References

Burns, Kate, Serge Male and Daniel Pierotti (2000), "Why Refugees Need Reproductive Health Services", *International Family Planning Perspectives*, Vol. 26, No. 4, December, pp. 161–92.

Dolan, Christopher G., Stephen M. Tollman, Vusimuzi G. Nkuna and John S.S. Gear (1997), "The Links between Legal Status and Environmental Health: A Case Study of Mozambican Refugees and their Hosts in the Mpumalanga (Eastern Transvaal) Lowveld, South Africa", *Health and Human Rights*, Vol. 2, No. 2, pp. 62–84.

Foundation House (2004), "Towards a Health Strategy for Refugees and Asylum Seekers in Victoria", Foundation House, Australia.

—— (2007), "Promoting Refugees Health: A Guide for Doctors and Other Health Care Providers for People from Refugee Backgrounds", Foundation House, Australia.

Gallagher, D. (1989), "The Era of Refugees: The Evolution of the International Refugee System", Refugees Policy Group, Centre for Policy Analysis and Research on Refugee Issues, Washington DC, pp. 1–2.

Hakovirta, Harto (1993), "The Global Refugee Problem: A Model and Its Application", *International Political Science Review*, Vol.14, No. 1, International Political Economy and the Global Environment, pp. 35–57.

Hynes, M. (2002), "Reproductive Health Indicators and Outcomes among Refugee and Internally Displaced Persons in Post Emergency Phase Camps", *Journal of the American Medical Association* 288 (5): pp. 595–603. Available at: http://jama.ama-assn.org/cgi/reprint/288/5/595.pdf.

International Organization for Migration (2004), "Migration Health Policies: Shifting the Paradigm from Exclusion to Inclusion", Seminar on *Health and Migration,* 9–11 June.

Ito, Karen L., (1999) "Health Culture and the Clinical Encounter: Vietnamese Refugees' Responses to Preventive Drug Treatment of Inactive Tuberculosis", *Medical Anthropology Quarterly,* New Series, Vol. 13, No. 3, pp. 338–364.

Mann, Julia Hauser (1985), International Protection Refugees and Displaced Persons: An Analysis of Lacunae and Weaknesses in the Legal and Institutional Framework for the International Protection of Refugees and Displaced Persons and Recommendations for its Strengthening, The Independent Committee on International Humanitarian Issues, pp. 1–2.

New Zealand Diversity Action Programme (2006), "Wellington Regional Action Plan for Refugee Health and Well-Being", Human Rights Commission, New Zealand.

NSW Health (1999), "Strategic Directions in Refugee Health Care in NSW", NSW Health Department, Australia.

Palinkas, Lawrence A., Sheila M. Pickwell, Kendra Brandstein, Terry J. Clark, Linda L. Hill, Robert J. Moser and Abdikadir Osman (2004), "The Journey to Wellness: Stages of Refugee Health Promotion and Disease Prevention", *Journal of Immigrant Health*, Vol. 5, No. 1 , pp.19–28.

Pross, Christian (1998), "Third Class Medicine: Health Care for Refugees in Germany", *Health and Human Rights,* Vol. 3, No. 2, Fiftieth Anniversary of the Universal Declaration of Human Rights, pp. 40–53.

Strand Paul J. and Woodrow Jones, Jr. (November, 1983), Health Service Utilization by Indochinese Refugees", *Medical Care,* Vol. 21, No. 11, pp. 1089–98.

UNHCR (2006), State of the World Refugees, United Nation, High Commissioner for Refugees Geneva.

Young, Rosalie F., Allen Bukoff, John B. Waller, Jr. and Stephen B. Blount (1987), Health Status, Health Problems and Practices among Refugees from the Middle East, Eastern, Europe and Southeast Asia", *International Migration Review,* Vol. 21, No. 3, Special Issue: Migration and Health, pp. 760–82.

Section IV

Health Status and Health Security

17

Population Ageing in India

Emerging Health Issues

K.E. VAIDYANATHAN

Population ageing is defined as the process by which the proportion of elderly persons in the population increases as a result of continuous decline in fertility and mortality over the years. In 1990, the proportion of population over 60 years of age was only 6.8 per cent, which is likely to increase to 20.1 per cent by 2050. Moreover, the oldest old (80 years and over) is also expected to increase to 3.1 per cent in 2050 from about 0.4 per cent in 1990. In absolute terms the elderly population in India (60+) will increase from 76.7 million in 2000 to 302.5 million in 2050, which is a fourfold increase. The population of very old (80+) will increase from 6.1 million in 2000 to 47 million in 2050, almost an eightfold increase. This paper addresses the health consequences of the ageing process in India and its implications for policy. At the outset, the paper tries to give a global perspective by comparing the situation in India with the situation in China and countries with more advanced ageing. In the following sections, the ageing trends in India are examined, along with the inter-state differentials in ageing. At the same time attempt has been made to look at the situation in states like Kerala and Tamil Nadu which are ahead of the rest of the states in the ageing process. The paper draws upon the 2000 revision of United Nations Population Projections up to 2050 for the national level trends, the Census of India, 2001 and the projections based upon these results for inter-state differentials. Other sources of data utilized in the study include the health data from the National Sample Survey (NSS) and the Survey of Causes of Deaths in rural areas that allow comparisons between states in their health situation.

The commonly used indicators of ageing are the proportion of population above 60 years of age and the median age of the population (United Nations, 2002). Another indicator that is widely used is the percentage of population over 80 years of age, which is meant to reflect the extent of ageing among the elderly. The median age of the population is that age which divides the population into two equal parts, and is regarded as an indicator of the shift in population structure towards older ages. These indicators derived from the United Nations population estimates provide an indication of the global trends in ageing.

Global Trends in Ageing

During the period 1950–2000 the proportion of elderly (60 years and above) in the world had increased from 8 per cent to 10 per cent, while the proportion of children under 15 years of age has declined from 34 per cent in 1950 to 30 per cent in 2000. The median age for the world had increased from 23.6 in 1950 to 26.4 in 2000, an increase of 2.8 years. Table1 presents the comparative trends in population ageing in India, China and more developed countries. In India, the proportion of elderly (60+) has increased from 5.6 per cent in 1950 to 7.5 per cent in 2000, and in China the increase has been from 7.5 per cent in 1950 to 10.1 per cent in 2000. It is obvious that China is ahead of India in the ageing process. The proportion of elderly in the more developed regions (MDR) in 2000 was 19 per cent, which is greater than the proportion of children (18%), while in 1950 the proportion of children (27%) exceeded the proportion of elderly (12%). During this period the median age rose from 28.6 years to 37.3 years, an increase of 8.7 years. It is obvious that the more developed regions are leading in the process of population ageing.

The population projections of United Nations provide an indication of the future trends in ageing, subject to the realization of the assumptions regarding the changes in fertility and mortality implied in these projections. Over the next fifty years (2000–50), the proportion of elderly (60+) in the world is likely to double to 21 per cent, while the proportion of children (0–14) is likely to drop by a third to 20 per cent. In India, the proportion of elderly will increase to 20.1 per cent in 2050 from 7.5 per cent in 2000, while in China the increase will be 30 per cent in 2050 from 10.1 per cent in 2000. In the more developed regions the proportion of elderly in 2050 is expected to be double that of children (32% as against 16%).

Table 1

Trends in the Ageing of Population in India, China and More Developed Regions

Year	India			China			MDR		
	% 60+	% 80+	Median Age	% 60+	% 80+	Median Age	% 60+	% 80+	Median Age
1950	5.6	0.3	28.4	7.5	0.3	23.9	11.7	1.0	26.6
1960	5.7	0.3	20.4	7.2	0.4	21.9	12.6	1.3	29.6
1970	6.0	0.3	19.9	6.8	0.5	19.7	14.5	1.6	30.6
1980	6.5	0.3	20.6	7.4	0.4	22.1	15.5	2.0	31.9
1990	6.8	0.4	21.8	8.6	0.7	25.3	17.6	2.7	34.4
2000	7.5	0.6	23.4	10.1	0.9	30.0	19.4	3.1	37.3
2010	8.6	0.8	25.8	12.3	1.3	34.6	21.8	4.2	40.0
2020	10.8	1.1	28.7	16.8	1.9	37.4	25.8	5.1	42.2
2030	13.8	1.5	31.9	23.6	2.7	40.8	29.1	6.3	44.2
2040	16.7	2.2	35.0	27.6	4.4	43.0	31.0	8.1	45.4
2050	20.1	3.1	37.0	30.0	7.0	43.8	32.3	9.2	45.2

Source: United Nations, World Population Prospects: The 2002 Revision, Vol. I Comprehensive Tables, New York, 2003. MDR refers to more developed regions comprising Europe, Northern America, Australia, New Zealand and Japan.

Population ageing in the less developed regions including India had been rather slow in the past due to the high levels of fertility. The proportion of elderly persons increased from 6 per cent in 1950 to 8 per cent in 2000 and the proportion of children declined from 38 per cent to 33 per cent during this period. United Nations projections indicate that more rapid population ageing may be expected in the future. By 2050, the proportion of older person in the less developed regions will rise to 20 per cent, whereas the proportion of children will decline to 21 per cent. The median age, which had undergone only a small change during 1950 to 2000, is projected to increase by almost 12 years to 35 years in 2050. It may therefore be expected that by 2050 the less developed regions are likely to have an age structure similar to that of today's developed regions (United Nations, 2003).

Population ageing will result in a rapid increase in the number of people aged 60 years and over. At the global level, the number will rise from 606 million in 2000 to 1.9 million in 2050. The absolute increase will be substantial in the less developed regions, where the elderly population will more than quadruple, from 375 million in 2000 to 1.5 billion in 2050. In India, the elderly population will increase from 76.7 million in 2000 to 302.5 million in 2050, a fourfold increase. In China the elderly population will increase from 130.8 million in 2000 to 391.5 million during the period 2000–50. The absolute increase will be less marked in the more developed regions, where the number of elderly persons is projected to rise from 232 million in 2000 to 394 million in 2050.

The very old (80+) population will be the fastest growing segment of the population. Their numbers in the world will increase from 69 million in 2000 to 377 million in 2050, a more than fivefold increase. In 2000, China had the largest number of persons aged 80 years and over (11.4 million) and India with 6.1 million came third after USA. The number of very old persons in 2050 in China and India is expected to reach 98 million and 47 million respectively. The number of older persons declines rapidly as the age increases. The octogenarians (80–89) will outnumber the nonagenarians (90–99) by a large margin. At the same time, the rate of increase in the number of nonagenarians will be greater than the rate of increase in the number of octogenarians.

Trends in Ageing in India

The elderly population (60+) in India is growing at a considerably faster rate than the total population. While the annual growth rate of total population had declined from 2.0 per cent during the 1940s to 1.5 per cent in 2000–05 and is projected to decline further to 0.4 per cent during 2045–50, the growth rate of the elderly population will increase until 2030 before declining. In absolute terms the number of elderly persons (60+) in India has increased 3.8 times over the last 50 years and is expected to increase 4.2 times during the next 50 years to touch 324 million by year 2050.

In relative terms the proportion of population 60 years and above had increased from 5.6 per cent in 1950 to 7.6 per cent in 2000 and is projected to increase almost three times to 20.6 per cent in 2050. For the (80+) age group, the increase in proportions will be even greater and it is estimated that the growth could be as much as five times during the next half century. Nearly the same pattern of increase is observed for males and females. As in the case of other developing countries the change in age distribution had been slow in the past, but it is expected to accelerate during the next half century. The median age of India's population which has been around 20 years during the sixties and seventies increased slightly to 23.7 in 2000 and it is projected to increase to 38 years in 2050. This will amount to an increase of 14 years in the median age in the next half century indicating a major shift in the balance between the young and the old.

An important feature of the ageing process is the ageing of the older population itself. The population 80 years and over is currently 0.6 per cent of the population. This proportion is projected to increase to 3.1 per cent by 2050. The average annual growth rate of persons aged 80 years and over during 2000–05 is 4.7 per cent as against a growth rate of 2.7 per cent for 60 years and over. In 2050, the growth rate of the 80+ age group is likely to be 3.5 per cent; while the growth rates of the (60+) age group is likely to be 2.2 per cent.

In 2000, India had about 6 million very old (80+) persons and occupied the third place (after China and USA) for the number of very old persons. By 2050, the number will increase to 48 million and India will move to the second position (after China). The number of centenarians in India is currently about 3200, but the number is expected to increase to 1,41,600 by 2050.

The femininity ratio for the age group (60+) is projected to increase only slightly from 109 per cent in 2000 to 110 in 2050. However, the femininity ratio for the age group (80+) will increase from 122 in 2000 to 140 in 2025 and marginally decline to 136 in 2050. By the end of the century, older women will greatly outnumber older men, and this will be more so in the oldest old population. The "feminization of ageing" has great implications for social security in old age.

Table 2

Trends in Fertility and Mortality in India

Period	*Total Fertility Rate*	*Life Expectancy at Birth*
1950–55	5.97	38.7
1960–65	5.81	45.5
1970–75	5.43	50.3
1980–85	4.48	54.9
1990–95	3.60	59.9
1995–2000	3.48	62.1
2000–2005	3.01	63.9
2010–15	2.46	66.3
2020–25	2.14	67.8
2030–35	1.92	70.0
2040–45	1.85	72.6
2045–50	1.85	73.8

Source: United Nations, *World Population Prospects: The 2002 Revision*, Vol. 1, Comprehensive Tables, New York, 2003.

Ageing is the result of the demographic transition in which both mortality and fertility decline from higher to lower levels. Table 2 presents the trends in fertility and mortality for the period up to 2000 and the projected trends up to 2050.

The total fertility rate of India had declined from 6 in 1950 to 3 in 2000 and is expected to decline further to 2.1 in 2025–30. In India fertility decline had started later than in several developing countries such as China, and is proceeding at a slower pace. At the same time the expectancy of life at birth for both sexes had increased from 38.7 years in 1950–55 to 64.2 years in 2000–05 or at the rate of over half year per year. It is expected to increase further to 75.4 years at the end of the century at the rate of 0.25 years per year. In other words the annual increase in life expectancy during the next half century is likely to be slower than the increase during the last half century.

Under the conditions of mortality of the period 2000–05, 64.2 per cent of the new born are expected to survive to 60 years and 27.8 per cent will survive to 80 years. Under the projected conditions of mortality for the period 2045–50, around 75.4 per cent of the new born will survive to age 60 and 48.4 per cent will survive to 80 years of age. There is thus a shift in the survival curve towards older ages. Those surviving to old age are also tending to live longer. The average expectancy of life in India at age 80 is expected to be 7.7 years in 2045–50, which is an increase of 24 per cent in the next half century. This is in contrast to the anticipated increase of 22 per cent for age 60 and 17 per cent at birth.

Inter-state Differences in Ageing

Table 3 presents the estimates of ageing for states classified according to their current levels of ageing. For this analysis, states have been grouped into four categories—those of relatively high, moderate, low and very low ageing—based on the proportion of population 60 years and over in 2001. There are differences in the extent of ageing in different states of India arising from differences in the past fertility and mortality regimes among the states. Only one state Kerala, which had 10.6 per cent of population in the age group 60 years and over in 2001 qualifies to be included in the relatively High ageing category. Four states (Tamil Nadu, Himachal Pradesh, Punjab and Maharashtra) which had proportions of (60+) population ranging between 8 and 10 per cent are included in the moderate ageing category. Seven states (Orissa, Uttaranchal, Karnataka, Andhra Pradesh, Haryana, Gujarat, West

Bengal), which had proportions of (60+) population ranging between 6.6 and 8.0 per cent are included in the Low ageing category. The Very Low ageing category includes ten states (Chhattisgarh, Jammu & Kashmir, Madhya Pradesh, Uttar Pradesh, Rajasthan, Bihar, northeastern states, Assam, Delhi and Jharkhand) that had proportions ranging from 5 per cent to 6.5 per cent.

Table 3

Trends in the Percentage of Population 60 Years and Over across States of India (High, Moderate, Low and Very Low Ageing States)

Level of Ageing/State	*2001*	*2006*	*2011*	*2016*	*2021*	*2026*
High						
Kerala	10.6	11.2	12.3	14.0	16.0	18.3
Moderate						
Tamil Nadu	9.0	10.0	11.2	12.9	14.8	17.1
Himachal Pradesh	8.8	9.4	10.3	11.5	12.9	14.7
Punjab	8.7	9.1	9.7	10.9	12.6	14.6
Maharashtra	8.3	8.6	8.0	9.9	11.2	12.9
Low						
Orissa	7.8	8.3	9.0	10.1	11.8	13.8
Uttaranchal	7.3	7.9	8.5	9.3	10.4	11.7
Karnataka	7.3	8.1	9.2	10.7	12.5	14.5
Andhra Pradesh	7.2	8.0	9.1	10.5	12.2	14.2
Haryana	7.0	7.2	7.6	8.7	9.7	11.4
Gujarat	6.7	7.4	8.4	9.8	11.6	13.7
West Bengal	6.6	7.5	8.5	10.0	11.9	14.2
Chhattisgarh	6.5	7.2	7.9	8.8	10.0	11.6
Jammu & Kashmir	6.2	6.9	7.7	8.9	10.5	12.4
Madhya Pradesh	6.2	6.7	7.1	7.8	8.9	10.4
Uttar Pradesh	6.1	6.6	7.1	7.8	8.7	9.8
Rajasthan	6.0	6.7	7.3	8.2	9.4	10.8
Very Low						
Bihar	5.5	6.3	7.2	8.2	9.5	11.0
N E States (Excl Assam)	5.3	6.2	7.3	8.7	10.4	12.4
Assam	5.2	5.8	6.5	7.6	9.1	11.0
Delhi	5.1	5.7	6.5	7.5	8.7	10.0
Jharkhand	5.0	6.0	7.1	8.3	9.7	11.3
India	6.9	7.5	8.3	9.3	10.7	12.4

Note: The states have been grouped into High, Moderate, Low and Very Low ageing categories based on the percentage of population in the (60+) age group as follows: 10+, 8–10, 6–8 and below 6.

Source: Government of India, Technical Group's Population Projections (RGI, 2006), Table 1.

According to these projections the proportion of (60+) population in India will increase from 6.9 per cent in 2001 to 12.4 per cent in 2026, an increase of 5.5 percentage points. Kerala State, which has the highest level of ageing in 2001 (10.6%), will gain 7.7 percentage points. Tamil Nadu which comes next in ageing in 2001 (9.0%) will gain 8.1 percentage points. At the other extreme Jharkhand, which has the lowest level of ageing (5.0%), will gain 6.3 percentage points. Table 4 compares the index of the pace of ageing in the four groups of states.

Table 4

The Pace of Ageing by States Grouped According to their Level of Ageing in 2001

Year/Period	*High*	*Moderate*	*Low*	*Very Low*
Proportion 60+				
2001	10.6	8.7	6.7	5.2
2006	11.2	9.2	7.4	6.0
2011	12.3	9.8	8.1	6.9
2016	14.0	11.3	9.2	8.0
2021	16.0	12.9	10.7	9.5
2016	18.3	14.8	12.4	11.1
Pace of Ageing Index				
2001–2006	0.6	0.5	0.8	0.8
2006–2011	1.2	0.7	0.9	1.0
2011–2016	1.9	1.7	1.2	1.2
2016–2021	2.3	1.8	1.7	1.6
2021–2026	2.7	2.2	1.9	1.8

Source: Derived from Table 3. This index is computed by expressing the change in the level of ageing as a percentage of the maximum possible change.

The states in the Very Low ageing group will gain 5.8 percentage points in the proportion (60+), while the High category will gain by 7.7 percentage points. The Moderate and Low categories will gain 6 to 7 percentage points. The Index of pace of ageing confirms that the high ageing states are ageing faster than the rest and the speed of ageing declines with the level of ageing. This indicates that while all the states are undergoing the process of ageing, 25 years from now the disparities between states will be greater. Kerala and Tamil Nadu are and will remain far ahead in the ageing process and the states of Bihar, Assam, other NE states, Delhi and Jharkhand will remain at the lowest rung of the ageing process.

Health of the Elderly

Mortality and morbidity statistics in India are inadequate to draw any definitive conclusions about the health situation of the elderly population. Only a third of the deaths are registered, and the extent of registration varies in different areas of the country. Medical certification of causes of deaths covers the deaths occurring in the district and teaching hospitals in the country but the coverage is less than ten per cent of the registered deaths in most states. The medically certified deaths are recorded for 17 broad cause groups, but regrettably the data are not classified by age groups to enable analysis of causes of deaths among the elderly population.

Table 5

Percentage Distribution of Deaths for Persons Over 60 Years by Cause (top nine only) Rural India and Kerala, 1995

Cause of Death	*India (percentage)*	*Kerala (percentage)*
Bronchitis and Asthma	38.4	23.2
Heart Attack	19.6	32.2
TB of Lungs	8.7	2.3
Pneumonia	1.4	1.5
Cancer	10.5	12.3
Paralysis	12.5	24.9
Anaemia	6.2	1.8
Vehicular accidents	1.9	1.5
Suicide	0.8	0.3
Total	100.0	100.0

Source: Derived from Tables 19–28 of RGI, Survey of Causes of Death, Rural, India, Annual Report, 1995, New Delhi.

Another source of information is the Annual Survey of Causes of Deaths in rural areas carried out by the Registrar General of India. The annual publication provides the distribution of the deaths due to major causes according to age groups. The data requires considerable manipulation to obtain the distribution by cause of deaths. Table 5 provides a comparison of the cause of death distribution for India and Kerala for the year 1995, to provide an idea of the changing structure of causes of death as a result of the ageing process. This table shows that a state like Kerala with a more advanced ageing has relatively greater proportion of deaths from heart attacks, paralysis and cancer and relatively less proportion of deaths from respiratory ailments. Based on a comparison of the spectrum of causes of deaths in India with the countries like

China and Japan, it may be expected that the non-communicable and metabolic diseases will increase with the ageing process in India (Vaidyanathan, 2006).

Disabilities of the Elderly

The 2001 Census provides valuable information on the disabilities among the elderly according to type of disability (Table 6). According to this table there are 3.6 million elderly persons with disabilities, and this works out to about 5 per cent of the population 60 years and above. The disability ratio is slightly higher among males than among females. Visual disabilities account for over one-half of the disabilities among the elderly population.

Table 6

Number and Percentage of Disabled Persons 60 Years and Above by Type of Disability, India, 2001

Type of Disability	*Males (000)*	*Percentage of 60+ Pop*	*Females (000)*	*Percentage of 60+Pop*
Visual Disability	965	2.55	992	2.55
Speech Disability	65	0.17	57	0.15
Hearing Disability	233	0.62	242	0.62
Movement Disability	604	1.60	434	1.12
Mental Disability	95	0.25	87	0.22
Total	1963	5.19	1611	4.66

Source: Derived from RGI, Census of India, 2001, Disability Tables, Table C–20.

Table 7

Percentage of Physically Disabled Persons 60 Years and Above by the Extent of Physical Disability, Rural and Urban, 2002

Extent of Physical Disability	*Rural Males*	*Rural Females*	*Urban Males*	*Urban Females*
Cannot take self-care even with aid/appliances	17.7	20.8	17.5	21.8
Can take care with aid/appliances	29.1	23.4	28.6	26.2
Can take care without aid/appliances	43.6	44.7	48.0	45.3
Aid/appliances not available	9.4	11.0	5.8	6.3
Not Reported	0.2	0.1	0.1	0.4
Total	100.0	100.0	100.0	100.0

Source: National Sample Survey Report No 485, Disabled Persons in India, July – December 02.

The National Sample Survey provides some interesting information on the ability of the disabled elderly to carry on their lives independently or otherwise (Table 7). Nearly one-fifth of the disabled elderly cannot take self-care even with aids and appliances, and these are the most vulnerable among the elderly population.

Economic Consequences of Ageing

The decline in fertility and mortality will result in an increase in Elderly Dependency Rations (EDRs). In India the EDR is likely to increase from 6 per cent in the year 2000 to 22 per cent in 2050. The Elderly Dependency Ratio is the ratio of the elderly population 65 years and over and 80 years and over expressed as a percentage of population aged 15–64 years. It will increase even more in China and more developed regions, but this is no consolation for us. What this implies is that more and more elderly will need public support, since there will be fewer sons and daughters who could support them.

Another aspect of the ageing of population is that it is taking place alongside the epidemiological transition in the country as reflected in the changing pattern of causes of death. There will be a decline in the share of communicable diseases as we move from the nascent stage of ageing to an advanced stage of ageing. The relative share of infectious and parasitic diseases will decline and the relative share of non-communicable diseases will increase. Non-communicable diseases (NCDs) like malignant neoplasm, diabetes mellitus, cardiovascular diseases and nutritional and endocrinal disorders will increase with the ageing of population. As a result of the shift towards chronic and degenerative diseases, there is a greater risk of disabilities among the elderly. Even as countries like India are struggling with infectious diseases, malnutrition and complications from childbirth, they are faced with the rapid growth of NCDs. The shift from communicable to non-communicable diseases will escalate as the ageing process continues, and by the year 2020, the NCDs will constitute three-fourths of the burden of diseases. This "double burden" of disease is causing great strains to the already scarce resources of the developing countries. The expenditure for treating chronic ailments is far greater than treating the traditional ailments.

The extended longevity of the elderly will comprise of years with chronic illnesses, the most common ailments being cardiovascular diseases, hypertension, diabetes, visual and hearing impairment, mental illnesses etc. According to WHO estimates of Healthy Life Expectancy (HALE), 10 to 15 per cent of expectancy of life is lost in illness and disability (WHO, 2004). The elderly will have to cope with higher health expenditures alongside a fall in productivity. Presently, very few elderly are able to avail health insurance, and public health institutions are poorly equipped and poorly run, with the result that they are not suitable for providing the services required by the elderly. At the same time employment opportunities for the elderly is practically non-existent in India.

Less than 2 per cent of the older persons in India have old-age pension, provident fund or other benefits. Our health care system is unable to cope with even traditional ailments and health insurance system hardly covers a negligible proportion of population. At the same time, the number of elderly persons is increasing and the burden of dependency is also increasing. The number of elderly persons living alone in their homes and without support is increasing as a result of the breakdown in the joint-family system and the migration of our young ones to greener pastures elsewhere. In all our cities the number of old-age homes is increasing and many of them are commercial ventures lacking even basic amenities.

Geriatric care is lacking in government hospitals and primary health centres, and is available at very high cost only in a multi-specialty hospitals. Home and community based programmes for the elderly is practically non-existent in India. In India, most elderly persons are cared in their own homes by their kith and kin. However, with urbanization and industrialization and the break-up of the joint-family system, more and more elderly will be in need of public support systems. The mushrooming of "old-age homes" and the increase in the number of cases in family courts seeking support of their sons and daughters is an indication of the growing need for a public support system for the elderly in India.

Since women tend to live longer than men do, the number of women do surpass men among the elderly, often referred to as "feminization" of the ageing process. They are also likely to be more vulnerable to illnesses during old age. Women have special health needs arising from their role as mother, and caregiver to the family. Women's traditional roles as care givers may also contribute to their increased poverty and ill-health during older age.

It is not uncommon that women give up paid employment in order to fulfil their care giving responsibilities. Others never had access to paid employment because they were looking after their husband, children or old parents. Because of cultural reasons many of the elderly women are widows who depend upon their sons or daughters for support. Census and survey data clearly indicate higher level of illiteracy among elderly women than among elderly men, and poverty levels is also greater among elderly women. In a recent paper Ashish Bose argues that increased life expectancy does not automatically lead to a better quality of life for the elderly, especially the women. (Bose, 2008)

Way Forward

WHO has been advocating a policy of "active ageing", where active ageing is defined as the process of optimizing opportunities for health, participation and security in order to enhance quality of life as people age (WHO, 2002). The active ageing approach provides a framework for the development of global, national and local strategies on population ageing. Active ageing applies to both individuals and population groups enabling them to realize their full potential for physical, social and mental well-being throughout their life time according to their needs, desires and capacities. At the same time they should be provided adequate protection, security and care when assistance is needed. WHO recommendations include policy proposals in the areas of: (1) health, (2) participation, and (3) security.

The proposals for health include reduction of risk factors and enhancing protection through access to health care where and when required. The proposals for participation include opportunities for employment, education and social, cultural and religious activities in order to make a productive contribution in paid and unpaid activities as they age. The proposals for security include protection, security and care in the event they are not able to support and protect themselves. Since public support systems are inadequate, families and communities should be encouraged to provide care for their older members. Older persons should be viewed as a resource and not a burden or a welfare recipient.

Regrettably, the issue of ageing of population has not received due attention in India in the past. The Tenth Five-Year Plan document hardly mentions the issue of ageing. There is only a small section in the plan document about pensions for destitute. (Planning Commission, 2002). The same has been the case with the Annual Reports of the Ministry of Social Justice and Empowerment, The Ministry's website has two small sections on the National Policy on Older Persons (NPOP) and the Integrated Programme for Older Persons (IPOP). The Maintenance and

Welfare of Parents and Senior Citizens Act 2007 which was passed by Parliament last year is a step in the right direction. This Act makes it obligatory for an adult child or grandchild to maintain elderly parents and enable them to lead a normal life. The Act also provides for a maintenance amount of a maximum of Rs 10,000 per month that children are liable to pay in case they neglect their parents (senior citizens). It remains to be seen how this legislation will be implemented.

The Ministry of Social Justice and Empowerment of the Government of India is the nodal agency vested with the responsibility of implementing the National Policy on Older Persons (NPOP), the Integrated Programmes for Older Persons (IPOP) and the legislation mentioned above. This Ministry is almost entirely occupied with the issues of quotas for SCs, STs and OBCs, and there is a neglect of all other issues including issues of the elderly. The establishment of a separate Ministry for Senior Citizens Welfare could contribute to a positive and dynamic approach to ageing. Moreover, the institutional infrastructure for the support of the elderly at the state, district and local levels is currently non-existent except perhaps some non-governmental organizations.

There is an urgent need to establish the councils, geriatric institutions, ambulatory services for the sick, etc., at the state, district and local community levels. There should be a thorough review of the existing laws and schemes for older persons and the anomalies and inconsistencies should be removed. The laws and regulations governing life insurance and health insurance need to be adapted to the internationally acclaimed best practices. Institutions for the aged such as the old-age homes and geriatric institutions should be regulated and monitored to prevent exploitation of the elderly and their supporters. Universities and academic research institutions should undertake operations and evaluative research on social security issues resulting from ageing of population.

References

Bose, Ashish, (2008), "Increasing Life Expectancy and the Elderly", *Economic and Political Weekly,* August 9.

Ministry of Social Justice and Empowerment (MSJE, 2006), Annual Report, New Delhi.

National Sample Survey (NSS, 1996), The Aged in India: A Socio-economic Profile, 1995–96, Report No. 446.

Planning Commission of India, (2002), Tenth Five-Year Plan, "Labour Welfare and Social Security", Chapter 3.5, New Delhi.

Registrar General of India (RGI, 1990), Survey of Causes of Death (Rural), India, Annual Report, 1995.

Registrar General of India (RGI, 1996), Vital Statistics of India, 1990 based on the Civil Registration System, New Delhi, 1995.

Registrar General of India (RGI, 2006), Population Projections of India and States, 2001–2026, Report of the Technical Group on Population Projections, New Delhi.

UNFPA, (2002), "Population Ageing and Development, Social Health and Gender Issues", Population and Development Strategies, Working Paper No. 3, New York.

United Nations (2003), World Population Prospects: The 2002 Revision, Vol. I. *Comprehensive Tables,* Population Division, DESA, New York.

United Nations, (2002), "Policy Responses to Population and Ageing", *Population Bulletin, Special Issue*, Nos. 44/45, Population Division, DESA, New York.

United Nations, (2002), World Population Ageing, 1950–2050, Population Division, DIESA, New York.

United Nations, (2006), Population Ageing, 2006 Wall Chart, Population Division, DIESA, New York.

Vaidyanathan, K.E. (2006), "Ageing and Health in Developing Countries: The Emerging Scenario", paper presented at the National Seminar on Population Ageing, Sri Venkateswara University, March, 2006

WHO, (2002), Active Ageing: A Policy Framework, Geneva.

WHO, (2004), The World Health Report, 2004: The Changing History, Geneva.

18

Ensuring Health Services for the Poor through Sustainable Micro-Insurance

Experience of BISWA in Sambalpur, Orissa

B.S. MISHRA

According to the World Health Organization (WHO), greater than 80 per cent of total expenditure on health in India is private (figure for 1999–2001 (World Health Organization, 2004)) and most of this flows directly from households to the private-for-profit health care sector. Most studies of health care spending have found that out-of-pocket spending in India is actually progressive, or equity neutral; as a proportion of non-food expenditure, richer Indians spend marginally more than poorer Indians on health care. However, because the poor lack the resources to pay for health care, they are far more likely to avoid going for care, or to become indebted or impoverished trying to pay for it. On an average, the poorest quintile of Indians is 2.6 times more likely than the richest to forgo medical treatment when ill.

Given this scenario of failing public health system and priced health care provisioning by private providers, the only means of universalizing access to health care lies in generating the buying capacity of health care among the poor. Such buying capacity cannot be developed through any other means except through insuring them against such expenditures that is random but inevitable. However, the insurance solution for the poor is always seen as unviable for their inability to pay the required premium regularly. Despite this view there are several innovative approaches suggested in the arena of health insurance provisioning to bring the poor under the umbrella of insurance. The insurance landscape in the country can be described within a two-way spectrum of fully subsidized to non-subsidized as well as for profit to non-profit categories. There are Community Based Health Insurance (CBHI) schemes like Karuna Trust, SEWA, UPLIFT as well as Yeshaswini, which are not for profit as well as without any subsidy. On the contrary we have schemes like Arogyasri, Rashtriya Swasthya Bima Yojana (RSBY) as well as NRHM, which belong to fully subsidized, and for profit category. Apart from the stated schemes, Mediclaim is for profit and not subsidized at all. Despite the variety in the existing landscape of health insurance provisioning, the coverage in general is the least in our country as well as it excludes the poor at large.

Exclusion of the poor as well as catastrophic expenditure on health care among the non-poor compels the interpretation of insurance as a financial tool rather than as a larger health care reform measure. It does have financial implications involving the state, the health providers as well as the individuals. Hence, health insurance has to be considered as a part of the system rather than an aid to smoothen rising health expenditures. In this context, we present below a model of health insurance among the poor executed as an incentive of micro-finance initiative.

Health Insurance for the Poor: The BISWA Model

Health insurance is a need for both the people living below poverty line and those above it. Bharat Integrated Social Welfare Agency (BISWA)'s innovative approach of micro-insurance and services intends to expand a scheme for the entire population of Sambalpur district in Orissa. Pluralistic and innovative model to reach out to members of SHGs, Federations (clusters of SHGs), beggars and people with disability can be a sustainable development approach for pro-poor development in achieving MDG by 2015. Several NGOs and governments worldwide have started micro-credit schemes for vulnerable groups to break the vicious circle of poverty, malnutrition, disease, low productivity, and low income. Micro-credit is now considered not only an effective tool for poverty reduction but also used as an instrument for empowerment of the poor, particularly the women. This operation generates income to the poor by extending them small credits for self-employment and other economic activities. However, it was soon realized that loan repayments by these groups were much below the expected level. The experience suggested that ill-health and expenditure on treatment and associated consumption needs were the prime reasons for defaulting on repayments. To plug the erosion of income of borrowers on health care needs, some NGOs (such as Grameen Bank in Bangladesh and the Self-Employed Women Association (SEWA) in India) have introduced health insurance schemes for their members. The Grameen Bank Health Programme was started in 1994 with the objectives to adopt preventive measures against diseases, to arrange for treatment at minimum cost, and to build a non-profit primary health care system. Under this scheme the borrowers pay a fixed annual amount of 60 Taka per family as premium and a very trivial sum at the time of using the facility. The scheme over time has proven to meet the desired objectives (Rahman, 2000).

This project "Providing sustainable micro-insurance and services to the poor through effective model of BISWA in Sambalpur" specifies that micro-insurance is an effective tool for providing better health care against insurable risks for the people at the bottom of income hierarchy in Sambalpur district of Orissa. The project views the poor not as object of charity but as an untapped market, which is seeking products and services denied to them due to inefficient public health services, low penetration of private insurance, and market disconnect between demand, supply and affordability.

Poor do not buy health insurance due to their inability to pay on a regular basis owing to the seasonal nature of income flows, and ignorance about benefits of insurance. Admittedly, inadequate income is a barrier to receipt of self-financed health protection, which can be overcome with well-targeted subsidies or providing affordable doorstep medical services. The absence of comprehensive assessment of potential insurable risk makes private insurers choose to cover only certain medical risks leading to more expensive rating. On the contrary, the poor are vulnerable to certain local diseases, which require the support from primary health care centres. In majority cases the poor pays frequently for these seasonal diseases rather than those risks covered under the insurance. Consequently, the poor find private health insurance schemes less attractive. In addition, the lack of mutual confidence between the poor and the insurer along with a weak regulatory framework to redress grievances keeps the poor beyond the reach of insurance.

After reviewing the lessons from micro-insurance project implementation on health throughout BISWA's operational area of 14 states in India, BISWA advocates for a partner agent model of providing micro-insurance products and services catering the need of targeted market segment for the poor. The strategy will include promotion of community based drug distribution (CBD) centres at SHG level, providing out-patient department (OPD) facility for SHGs at village level in reimbursing the amount with the insurance companies, and providing health services at affordable cost to the people in disadvantageous conditions.

The innovative component of the proposed project is that BISWA will be promoting community based drug distribution centres at SHG level and establishing the OPD centres at SHGs cluster level. The CBD centres will be promoted in the villages having Self-Help Groups (SHGs) promoted by BISWA and selected members will be provided with necessary training on health issues and social marketing to run the CBD in a social entrepreneurial manner. Medicine for common ailments, equipment for childcare, etc., will be provided in the centres. Establishment of OPD centres will be professionally managed units by doctors, surgeons, pharmacists and pathologists, in providing 24 hrs services at SHGs cluster. The objective of OPD centres will be providing free services to the insured SHG members and providing services to the disadvantaged people at affordable prices.

As a result, people from rural area will be getting primary health services at doorstep at affordable cost through CBD centres, and primary medical facilities like (medicine charges, doctor consultation charges, investigation charges, blood test charges) through OPD centres at affordable prices. The direct economic impact will be wage saving, saving on transportation cost, avoidance of exploitation by intermediaries, and avoidance of higher prices for services. The direct social impact will be awareness among the SHGs and disadvantaged groups about health insurance and improved consciousness regarding utilization of health care. This is a replicable and self-sustainable approach for effective social marketing. Extra efforts will be taken for mitigating frauds, morale hazards, retentions, high transaction costs in the projects through emphasizing client education, peer pressure, communication, special promotional activities on promoting CBD centres and establishment of OPD centres.

Aside from cases where people believed that their illness was not serious, the main reason for not seeking care was cost. The richest quintile of the population is six times more likely than the poorest quintile to have been hospitalized in either the public or private sector. It is estimated that at least 24 per cent of all-India hospitalized category fall below the poverty line because they are hospitalized, and that out-of-pocket spending on hospital care might have raised by 2 per cent the proportion of the population in poverty. Given this context, health insurance appears to be an equitable alternative to out-of-pocket payments.

In recent years, community health insurance (CHI) has emerged as a possible means of: (1) improving access to health care among the poor; and (2) protecting the poor from indebtedness and impoverishment resulting from medical expenditures. The World Health Report 2000, for example, noted that prepayment schemes represent the most effective way to protect people from the costs of health care, and called for investigation into mechanisms to bring the poor into such schemes (World Health Organization, 2000).

BISWA Model of Health Insurance: Against the Odds of Typical Issues in Spreading Health Insurance

Common health insurance initiative begins by considering the optimal design of health insurance policies. Such policies must make trade-offs appropriately between risk sharing on the one hand and agency problems such as moral hazard (the incentive of people to seek more care when they are insured) and supplier-induced demand (the incentive of physicians to provide more care when they are well reimbursed) on the other. Optimal co-insurance arrangements make patients pay for care up to the point where the marginal gains from less risk sharing are just offset by the marginal benefits from less wasteful care being provided. Empirical evidence shows that both moral hazard and demand-inducement are quantitatively important. Co-insurance based on expenditure is a crude control mechanism. Moreover, it places no direct incentives on physicians, who are responsible for most expenditure decisions. To place such incentives on physicians is the goal of supply-side cost containment measures, such as utilization review and capitation. This goal motivates the surge in managed care in the United States, which unites the functions of insurance and provision, and allows for active management of the care that is delivered. The analysis then turns to the operation of health insurance markets. Economists generally favour choice in health insurance for the same reasons they favour choice in other markets: choice allows people to opt for the plan that is best for them and encourages plans to provide services efficiently. But choice in health insurance is a mixed blessing because of adverse selection – the tendency for the sick to choose more generous insurance than the healthy. When sick and healthy enrol in different plans, plans disproportionately composed of poor risks have to charge more than they would if they insured an average mix of people. The resulting high premiums create two adverse effects: they discourage those who are healthier but would prefer generous care from enrolling in those plans (because the premiums are so high), and they encourage plans to adopt measures that deter the sick from enrolling (to reduce their overall costs). The welfare losses from adverse selection are large in practice. Added to them are further losses from having premiums vary with observable health status. Because insurance is contracted for annually, people are denied a valuable form of intertemporal insurance – the right to buy health coverage at average rates in the future should they get sick today. As the ability to predict future health status increases, the lack of intertemporal insurance will become more problematic. We can relate health insurance to the central goal of medical care expenditures – better health. Studies to date are not clear on which approaches to health insurance promote health in the most cost-efficient manner. Resolving this question is the central policy concern in health economics. However, there continues to be endeavours at developing variety of models of providing health insurance that promises expansion in coverage and sustainability.

The proposed model by BISWA is one of them, which considers two vital elements of limitation hindering the spread or viability of health insurance expansion. Making health insurance accessible for the poor is primarily affected by their incapacity to pay as well as the timely payment of premiums owing to their irregular nature of earnings. The BISWA model is overcoming this particular limitation, given that the insurance premium is also paid as a part of the loan that they acquire through micro-finance initiative. Such an arrangement not only ensures timely premium payment from the perspective of the insured but also the insurance company of a certain receipt of premiums. When one considers insurance as a risk pooling exercise, one inherently assumes a larger collection of premiums with lesser and lesser risks of claims. This could always be true when the size of premium payer's domain increase substantially including the less vulnerable as well. BISWA's initiative could also be attractive to the insurance company with profit motive because of ensuring a larger premium collection with less of a transaction cost on their part and least default rate. In either ways an insurance initiative is sustainable provided both the insured and insurer have a win-win situation.

We present below the diagrammatic sketch of the pathway of insurance settlement operation for a particular SHG member (see Figure 1). Micro-insurance coverage of BISWA is given in Table 1 wherein we have provided the different schemes that are adopted from LIC of India, ICICI Lombard, Oriental Insurance as well as TATA AIG. In addition to this information, Table 2 elaborates on the magnitude of coverage and rates of claim settlement, which looks promising.

Concluding Remarks

The three contributing factors that will strengthen this partnership model are: Social capital, pre-existence of community institutions, and interconnectivity with other players (social capital refers to the affinity based relationships, financial support, and safety net that low income groups have with their immediate family, relatives, neighbours, and friends). Non-governmental organization that build on these social assets and have grass-root presence are able to reduce transaction costs, fraudulent claims, and adverse selection through this approach. In fact, taking insurance to the doorstep of the client is perhaps possible only through such initiative where in mutual trust ensures spread and continuity of insurance coverage. Hence, this might pave the way towards making universal health insurance a reality.

Table 1

Micro-insurance Coverage of BISWA

Insurance Company	*Details of Policy Coverage*	*Premium details by the SHG Member*	*Support Provided by BISWA*
LIC of India	Janashree Bima Yojana. 1. Sum assured amount for normal death is Rs 30,000 2. Sum Assured amount for accidental death is Rs 75,000. For permanent disability 100% and for partial disability 50% of the sum insured payable. 3. Scholarship for 2 children studying in 9th to 12th class @ Rs 100 per month.	Rs 100 per year.	To provide complete life insurance service to the SHG members. Moreover extending social as well as financial security service to them covering the risk towards loan.
ICICI Lombard	Health Insurance Scheme for SHG Members. 1. Family Floater group health insurance scheme. 2. Covers all hospitalization expenses as per the policy terms and conditions. 3. Sum insured amount is Rs 15,000 per family. 4. Accidental insurance sum insured is Rs 10,000. 5. Maternity benefit for normal delivery Rs 2,000 and for CS Rs 5,000 is the max amount payable.	Rs 350 per Family.	To provide complete health insurance service to the SHG members and their family. Moreover extending social as well as financial security service to them covering the risk towards loan.

Cont'd...

Cont'd...

Oriental Insurance Company Ltd.	(i) Health Insurance Scheme for SHG members. 1. Family Floater group health insurance scheme. 2. Covers all hospitalization expenses as per the policy terms and conditions. 3. Sum insured amount is Rs 15,000 per family 4. Accidental insurance sum insured is Rs 25,000 for the SHG member only. 5. Maternity benefit for normal delivery Rs 2,000 and for CS Rs 5,000 is the max amount payable. 6. Wage compensation of the member of Rs 40 per day up to 20 days at max. 7. Transportation charges to hospital for Rs 300 at maximum payable. (ii) Asset Insurance Scheme 1. Janata Personal Accident. 2. Kisan Package Policy. 3. Shopkeepers Insurance Policy. (iii) Live Stock Insurance Scheme.	(i) Rs 325 per family. (ii) Varies from Rs 64 to Rs 250 as per the loan amount. (iii) 5% of the loan amount + 12.36% Service tax for one year. 8% of the loan amt + 12.36% Service tax.	To provide complete health insurance service to the SHG members and their family. Moreover extending social as well as financial security service to them covering the risk towards loan. To provide complete asset and live stock insurance service to the SHG member. Moreover extending social as well as financial security service to them covering the risk towards loan.
TATA AIG LIC Ltd.	Sampurna Bima Yojana Sum assured amount is Rs 10,000	Varies from Rs 261 to Rs 1,002 as per the age of the member.	To provide complete life insurance service to the SHG. members along with a policy maturity value after 15 years. This enhances saving nature of the member. Moreover extending social as well as financial security service to them covering the risk towards loan.

Figure 1

The Process of Claim Settlement

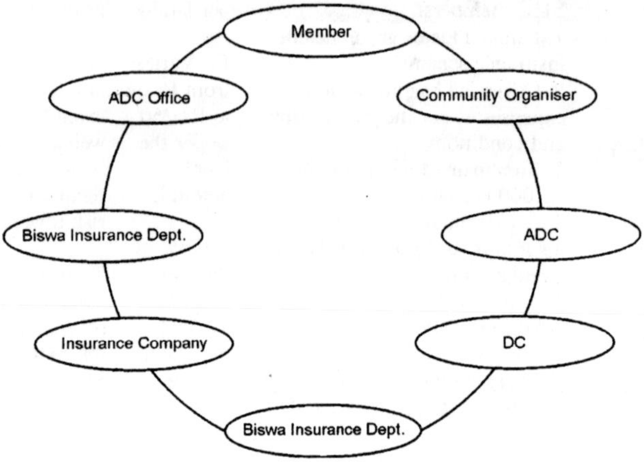

Table 2

BISWA Micro-insurance Achievements as on Date

Policy coverage	*Insurance company and year of commencement*	*Total members covered*	*Number of claims registered*	*Claim settled and payment received*
Life	LIC of India. Started in the month of March 2003.	74,228	135	105 amounting to Rs 27,80,000
Life	Tata-AIG started in the month of June 2007.	18,205	7	7 amounting to Rs 70,000
Health	ICICI Lombard started in the month of January 2006.	1,77,047	604	483 amounting to Rs 27,00,175
Health	Oriental Insurance started in the month of November 2007.	13,581	135	35 amounting to Rs 1,76,442
Asset	Oriental Insurance company started in the month of February 2006.	85, 700	55	31 amounting to Rs 33,00,742

References

Rahman, K., (2000), “Poverty, Micro Credit and Health: What Role can WHO Play?”, WHO Regional Health Forum, Vol. 4, Nos. 1 and 2, pp. 68–80.

WHO (2004): World Health Report 2004, WHO, Geneva.

19

Health Status of Elderly in Old-Age Homes

V. VIJAYALAKSHMI AND K. ANBU

Sociologically speaking, ageing is a series of transition from one set of social roles to another, which is structured by the social system rather than mere biological one. The age categories – infancy, childhood, adolescence, adulthood, middle age, and old age are the inexorable stages of human life, which are determined by both biological as well as socio-economic conditions. The concept of 'ageing' denotes three dimensions: biological, psychological and social. Prior to industrialization, the traditional Indian society bestowed the old age members with responsible leadership roles and powerful decision-making positions because of their vast experience and knowledge. However, the technological developments due to industrialization, westernization, and urbanization – under the purview of distorted form of modernity – have neglected these statuses by weakening the unity and integrity of the joint family and caste group. Moreover, the emergence of achieved properties like wealth, education, etc., has colonized the mindset of the youths by adopting the individualistic value of the West. As a result, the social support and respect for the elderly is in constant decay, today.

The Indian family has traditionally provided natural social security to the old people. However, in more recent times, the traditional role of the family is being shared by institutions such as old-age homes. Many of the elderly parents are compelled to leave their children and stay in old-age homes. The old-age homes, which were a rarity, have recently spread across the country, a fact that indicates the growing rift between the generations.

Old-Age Homes in India: A State-Wise Profile

Development of institutional care for the handicapped, infirm and aged persons in India has a long history. The first old-age home in India is supposed to have been started in the early 18th century but information is available only from 1782. Today, such services are provided mainly by non-governmental agencies, particularly the religious charitable organizations. The central and state governments still play only a very negligible role in providing care to the deprived sections of society. According to the survey conducted by the Madras Institute of Ageing, there were 529 old-age homes in India in 1995 (Nair, 1995). Helpage India has reported that there were 700 old-age homes in 1998 (Helpage India, 1998). Our discussion is based on data released by the Madras Institute on Ageing. India had only 96 old-age homes before 1950; another 94 were added in the next two decades (1951–70). During the next two decades, there was a rapid expansion in the number of old-age homes in the country. As of 1995, Kerala state led the rest of the country with 102 old-age homes, followed by Tamil Nadu (94) and Maharashtra (65). South India (Kerala, Tamil Nadu, Karnataka and Andhra Pradesh) accounts for 275 old-age homes forming 52 per cent of the total. The reason for the old-age homes flourishing in South India is nothing but, old-age homes are run by various agencies – secular organizations, religious groups (Hindu, Muslim, Christian), government and others. Taking the country as a whole, secular organizations run 224 old-age homes (42%), followed by Christian 12 agencies with 216 (40%) old-age homes. Of the 216 old-age homes maintained by Christian agencies, 82 are located in Kerala, 42 in Tamil Nadu and 21 in Goa. The government—central and state—is responsible for only 10 old-age homes in the entire country.

In keeping with the cultural and religious traditions prevailing in India, there are separate old-age homes for males and females while some old-age homes are meant for the poor aged and destitutes. Others concentrate on the sick and handicapped. There are 16 old-age homes catering exclusively to males, 4 are meant for aged, 13 for poor aged and destitutes and 3 for sick and handicapped. The institutions which admit both male and female elderly are large in number. Among the 306 homes in this category, 141 are run exclusively for aged, 136 for the poor aged and the destitutes and 29 for the sick and the handicapped. As discussed earlier, around 83 per cent of old-age homes in the country are managed by secular (non-religious) and Christian organizations. Interestingly, three-fourths of the old-age homes run by Christian organizations offer free accommodation as against one-half in 13 in the case of secular organizations. The number of old-age homes run on payment basis is much higher among secular organizations (45) than Christian institutions (27). Almost an equal number of both institutions (around 30) accommodate elderly on free as well as payment basis. Out of 376 old-age homes for which the relevant information is available, 62 per cent provide free accommodation. The Madras Institute of Ageing survey also reported the number of inmates of 398 old-age homes in India. Accordingly in 1995, 21,214 elderly lived in old-age homes. Around 1,120 males lived in homes exclusively meant for males, 2,759 females meant for females only and the remaining were taken care of in old-age homes where both males and female were admitted.

Health and Disability among Elderly

Old people in India, like those in other countries, suffer from a range of problems. However, of all the problems associated with an ageing population, health care demands the top priority. Ageing is a time of multiple illness and general disability. Along with the changes in the biological compositions, lifestyle factors are also important for disorders and diseases in old age. Old-age diseases are not always curable, implying a strain on financial as well as physical health infrastructure resources. However, the feeling of well-being can still override actual physical discomforts if the surrounding environment is nurturing.

Findings from Some of the More Reliable Studies

A study by Chanana and Talwar (1987) dealt with the growth rate of the aged population in India, the dependent population in the non-productive age groups, the old-age dependency ratio, sex ratio, marital status, literacy among males and females, and working and non-working aged. The health status of the aged was also analysed on the basis of the data collected in the 28th Round of the National Sample Survey in 1973. The analysis included measures of the prevalence of temporary illness and chronic diseases, the number of old people requiring medical assistance and the types of physical impairment from which they suffered, cross-classified by place of residence and sex. The study also threw light on the welfare programmes for the aged being implemented in different states of India.

A study of ageing in the state of Kerala (Irudaya Rajan, 1989) described factors contributing to population ageing, changes in age composition, dependency ratios and structural changes, that is, changes in the age and sex composition of the population aged 60 years and above over a period of three decades to 1981. The findings of another study of the population aged (60+) in the state of Kerala (Gulati and Rajan, 1990) were very similar to those of Rajan (1989). After analysing the socio-economic and demographic characteristics of the aged, the study described the current welfare programmes for them in Kerala, including the Kerala Agricultural Workers Pension Scheme, 1980.

In a study of 460 persons aged (60+), of whom 130 men and 100 women were from 30 villages, and 140 men and 90 women were from two urban centres in Chittoor district of the state of Andhra Pradesh, Kumar (1991) focused his analysis on familial and socio-economic problems, including health problems. Joseph (1991) made a comparative study of 411 persons: 207 men and 204 women over 60 living with families; 48 men and 44 women aged (60+) living in homes for the aged; and 257 people, 127 men and 130 women, aged 20–50 years in Kottayam district in Kerala. Joseph (1991) identified stereotypes of the aged, attitudes of the young towards them, their problems, including health problems, and their personality and religiosity. A study by Nair (1989) of 745 persons aged (60+), 375 men and 370 women, from the rural areas of four districts in the state of Karnataka, investigated their socio-economic and health problems. Although the main objectives were different, a study of demographic change in South India, employing micro approaches, enquired into support for the aged (Caldwell, Reddy and Caldwell, 1988: 187–95).

Mishra (1993) found that all the inmates felt dissatisfied residing in old-age homes as they felt segregated from the family and the wider community. They all wanted to go back to their families to spend the rest of their lives with their near and dear ones. Bagga (1997) in her study of all-female old-age homes showed that younger entrants to the old-age homes feel more depressed than their senior counterparts. Further she added that the residents felt more lonely and depressed in old-age homes where they stayed as guests and did not prepare food themselves. Kanwar and Chadha (1998) have also mentioned in their study that the institutionalized aged feel lonelier and depressed as they lack social network support and do not feel "the level of kinship" felt by non-institutionalized aged. By providing the findings of the various literatures made on the health status of elderly, it could able to understand the need for the study and the present paper attempts to find out the health status of elderly in an old-age home named "Volantariat" in Pondicherry.

An Overview of Volontariat

Volontariat is a non-profit, non-political, secular, registered Indian organization that was created in order to help the poorest of the poor. Founded in 1962 in the suburbs of Pondicherry, it is staffed by Indians and mainly financed by European humanitarian associations. It has been registered at Pondicherry since 1966. In Belgium and France, friends of Volontariat have started Associations. These groups took the responsibility of raising funds for sponsorship and other requirements; they also provided informal marketing outlets for the fabric woven at Atelier Shanti, the weaving unit set up with rehabilitated leprosy persons. The money raised is used for providing health care and education to children and adults, training of youth for carpentry and other skills, the rehabilitation of handicapped persons, the care of resourceless aged people and for the needs of the farm.

Volontariat has come a long way since the sixties, but friends and supporters are always needed. Today, your friendship, support and your donations will be welcome for the present following programmes:

- sponsorship of children
- social work
- sale of fabrics and handicraft
- heart surgeries
- home care for the aged
- homes for street children, abandoned, gypsy's children and the programmes to be developed in the future

Volontariat was created in 1962 by Madeleine de Blic at Pondicherry in order to help the poorest of the poor. It has been registered as a non-profit, non-political organization since 1966.

History of Volontariat

1962 Creation of Volontariat.

Mobile dispensary was inaugurated. People in the village meet to discuss problems. Construction of huts with help from young students in France.

1966 Weaving centre for cured, but handicapped former leprosy patients.

The Registration of Volontariat Association at Pondicherry.

1968 Touttipakam farm started for self-reliant food production.

The Community Centre was established in the heart of the village with a dispensary, kitchen, room for milk distribution, crèche and nursery school.

1977 A sewing section comes into being. Bags and patchwork quilts are made.

1978 New buildings are constructed on the farm to store grain, fertilizers and tools.

1981 The weaving and sewing centres are registered as an autonomous institution atelier Shanti. An embroidery section is created.

1982 Selva Nilayam was opened.

The centre contains a large dining room with a kitchen, a library, rooms for evening classes and workrooms.

Sponsorship system was introduced. A sponsor would finance a child's education and health costs.

1991 Shakti Vihar was built with the help of an European project. Evening classes and craft apprenticeship classes have been conducted there.

1997 A programme to finance children who need heart surgery was started.

2000 Inauguration of Amaidi Illam for the elderly and a small group of physically handicapped person. It contains a clinic.

Inauguration of Thendral Illam for aged resourceless persons cured of leprosy.

At this time, more than 1,200 children benefit from our programmes, 800 of whom are sponsored.

Our Focus is on the Inmates of Amaidi Illam

Amaidi Illam

Aim: Caring the Aged and Giving them Human Touch

A new centre was opened in 2000 to welcome destitute aged women and men, many of them coming from the pavement. The centre is called Amaidhi Illam, which means: *the home of peace and rest,* in Tamil and was born thanks to the help of a generous donor, Mr Bernard Aubé. In those days, Indian people were living in the "joint family" system which looks and cares for everybody, so grand parents were never abandoned. Today, especially in the urban environment, the Indian society moves to a nuclear model (father, mother and their children) and the aged generation is rejected. If they have no pension and no properties, they quickly become destitute people who, even, live in the streets and beg (or die) for thêir subsistence. It is the reason why Volontariat distributes the mid-day meals to many aged people of Uppalam and Dubraypet, it is also why Amaidhi Illam and Thendral Illam were opened.

The Amaidhi Illam centre tries to care for their health, to give them affection until the last moment of their life. The centre has 25 rooms, single or double, with bathroom and toilet attached. The priority is given to the poorest and alone in life, after an enquiry made by a social worker. The doctor and nurses are looking for their health problems at any time; dentist is available during his regular visits. From January and October 2006, 6 inmatés passed away, peacefully, among the affection of every one, other inmates, staff and employees. After a short ceremony which is attended by all, they go to the cemetery. One of the inmates was a Sikh, speaking Hindi only, travelling and begging for more than 20 years. He was found on the pavement of Pondicherry. Through the information he gave to a social worker speaking his language, they traced his family, in Bihar and they organized his return home, after so many years! Likewise, the service of the Amaidhi Illam under Voluntariat is well known and this study attempts to bring out the health status of elderly in the old-age home under "voluntariat", The Amaidhi Illam.

Methodology

The present paper is descriptive in nature. It tries to bring out the health status of elderly in the old-age homes. The method adopted for the study is census method, since the study is conducted with all the 25 respondents in the old-age home. All the details and information with regard to their socio-economic and health status are collected. The collected data are codified and analysed using appropriate statistical tools like SPSS and so on. While conducting the research, the researchers had few difficulties due to the physical health problems of respondents due to their old age like dementia, visual problem, etc., which the researcher could cope up and were able to get reliable data.

Findings

- Among the respondents, majorities (64%) are females and 36 per cent of them are males, which show the high prevalence of female population in the old-age home.
- All the respondents are above 60 years of age. Most of the respondents (32%) in the old-age home are above 75 years, 20 per cent of them are in the age group of 60–64 years, 16 per cent each are between 70 and 74 years and below 60 years and 8 per cent of the respondents are within the age 65–69 years.
- More than half of the respondents (56%) are widow/widower, 28 per cent of them are unmarried and 16 per cent are married, which shows there is high prevalence of widows and unmarried in old-age home and among those married (16%) only 8 per cent are living along with spouse.
- Higher percentages of respondents are illiterates and few have studied till primary education.
- With regard to previous occupation, majority of respondents are unemployed, few are housewives and few others are skilled workers, handling petty business and ordinary labourers.
- Most of the respondents (88%) are engaged in some gainful employment presently and remaining (12%) are unemployed.
- Higher share of 80 per cent the respondents belong to Hindu religion and the remaining (20%) belong to Christianity.
- It is a significant fact that, none of the respondents have independent source of income, which shows their economic dependence.
- As discussed earlier, only 8 per cent of the respondents in the old-age home are staying with their spouse, all others are staying alone.
- Duration of stay in old-age home differs from respondent to respondent. Twenty-four per cent of the respondents are staying in old-age home for past 7 years and above, 24 per cent are staying for past 1 to 3 years, 40 per cent for above 3 years to seven years and 12 per cent are living within 1 to 3 years.

- With regard to the place of stay where they spent most of their life, 60 per cent of the respondents was from city area and 40 per cent are from village area, which shows the high percentage of mobility towards old-age home from city area:
- The following are the health problems specified by the respondents:
  - 36 per cent suffer from visual problem and weakness of muscles
  - 24 per cent suffer from arthritis/joint pain
  - 20 per cent suffer from gastric/acidity problem
  - 16 per cent from depression
  - 12 per cent from back pain
  - 8 per cent from piles, loss of appetite, sleeplessness and diabetes
  - 4 per cent suffer from problems of mobility, speech difficulty, respiratory/asthma, low blood pressure and mental disease
- Majority (88%) of the respondents are availing the treatment currently availing in the old-age home, while the other (12%) are not availing it. Among those availing, 80 per cent are towards homeopathy and 8 per cent are towards allopathy, which shows their inclination towards the homeopathy medicine.
- In considering the inmates opinion about their health, though 48 per cent of the respondents felt that their health is somewhat good but still 52 per cent felt that they are not healthy.
- It is very significant that in considering the satisfaction level expressed by the inmates with the services provided at the old-age homes, all the respondents are satisfied with the services provided at the old-age home and reasons specified for their satisfaction is ranked as follows:
  - Services are free/at low cost
  - Food is good/wholesome food/find food suitable
  - Accommodation satisfactory
  - Good medical facility/medical care is good
  - Entertainment/library facility is good
  - Have freedom/facility to participate in religious activities
  - All services are good/good behaviour of the staff
  - Have no choice/have to be satisfied with services
- With regard to the preference of stay, if provided a choice, to the surprise that all the respondents have specified the old-age home as their preferred place, which shows their likeness and satisfaction with respect to the stay in old-age home and the reasons specified by them for their liking is ranked as follows:

- — Lack of economic support
- — Lack of affection in family/no familial support
- — For self-respect/peace of mind/away from familial conflict/more freedom/this is the best option at this age
- — Do not want to be a burden on any-one
- — Have no one to take care/absence of close family members
- — Fulfilment of all needs/requirement/do not have to depend on any-one
- On account of the feel of loneliness in old-age home, higher percentage (82%) expressed that they did not feel lonely being in old age and only 12 per cent expressed that they could feel lonely and specified the reason for loneliness as is natural to miss children and family and to feel isolated from social life.
- Those respondents who did not feel lonely, ranked the reasons as follows:
- — We are in contact with children and relatives; children and relatives come to visit us and we can also go to visit them
- — Have freedom to do what we want
- — Staff takes care of us/staff is good to us/services and facilities are good
- — Have no close family; used to living alone, not having married
- — Have made friends here/have company here
- — Have come to terms with our life/have made our life/this is our home
- — Do not miss children because they have no love or respect for us/they are self-centred
- — With regard to their stay in old-age home, it's elegant that all the respondents are very happy to stay in old-age home, which shows not only their inclination towards old-age home, but also their detachment towards their family.

Summary and Conclusion

It is found from this study that the residents of the old-age home are enjoying good health with satisfaction being away from their home. They are quite satisfied with their life in the old-age home and, even saying that they are happier here than at home. The residents do not experience either social isolation or desolation or any other health problem. This is due to the regular mutual visits of the residents and family members and the effort on the part of the old-age home officials and residents to take proper care of themselves and their health in particular and also engage themselves in various activities.

It is very difficult to arrive at a generalization from this study as it draws upon a small number of respondents. Since the study did not look at other types of old-age homes such as old-age homes managed by the government or by some other voluntary agencies, it is not possible to generalize that the health status of elderly residents in all old-age homes in India are good. My findings also differ from earlier studies, especially those which were carried out in other types of old-age homes, particularly run by government where proper medical care is not available. Nevertheless, the findings point to a significant trend that can be taken up in further studies. It needs to be investigated if the presence of the same set of variables, such as proper health care, regular contact with family and friends, good relationship with co-residents and engaging them in work inside the old-age home, facilitates for good health among the residents of old-age homes. Thus, to conclude, this old-age home plays a tremendous role in its service and care for the health of the elderly.

References

Bagga, A. (1997), "A Study of Women in Old-Age Home of Pune", *Life in Twilight Years*, Calcutta, Kwality Book Company.

Caldwell, John C., P.H. Reddy and Pat Caldwell (1988), *The Causes of Demographic Change: Experimental Research in South India*, Madison, University of Wisconsin Press.

Dandekar, K., (1993) "The Aged, Their Problems and Social Intervention in Maharashtra", *Economic and Political Weekly*, Vol. 27 (23), June 5, pp.1188–94.

Das, N.P. and Urvi Shah, (2001), "The Social and Health Status of the Elderly in India: Evidence from Recent National Level Data". A special report prepared as a part of the research initiative at the Population Research Centre, Baroda for the MOHFW, New Delhi.

Government of India, (1991), "Socio-Economic Profile of the Aged Persons", NSS 42nd Round, (July, 1986 – June 1987), *Sarvekshana*, Vol. 15, No. 2, Issue No. 49, Oct. – Dec. 1991, National Sample Survey Organization (NSSO), Department of Statistics, Ministry of Planning, New Delhi.

——, (1998), "The Aged in India: A Socio-Economic Profile, NSS 52nd Second Round, (July 1995–June 1996), NSSO, Department of Statistics, Ministry of Planning and Programme Implementation.

——, 2000, "Elderly in India Profile and Programmes 2000", Central Statistical Organization, Ministry of Statistics and Programme Implementation. New Delhi.

Gulati, Leela and Irudaya Rajan, S. (1990), "Social and Economic Implications of Population Aging in Kerala, India", *Demography India*, 19(2).

Helpage India, (1998), "Directory of Oldage Homes in India", Research and Development Division, Helpage India, New Delhi.

Irudaya Rajan, S. (1989), "Aging in Kerala: One More Population Problem", *Asia Pacific Population Journal*, (4(2).

Irudaya Rajan, S., U.S. Mishra and P.S. Sharma, (1999), India's *Elderly: Burden or Challenge*? Sage Publications, New Delhi.

——, (2000), "Ageing in India: Retrospect and Prospect", *Indian Journal of Social Science,* Volume 2, No. 1.

Joseph, James (1991), *Aged in India: Problems and Personality*, Allahabad, Chugh Publications.

Kanwar, Priya and N.K. Chadha (1998), "Psycho-Social Determinates of Institutional Elderly: An Empirical Study", *Indian Journal of Gerontology*, 12(1&2) 27-39.

Kumar, S. Vijaya (1991), *Family Life and Scio-Economic Problem of the Aged*, Delhi, Ashish Publishing House.

Misra, S. (1993), "Scenario of Segrefated Seniors", *Indian Journal of Gerontology*, 3: 104–110.

Nair Krishnan (ed.), (1995), "Care of the Elderly: Directory of Organisations Caring for the Elderly in India", Centre for the Welfare of the Aged, Madras Institute of Ageing.

Rao, V.A., P.M. Vasudevan and T. Madhavan, (1982), "Psychosocial Aspects of Geriatric Population", in A. Kiev and A. Venkoba Rao (eds.), *Reading in Transcultural Psychiatry*, Madras: Higginbothams.

Sharma, S., (1999), "Elderly in India: Their Mental Health Problems", in Arun P. Bali (ed.), *Understanding Greying People of India*, Inter-India Publications, New Delhi.

Sharma, S.P. and Peter Xenos, (1992), "Ageing in India: Demographic Background and Analysis Based on Census Materials. Occasional Paper No. 2, Office of the Registrar General and Census Commissioner, Government of India, New Delhi.

United Nations, (1987), "Population Ageing: Review of Emerging Issues", Asian Population Studies, Series No. 80, Economic and Social Commission for Asia and the Pacific, Bangkok, Thailand.

20

The Politics of Health Security: Challenges of Neo-Liberal State

An Indian Perspective

SABU THOMAS

The study of politics essentially deals with human individual and hence, his being and well-being are of immediate concern to the subject. In the political grouping, namely, state, health security of its individual members becomes a major parameter for measuring the system's success. With the pre-welfare state, health security was more or less a commodity that follows laissez-faire market rules. Differing from the laissez-faire state, the post-world war welfare state highly promoted social welfare ideals. As a result, health security also became a-priori state concern, patronized and promoted by the government and its agencies. This period is also marked by pro-poor, pro-public policy outputs in health sector. Many social and health security schemes and institutions were designed and implemented. Health care was considered as one of the three pillars of social policy, along with education and social welfare and it was mainly funded through taxation. Governments and international organizations have widely recognized the need to improve the health of the poor. In the 1970s, for instance, the World Health Organization led a global effort to achieve "Health for All" by the year 2000. Representatives from more than 130 governments met in 1978 in Alma Ata (now Almaty, Kazakhstan) and signed a declaration stating that "inequality in the health status of people, particularly between developed and developing countries as well as within countries, is politically, socially, and economically unacceptable".

Globalization and Neo-Liberal State

The emergence of globalization undermined the very notion of a welfare state and replaced it with a soft state. This new state is characterized with liberalization, privatization and public private participation. It is mainly conditioned by the themes of international funding agencies. A major challenge of globalization is the balancing between state as a corporation and state as a guardian. The soft state is a service provider; a business concern – levying the services whenever and wherever possible.

Public health also joined other social services in being recast within a market framework. Across the Third World, frayed but tangible social safety nets were replaced by things somewhat less concrete than nets: ideas and promises, framed in a model presented as the only remaining option. One of the tenets of the new consensus was the efficient provision of social services, which included an opening for the private sector into what was previously, in many instances, principally or entirely a public domain; the incorporation of competition into the provision of social services; and the application of user fees. Under the new framework, the commitment to primary health care was stripped bare, replaced by a much more limited strategy that sought to address a narrow range of health interventions while ignoring the broader health context.

The major themes of globalization are generally regarded as threefold: (a) the necessity of free market, (b) individualism, and (c) the pursuit of narrow self-interest rather than mutual interest. This mood is evidenced in the views of World Bank.

> Far from supporting a minimalist approach to the state the world's development success stories) have shown that development requires an effective state, one that plays a catalytic, facilitating role, encouraging and complementing the activities of private business and individuals.

However, by the early 1990s, many began to question the uneven economic outcomes that accompanied the neo-liberal framework. The World Bank initiated a series of programmes to address issues of equity, such as the Heavily Indebted Poor Countries (HIPC) debt reduction initiative and micro-credit lending. In the area of health security also neo-liberalism made negative impacts. The world food crisis in 2008 and the international finance crisis in September 2008 forced the policy makers to recast their priorities and even fundamentals. It is in this context the present paper tries to analyse the challenges of neo-liberalism and policy alternatives in a political framework.

Indian Position

The welfarist impact of modern state was reflected in the post-independence Indian polity. The new Indian Constitution incorporated principles of health security in the fourth chapter of the constitution, i.e., directive principles of state policy. Article 47 of the Indian Constitution says that "the State shall regard the raising of the level of nutrition and the standard of living of its people and the improvement of public health as among its primary duties ...". Later, the Supreme Court of India moved this proposition to the third chapter of the constitution, i.e., fundamental rights. The honourable court observed that the "Right to Life" (a fundamental human right under Article 21A) means a right to life with dignity, and indicated that access to basic education, health and food were part of a citizen's claim to a right to life with dignity. Healthy and dignified life is now a basic right of every Indian citizen. The later governments were guided by these principles and evolved a model health policy and initiated many health schemes. During this period Indian health policy focused on infrastructure development and resource management. Large number of primary health centres were established, health personnel trained and deployed and health programmes implemented. In fact, the state adopted a charitable approach to health care.

> During the last three decades and more, since the attainment of Independence, considerable progress has been achieved in the promotion of the health status of our people. Smallpox has been eliminated; plague is no longer a problem; mortality from cholera and related diseases has decreased and malaria brought under control to a considerable extent. The mortality rate per thousand of population has been reduced from 27.4 to 14.8 and the life expectancy at birth has increased from 32.7 to over 52. A fairly extensive network of dispensaries, hospitals and institutions providing specialized curative care has developed and a large stock of medical and health personnel, of various levels, has become available.

During this period the makers of Indian health policy were guided by the social democratic principles enshrined in the constitution. A policy shift became inevitable when the global economy settled into the hands of Chicago School of Economics, in the early 1980s. The health sector was one of its major prey. The field of health services and health policy were deeply impacted. The shift in health policy exemplified the era's general migration from Keynesian social democracy to the market hegemony of the Washington Consensus. The dearticulation of the state in the area of health care, replaced by the primacy of the market and privatization of the sector, would have profound impacts in India, especially on the marginalized.

The consequent pay-use policy, when implemented to health sector may result in many far-reaching consequences. In the absence of a strong social security system the less capable may become a prey to the health corporations. Even though the support of international agencies resulted in enhanced infrastructure, in the long run they cannot be maintained if they are not rewarding. Neo-liberal policies are generally market oriented and promote consumerism. The advocates of this new gospel believe in the infallibility of economic growth which in turn uplinks welfare and social security with privatization and corporatism.

> The historical record is clear: the single, most effective way to reduce world poverty is economic growth. Western countries began discovering this around 1820 when they broke with the historical norm of low growth and initiated an era of dramatic advances in material well-being. Living standards tripled in Europe and quadrupled in the United States in that century, improving at an even faster pace in the next 100 years. Economic growth thus eliminated mass poverty in what is today considered the developed world.

Neo-liberalism is not an evil in itself, but the world food crisis of 2008 and the great economic crisis that erupted during September 2008 clearly invalidated many of the basic principles of the new theory. The denial of welfarism and social democracy are now acknowledged as cardinal sins. In this context the Indian policy shift towards neo-liberalism, especially in the area of health care should be subject to immediate revision and renewal.

The Major Challenges

In the Indian perspective the policy shift towards neo-liberalism essentially results in a confrontation with the social democratic model. This confrontation in the health sector develops crisis in three levels. They are:

1. Input crisis,
2. Management crisis, and
3. Output crisis.

Input Crisis

The crisis in input is a recent development in the area of health security. The major advocates of neo-liberalism include the developed first world countries and the international funding agencies controlled by these countries. These states and funding agencies pump large amounts to the needy states, especially for infrastructure development.

> India is also now "a priority destination" for ADB's private sector operations, with direct investments increasing significantly since 2003; after five years, it has invested $177 million in four projects. Going forward, the ADB said private sector investments and public-private partnerships would continue to focus on infrastructure and the financial sector. The financial sector would include investments in asset reconstruction companies and financing or guarantees for municipalities and infrastructure funds. Its 2005–07 loan programme is focused on infrastructure investments.
>
> On the issue of the government's poverty reduction strategy, the ADB said that while the latest available data suggest significant improvements in several education and health indicators, India still lags behind in other indicators, especially gender-sensitive ones such as maternal mortality or the gender gap in secondary education and the high incidence of Human Immuno-deficiency Virus/Acquired Immune-Deficiency Syndrome (HIV/AIDS) and other infectious diseases.

Presently, with the intervention of international funding agencies more and more funds are available for infrastructure development in health sector. At the same time state funds were also diverted in this direction. The result is more buildings, more operation theatres, more computers and more and more amenities. But these investments are on the peripheral structure. Supportive and subsequent structures were disregarded. A Government of India release clearly evidences this situation. Accordingly in the state of Chhattisgarh 33 per cent of primary health centres are without motorable approach roads. In Mizoram it is 70 per cent and in Uttar Pradesh the figure is 56 per cent. In Mizoram, according to the latest survey 100 per cent PHC are without regular water supply. In Chhattisgarh the figure is 64 per cent, Uttar Pradesh 59 per cent, Kerala 25 per cent and Orissa 43 per cent. There is a shortfall of 5 per cent doctors in PHC all over India. More than 10 per cent of health centres are functioning without a pharmacist, 50 per cent CHC are working without a surgeon. The data shows that the shortfall is heavy in the backward areas. The infrastructure revolution does not attend these problems.

According to a Planning Commission report, India is short of six lakh doctors, 10 lakh nurses and two lakh dental surgeons. India has a dismal patient-doctor ratio. According to the report, for every 10,000 Indians, there is one doctor. In contrast, Australia has 249 doctors for every 10,000 people, Canada has 209, UK has 166 and US has 548. India also faces an acute shortage of dental surgeons. At present, the number of dental surgeons registered in India stands at just over 73,000 against a requirement of 3 lakh. Similarly, the health ministry estimates that there needs to be one nurse for every 500 people. According to this, India required 21 lakh nurses in 2007. But only 11 lakh nurses were available.

This problem is not a matter of policy absentism. It is a part of neo-liberal policy initiatives. Infrastructures are provided in places where there is an anticipation of returns. The marginalized areas and populations are consciously disregarded. Further investments only in peripheral infrastructures without attention to supportive structures may undermine the very purpose of these reforms. This crisis may lead to a failure of the long established health system and result in a debt trap. Finally, the compulsion may be directed to complete privatization and commercialization of health sector.

Management Crisis

Neo-liberalism rests upon the three pillars of liberalization, privatization and globalization. In the matter of health security in India these fundamentals direct us to a management crisis. In the case of globalization its evident results are health tourism and health outsourcing. These may be a boost to our economy in a peripheral view. But in the long run it may undermine the very concept of social equity. Health tourism and health outsourcing are the result of comparative difference in health cost. The Indian doctors and services are comparatively less expensive to a western health tourist or corporation. Subsequently, many outsiders demand Indian health services and new avenues will be open to our economy. The services will get higher remunerations. However, the crisis is that these cheap hiring is in fact high above the hiring capacity of a majority of native beneficiaries. They may remain unattended and the public service will no more become a destination to the new professionals. The present policy regime is diverting their attention to these exchange benefit of globalization and less attentive to the issue of downtrodden and social equity. The management crisis is also associated with the policies of liberalization and privatization. Health becomes a commodity that is to be sustained by the rules of market. The function of state becomes supervision and facilitation.

> The neo-liberal policies that gained ascendancy in the 1980s spurred a strong wave of economic liberalization, privatization of state enterprises and services and deregulation of the economy. The intensification of globalization, technological change and competition led to further pressures for containing public expenditure and reducing tax rates. Over the past two decades this has resulted in many countries dismantling key social programmes and reducing the scope, level and range of benefits. There is also a trend towards privatizing social security – replacing or supplementing government schemes by private schemes or contracting private agencies to manage existing schemes.

This market determinism is a corollary of the policy shift. But it tends to become manipulative determinism contracted by multinational drug insurance and institutional groups. The older general practitioner family doctor had already vanished into the world of superspecialization. At this end the producer monopoly, i.e., doctor-druggist-technologist trinity is highly beyond the rules of regular market. The lack of transparency, accountability and professional ethics become the rule rather than the exception. The entry of multinational health insurance corporates in India inaugurated a paradigm shift in health security. It is now a consumer product at the choice of the haves. Rules of demand and supply regulate the market. Here, maximum demand is the target of the market. Consequently, the diseases are not treated but managed by the professionals. The benevolent paternalism of doctor is replaced with profit orientation of professionals, which also includes druggists and technicians.

Another outcome of commercialization of health security is the bundle of vulnerable policy outputs. Communicable diseases and disasters were handled in terms of market determinism. The result is the subjection of the marginalized both to the diseases and health corporates. The implication of user-fee policy transforms the very attitude of the vulnerable groups. They may avail the services only if they can pay. There are freebees but there are many formalities and limitations to avail the same. In short, you may live as long as you can buy the health service.

Output Crisis

The neo-liberal policy shift may finally result in an output crisis. This includes both social and political costs. Socially, the present social structure will be fractured internally and externally. The social equity will be displaced with market equality. The neo-liberal equality caters only for the payers. Thus, in the case of developing countries like India the socially backward and neglected sectors will be at a larger disadvantage. The absence of firm social service networks also complicates this crisis. After the adaption of LPG pattern the state will not be in a position to regain its earlier position. Necessarily the social fabric will be damaged, questioning the basic purpose of a social structure.

On the other side, the political costs of the crisis are heavy. As a result of the failure in social structure the legitimacy of the relevant political structure will be questioned. A legitimacy crisis will necessarily follow. The existing political systems and structures will be questioned. The prevailing political obligation chord will be broken. The citizenry may feel distanced from a state which cannot secure their health security and leave them at the mercy of market forces. Political violence may erupt and political apathy may become a common ideology. This is not only a theoretical assumption but a real position faced by many of the present Third World heavily indebted poor countries. In the Indian context this may pose a great threat considering the relatively younger status of our democracy and the so-called diversities in our polity. This three-level crisis forms the basic of any future political discourse on health system in a neo-liberal state. This is necessarily an outcome of globalization and can be remedied with a firm approach. The main remedial approaches suggested are:

1. Protective Guardian Community Approach
2. Alternative Choice Approach
3. Public-Private Partnership Approach

Protective Guardian Community Approach

The protective guardian community approach postulates the community as the guardian of individual concerns. Health security can be achieved by the decentralized activities of these communities. This decentralization is an autonomous redirection to the grass-roots. Present neo-liberalism also postulates decentralization, but it is activated without adequate resources and political power. The local governments struggle with the new burden of powers. They are without necessary capability and technical support. The projected approach on the other hand replaces the bureaucratic governance structure with a participatory community model. For example the self-help groups are active in many developing countries. They possess immense potentials and can effectively manage the health security of local communities. The concerned people are of better knowledge about their health requirements. The physician-druggist-technician trinity can be easily replaced with the doctor-patient concept by the intervention of the community. The community can effectively make prescription and facility auditing and ensure transparency and accountability in the field.

Alternative Choice Approach

New alternative choice should replace the traditional dependence system. The disease burden can be subjected and fought with alternative choices. Against the rules of market, people may take their own choice. For this the health consumer is to be redesignated as a patient who deserves a remedy inextricable from his environment. The health machines and health supermarkets need not be the priorities of our prescriptions. The proved local alternatives should be strengthened against the multi-nationalist health menu. For example in the Indian context 'Ayurveda' gained wider acceptance among the health tourists but not among the natives. In every area of health care these alternatives should be found out and popularized.

Public-Private Partnership Approach

Public-private partnership is a basic theme of neo-liberalism. But this partnership is more in favour of the private element rather than the public. For them it becomes a chance for the private to encroach and acquire public resources. In matter of a future health policy the focus should be more on public. Governments may opt for alternatives to the direct delivery of services by developing partnerships with non-governmental providers. In many countries non-governmental organizations receive public support to deliver health services to poor and vulnerable segments of society. Since many NGOs already work closely with the poor, they may be better equipped to identify and serve the poor than governments. In some countries, NGOs may also have greater flexibility and accountability than centralized, hierarchical bureaucracies. For example the Janani programme, operating in India, has mobilized private and other resources to provide family planning services to low-income families in Bihar, Jharkhand, and parts of Madhya Pradesh. The private sector at times possesses new technologies and facilities. The government on the other hand possesses wider acceptance and coverage. A partnership can combine these two elements for the benefit of the marginalized.

Summary

Health security is essentially a state concern that needs direct attention and intervention of the government and its machinery. The neo-liberal policies tend to transform it into the hands of market forces, leaving the vulnerable sections under the mercy of profit-motivated cartels. This policy shift results in many socio-political crisis. Governments may face legitimacy and obligation crisis. The marginalized groups may become a prey to the profit-motivated user-fee regime. Such a crisis can be effectively met with the support of community acting with autonomous authority. They have to develop alternative choices. Finally, the public should forge a partnership with the reliable private operators. This mutual sharing will compensate for the maladies of both sectors.

References

Carr, Dara, "Improving the Health of the World's Poorest People", *Health Bulletin* 1, Washington, DC.

McGregor, Sue L.T., "Neoliberalism and Health Care", *International Journal of Consumer Studies*, Special edition on 'Consumers and Health', 25 (2), 2001, 82–89.

Singh Manasi and Swati Sahi, "Most Indians Spending from Pockets on Health", *One World South Asia*, 09 April 2008.

Sinha Kounteya and Mahendra Kumar Singh, "India Short of 6 Lakh Doctors", *The Times of India*, April, 2008.

Srinivasan G., *Businessline Financial Daily*, Saturday, October 9, 2004.

Ursula Grant Rachel Marcus, "Chronic Poverty and PRSPs: A Desk Study", Background Paper for the Chronic Poverty Report 2008–09.

Wolfensohn D., World Bank President, "Foreword to the State in a Changing World" http://www.popfound.org/wallindex.htm accessed on 15–10–2008.

Index